PSYCHODYNAMIC NURSING

A BIOSOCIAL ORIENTATION

Fourth Edition

MARTHA MONTGOMERY BROWN, R.N., Ph.D.
Professor of Nursing, and
Director of Nursing Care Research Center,
University of Nebraska School of Nursing,
Omaha, Nebraska

GRACE R. FOWLER, R.N., M.A.
Director, Graduate Psychiatric Nursing
and Professor of Nursing,
University of Missouri School of Nursing,
Columbia, Missouri—Extended Campus,
St. Louis, Missouri

W. B. SAUNDERS COMPANY   PHILADELPHIA   LONDON   TORONTO

W. B. Saunders Company: West Washington Square
Philadelphia, Pa. 19105

12 Dyott Street
London, WC1A 1DB

1835 Yonge Street
Toronto 7, Canada

Psychodynamic Nursing: A Biosocial Orientation   SBN 0-7216-2162-7

Print No.:   9   8   7   6   5   4   3   2

Preface

Psychodynamic Nursing—A Biosocial Orientation is addressed to the professional student in psychiatric-mental health nursing and is divided into five major sections: *Low-Visibility Functions in Nursing; High-Visibility Nursing Functions in the Care of Psychiatric Patients; The Psychiatric Patient and His Socio-Environmental Milieu; Psychiatric-Mental Health Nursing in Community Settings;* and *The Teaching-Learning Milieu for Psychosocial Nursing.*

The *Introduction,* in Part I, is intended to present the conceptual schema for understanding the broad functions of the nurse in terms of three main categories: the biologic and psychologic requirements of all individuals, as well as those characteristics in a patient with a given socioeconomic status and from a specific cultural group. These nursing requirements or needs are then viewed from their degree of visibility with respect to the functions of the nurse. The student will find that, for the most part, Part I, *Low-Visibility Functions in Nursing,* is applicable to the psychosocial nursing requirements of all patients; therefore, it is recommended for all students early in the nursing curriculum. Special mention should be made of the fact that Part I takes a developmental approach which begins with normal childhood and continues through the life span.

Part II, *High-Visibility Functions in the Care of Psychiatric Patients,* is intended to introduce the student to psychiatric nursing through a presentation of content that is easily learned because of its high visibility. Thus, the student should have a feeling of accomplishment early in the course.

Although Part III, *The Psychiatric Patient and His Socio-Environmental Milieu,* is concerned primarily with patients in residential arrangements that set them apart from the rest of the community, the student will find that much of the content in this section is also applicable to the nursing care of psychiatric patients in the community. The nurse's functions as she cares for psychiatric patients are primarily of a low-visibility nature.

The effectiveness of the care of a specific patient depends on how meaningful his interaction and communication is to the nurse. Within a broad frame of reference, the dynamics of particular patterns of behavior is explained and is related to the needs expressed by the patient. With this understanding, the nurse may then identify what is unique about her patient and, within a total framework, determine her action on the basis of needs. If the student of nursing develops the understanding and skill relevant to selected broad nursing problem constellations, she will then be able to give therapeutic care to a psychiatric patient with any given diagnosis.

Psychiatric-Mental Health Nursing in Community Settings, Part IV, focuses primarily on community care. Since the value system of a group often reflects the goals for treatment, consideration has been given also to the development of beliefs of the past as a basis for their influence on practice within the community. This section focuses on care for groups rather than care designed for the individual. Community services are described in terms of both sick and well groups of people.

Part V, *The Teaching-Learning Milieu for Psychosocial Nursing,* gives consideration to the climate conducive to creative endeavors in learning. The alleviation of stress in the student's learning situation may be perceived as a form of psychosocial intervention. The psychosocial interchange in the student-teacher-patient triad is a most important type of learning experience for the student.

The authors wish to thank their many colleagues and students, both graduate and basic, who have criticized the material of this text and have offered valuable suggestions and comments. Special mention should be made of the helpful comments made by students of the schools of nursing at the University of Missouri and Washington University. We are especially indebted to our former psychiatric nursing instructor, Miss Irene Bower, who did much to stimulate our thinking so many years ago.

We gratefully acknowledge our debt to Miss Jean Lagerstrom, Assistant Professor of Psychiatric Nursing, Dr. Mary M. Spelman, Associate Professor of Nursing, University of Missouri School of Nursing, and Dr. Patricia R. Brown, former Associate Professor and Chairman, Department of General Nursing Science, Washington University School of Nursing, who gave invaluable assistance in making suggestions for supplementary reading materials, in locating and checking bibliographic sources, and in the tedious and laborious reading of the manuscript.

MARTHA MONTGOMERY BROWN
GRACE R. FOWLER

Contents

Part Two   High-Visibility Nursing Functions in the Care of Psychiatric Patients

Part Three   The Psychiatric Patient and His
              Socio-Environmental Milieu

Part One   Low-Visibility
Functions in Nursing

Chapter 1 Introduction

The student may first ask why the writers have designated the title of this book as *Psychodynamic Nursing—A Biosocial Orientation.* What is psychodynamic nursing and what is meant by the term biosocial? What is nursing and how does it differ from the practices of other occupational or professional groups in the health field? Is nursing a profession or is it an occupation? What are the characteristics of the nurse? What does the nurse do and how does she do it? Who is the recipient of nursing? These are but a few of the questions that are raised in thinking about a very complex situation—nursing as it is and nursing as it could be.

It seems that nurses, eager to build a body of knowledge and hungry from the lack of it, reach out to other disciplines for almost anything that might reflect light on the present state of development. While other disciplines do have much to offer nursing, there is a pressing need for more research in the clinical nursing field if nursing is to reach full professional status.

When exploring solutions to nursing problems, it is essential to make an explanation of pertinent terminology, a tedious but often fruitful task. Let us turn, now, to that task.

DEFINITION OF TERMS

Weiss defines the term *psychodynamic* in the following manner: "Psychodynamics is the science which describes and explains the manifestations and consequences of the interaction of mental forces within the human being."[1] We are concerned, then, with the psychologic forces or energy within the human being, such as feelings and emotions, that impel the individual to act in a certain manner, the forces that restrain or inhibit his behavior, as well as the interaction of these forces, which results in either integrated or ineffectual behavior.

Inherent in all of us is the desire to understand the behavior of others. We want to know why a person acts and feels as he does in a given situation. What motivated him to act that way? Why does he feel that way?

Psychologic phenomena, unlike physical phenomena, are experienced only by the subject. One comprehends the mental phenomena of another only indirectly in that he, too, at some time or other has lived through similar situations and has experienced comparable desires, feelings and emotions. Each of us may describe these psychologic phenomena with different terms. However, if we begin with the same background, we will have a common basis for understanding the behavior of patients, and for solving nursing problems and expanding or changing the theoretic formulations as new data are acquired.

The term *biosocial* is used by Cameron, who says that we call the individual "biosocial to indicate that his biology has been made to operate socially, in terms of others' needs and others' interests, as well as his own."[2] Man is born with certain anatomic equipment that carries on physiologic processes, and the environment in which man lives provides certain substances necessary for his body to maintain these biologic functions. For example, man must have air, food and water to provide the necessary energy for survival; however, the way other individuals in his environment cooperate to meet these needs or requirements, whether they be biologic or psychologic in nature, is social.[3]

As the student reads other chapters and gains experience with patients, the above definitions will become more meaningful. Thus, we shall continue the discussion of terminology by examining the term nursing.

---

[1] Edoardo Weiss: *Principles of Psychodynamics.* New York, Grune & Stratton, Inc., 1950, p. 1.

[2] Norman Cameron: *The Psychology of Behavioral Disorders; A Biosocial Interpretation.* Boston, Houghton Mifflin Company, 1947, p. 16.

[3] M. F. Ashley Montagu: *The Direction of Human Development.* New York, Harper & Brothers, 1955, p. 32.

If nursing is to build a systematized body of knowledge validated by research, then the concept will be one that can be measured and tested in research situations. For present purposes, the writers have defined *nursing* as a process of verbal and nonverbal interaction directed toward the healthful status of the recipient within an institution, an agency or the community. The nurse does something with the individual recipient or perhaps to groups of persons so that they can get well or stay well. What the nurse does from day to day may depend on the response that the recipient makes to the nurse's previous action. The nurse, in turn, evaluates this response, and then acts accordingly. These dynamic forces between the nurse and the patient constitute an ongoing process directed toward the patient's getting well and keeping well. What the nurse and the patient do in response to each other may be either verbal or nonverbal. This process of interaction is defined by Homans as "a unit of one man's activity which follows or is stimulated by some unit of activity of another person."[4]

Verbal and nonverbal interaction not only occurs between the nurse and the patient, but includes other members of the health team and others such as the patient's family and friends; however, all of the interaction is goal-directed in the area of the subject's health. The concept of nursing is elaborated in Chapter 9, *Nurse-Patient Interaction Analysis*.

FUNCTIONS OF THE NURSE

The nurse's verbal and nonverbal components of interaction seem to cluster logically around three main categories.[5] First, there are those functions centered on the *biologic* needs that are common to all people, as exemplified by hunger and thirst. Here, too, fall those biologic needs that must be met by the nurse in special ways because of the patient's biologic health problem, disability or condition. An example might be to feed a patient through a tube, to cut meat for a patient who has an injured arm, or to give a bottle of formula to an infant who cannot assimilate other foods. In addition, this area also contains those functions which an average individual can normally carry out for himself, as, for example, combing his hair and dressing himself.

The second cluster of functions is related to meeting common *psychologic* requirements, such as giving love to an infant. In this cate-

---

[4]George Homans: *The Human Group*. New York, Harcourt, Brace and Company, 1950, p. 36.

[5]James M. A. Weiss (ed.): *Nurses, Patients, and Social Systems*. Columbia, Mo., University of Missouri Press, 1968, p. 62.

gory, too, fall the consideration of individual preferences expressed by the patient, such as giving him the opportunity to select his own clothing. Just as with biologic health problems, there are those special ways in which the nurse meets the patient's psychologic health problems manifested by exaggerated feelings and emotions.

The third area in which the nurse functions is that concerned with the patient's given *socioeconomic* status. How does the nurse explain the diet to a patient with a low socioeconomic status? There may be differences, too, because of the patient's membership in a certain cultural group; for example, in some cultures specific foods are not sanctioned, and the nurse may, in such cases, find other foods that are acceptable to the patient.

Degrees of Visibility in Nursing Functions.   Let us look further at these three areas in which the nurse functions. A continuum which runs through all areas of functioning is the degree of visibility. That is, these functions can be observed by others, but the degree to which they can be observed differs. For our purposes, we shall designate those functions that are easily seen as having high visibility, and those that are not easily seen as having low visibility. In comparing the visibility of the performance in the clusters of functions, those related to the patient's biologic functions are highest, while those functions related to the psychologic, social and cultural requirements are lowest.

If the characteristics of high-visibility functions are examined more fully, the question is raised as to what makes them easily seen. A patient's relative, for example, may walk down a hospital ward, and see one nurse making a bed, another passing medications from a tray, and still another handing an instrument to a physician. The relative may also see rows of neatly made beds which appear fresh and clean, or rows of food-smeared faces peeking from beneath dark gray blankets. Why does the casual observer notice these things so readily?

In high-visibility functions, objects and tools are employed with a degree of manual skill. Thus, the nurse employs a syringe, her tool, in giving a hypodermic injection, and she uses manual skill in manipulating the tool. The high visibility of material goods such as tools and objects manipulated by the nurse may be also related, in our culture, to the high value that society places on the material aspects. Involved, too, in the high-visibility functions are the patient's anatomic structures and processes which are visible sometimes to the casual observer and sometimes only by microscopic means or other refined tests. American culture seems to emphasize the dichotomy of the mind and the body in that somatic disorders are more easily perceived and tolerated than mental illness.

The intended general or meaningful purpose of high-visibility functions is usually more discernible to the observer than the intended purpose in low-visibility functions. It is usually assumed, when one sees a nurse make a bed, that she is performing this function so that a patient may rest or sleep; however, if the nurse is sitting with a patient to provide him with emotional support, the action may be interpreted to mean that the nurse is pampering the patient or merely resting her feet.

Since high-visibility functions are more easily seen, the steps involved in completing the action are more readily identified. Thus, we have a host of procedure books in hospitals describing these steps in detail. Then, too, something that is easily explained in steps is usually easier to teach to others. Perhaps this is the reason many technical functions are delegated to nursing assistants.

When steps are identified, and the manipulation of material objects is employed for meeting the patient's biologic needs, any deviations in the procedure are easily observed. If a nurse withholds fluids from a patient, it soon becomes evident; but it is not so discernible when she withholds respect for the human dignity of an elderly man as he goes mumbling down the corridor.

Another characteristic of high-visibility functions is that they are usually nonverbal in nature. The nurse, for example, may make a bed, a nonverbal function, without uttering a sound. That is to say, it may be desirable to talk with the patient, but talking is not an absolute requirement in accomplishing the task of bedmaking.

The fact that objects are involved in high-visibility functions leads us to another characteristic—routinization into a mass-productive and assembly-line function. If high-visibility functions are performed in this manner, then they tend to become staff centered rather than patient centered. That is, they are organized in a manner convenient for the staff, thus meeting their needs in preference to the individual patient's desires and feelings.

High-visibility functions are an important segment of first impressions, and hospitals, so much in the public eye, seem to like making everyone look busy. However, these first impressions made by the performance of high-visibility functions often give way to a more lasting impression made by the performance of low-visibility functions.

Since the steps involved in high-visibility functions are easily identified, they are more easily controlled by power figures, such as the nursing supervisors or administrators. When complaints come in, administrators can send out edicts on how such situations are to be handled in the future. It is difficult, however, to send out such pronouncements about what a nurse should say to a patient, a low-visibility function. Nursing supervisors seem to praise the nurse for tasks that are easily observed, such as maintaining neat bedside units, but may criticize the nurse for talking with a patient unless it is for a special purpose. Thus, one might hypothesize that reward by high-status personnel, such as administrators and supervisors, tends to reinforce the performance of high-visibility functions, and to extinguish the performance of low-visibility functions. If this be true, it is little wonder that nurses tend to place the task of the administration of an aspirin or sleeping medication above the task of talking with a patient.

Low-visibility functions in nursing can be summarized as follows: (1) they are not easily seen by others; (2) they do not require the employment of material goods with a high degree of manual skill; (3) they are related to the psychologic functions and processes of the individual; (4) they are both verbal and nonverbal in nature; (5) they do not tend to become routinized; (6) they tend to provide the basis for more lasting impressions on others; (7) their intended or general purpose is often misinterpreted by others; (8) they usually cannot be broken down into steps that are identifiable without considerable thinking, and thus are difficult to teach to others; (9) they are less easily controlled by high-status personnel in that results of the performance are not easily seen; (10) they probably are less highly rewarded by high-status nursing personnel. High-visibility functions, in general, are the opposites of the criteria mentioned above.

While nursing functions seem to cluster in three main categories, it does not mean that each is carried out without consideration of the others, for the skillful nurse often performs these functions in combination with one another. For example, the nurse may explain to a newly admitted patient who is soaking his foot what he may expect when he goes to the x-ray department the next day.

UNIQUENESS OF NURSING

What makes nursing different from medicine or psychology? Can't a clinical psychologist give a patient orange juice? Can't a physician help a patient to dress? The psychologist can give orange juice providing he knows *when* to give it and *when* to withhold it. Because of the nature of the patient's illness, as in hypoglycemic shock, it may be necessary to give this certain patient orange juice immediately before doing anything else for him. The physician, too, may help the patient to dress; however, not being familiar with the patient's intimate life situation in carrying out the daily activities of living, he may do considerable fumbling before the task of dressing is completed. Physicians, psychologists, and other members of the health team are usually accustomed to working in a more structured situation than the nurse. That is, they may be in an interview situation either at the patient's bedside or in an office, but seldom do they achieve their goals of diagnosis and therapy through the patient's response to the activities of daily life, such as eating, sleeping, defecating, dressing, and the like. In fact, the physician calls the nurse when the patient has to go to the bathroom or needs assistance in carrying out such intimate activities of daily life. Since the activities of daily living go on twenty-four hours a day, day after day, nursing is also said to be continuous. It is believed that if nursing is to be goal-directed, and if changes in patient behavior are to be effected and evaluated by the nurse, it should be administered to the same recipient by the same person over a period of time.

THE STATUS OF NURSING

The student is referred to Chapter 10 of *Twenty Thousand Nurses Tell Their Story*[6] for a discussion of the criteria of a professional group and the ways nurses meet or do not meet these criteria. Notwithstanding the fact that there are nurses whose practice of nursing is of professional quality, it is the opinion of the writers that nursing at present is an occupation rather than a profession, although it does seem to have potentials for achieving full status as a profession.

A DIFFERENT PATTERN OF CARE

If the nuances indicative of change in a patient's behavior are to be observed in relation to the performance of low-visibility functions, then perhaps a different pattern of care than that of the present "rotating shifts" will be instrumental in bringing about the degree of desired change in the patient. It is conceivable that nursing could have a method of practice similar to that used by medicine or other professional disciplines on the health team. What would happen if physicians referred their patients to a clinical practitioner of nursing (the clinical nursing expert) who would, in turn, employ general practitioners of nursing, students and nursing assistants to help her care for these patients over a twenty-four-hour period, day after day? Such a pattern of care, once implemented, would not require the services of the nursing hierarchy, that is, the head nurse, the supervisor and the ward instructor, but only a nursing administrator in each broad clinical area who would make clinical judgments in relation to patient care. Perhaps, then, prestige would shift from that now acquired by going up the administrative ladder to prestige so rightly deserved by the clinical

---

[6]Everett Hughes, Helen MacGill Hughes, and Irwin Deutscher: *Twenty Thousand Nurses Tell Their Story*. Philadelphia, J. B. Lippincott Co., 1958, pp. 232-250.

nursing expert What would happen if the monetary rewards were higher for clinical expertness than for the present high-status nursing personnel? What would happen to the doctor-nurse relationship if both were to focus on the patient and communicate directly without going through the present nursing channels? What would happen to the nursing student freed from the trap of pleasing personnel from both nursing service and nursing education? More research is needed to establish a pattern of care that will maximize nursing functions.

Although nursing has assisted with medical research, little has yet been done in the way of clinical nursing research, and so it is impossible to say to a student that, if one performs in a given manner, one can predict the exact limits of the outcome.

We *wonder* why nurses are so dissatisfied, we *wonder* why patients complain that they never see a nurse, and students *wonder* why they are taught all the little details of patient care when they cannot or are not given the opportunity to carry them out in actual practice. Often the student is caught between her instructor, who advocates one thing, and the head nurse in an actual situation, who advocates something else. At any rate, the student often feels that these two immovable objects, the head nurse and the instructor, must eventually "get together and give a little" if she is to learn to give adequate patient care and gain some satisfaction from it. Students *wonder,* too, *why* the head nurse and instructor do not agree. To wonder is a step in the right direction, for it is this curiosity that stimulates research.

Throughout this chapter the student has seen the term "behavior" used again and again. We shall turn to a clarification of this term in the next chapter. In order to perform low-visibility functions effectively, the student will need more understanding of terms and their interrelationship to broad areas of practice.

Summary

Nursing has been defined as a process of verbal and nonverbal interaction directed toward the healthful status of the recipient within either an institution, an agency or the community. Nursing has been discussed in relation to professional status, uniqueness and function of the nurse, in an attempt to offer suggestions which may be utilized in identifying and solving problems related to nursing and nursing situations.

Terms such as psychodynamic, biosocial, high- and low-visibility functions and others, which are used throughout the text, have been defined. The functions of the nurse have been discussed in relation to those concerned with the patient's biologic needs, those concerned with the patient's psychologic requirements and those concerned with the patient's socioeconomic status.

Degree of visibility has been discussed in relation to the above functions of the nurse. High-visibility functions are summarized as follows: (1) they are easily seen by others; (2) they require the employment of material goods with a degree of manual skill· (3) they are related to the anatomic functions and processes of the body; (4) they are nonverbal in nature; (5) they tend to become routinized and staff centered; (6) they tend to provide the basis of first impressions on others; (7) their intended or general purpose is usually correctly interpreted by others; (8) they can be broken down into steps that are easily identified and thus are comparatively easy to teach to others; (9) they are more easily controlled by high-status personnel in that results of the performance are more easily seen; (10) they probably are more highly regarded by high-status nursing personnel.

Low-visibility functions are, in general, the opposites of the criteria mentioned above and have been enumerated within the chapter. Some reasons why nursing is believed to differ from other professions on the health team have also been offered.

Suggestions were made in regard to a different pattern of care for patients, utilizing a clinical practitioner of nursing (the clinical nursing expert) who would employ general practitioners of nursing, students and nursing assistants to help care for patients over a twenty-four–hour period, day after day. The implications of such an innovation have also been discussed.

An attempt has been made through definition and discussion to give the reader some background in the terminology to be used in this book so that there will be a common basis for understanding the behavior of patients and for solving nursing problems and expanding or changing the theoretical formulations as new data are acquired.

Bibliography

Brown, Martha M.: "Nurse-Patient Relationships with Older Patients," Unpublished manuscript, 1958.

Cameron, Norman: *The Psychology of Behavioral Disorders: A Biosocial Interpretation.* Boston, Houghton Mifflin Co., 1947.

Caudill, Williams: *The Psychiatric Hospital as a Small Society* Cambridge, Harvard University Press, 1958.

Davis, Fred (ed.): *The Nursing Profession: Five Sociological Essays.* New York, John Wiley and Sons, Inc., 1966.

Dickoff, James, and James, Patricia: "Theory in a Practice Discipline." *Nursing Research,* 17:415-435, September–October, 1968.

Homans, George: *The Human Group.* New York, Harcourt, Brace and Co., 1950.

Hughes, Everett, Hughes, Helen MacGill, and Deutscher, Irwin: *Twenty Thousand Nurses Tell Their Story.* Philadelphia, J. B. Lippincott Co., 1958.

Kreuter, Frances: "What is Good Nursing Care?" *Nursing Outlook,* 5:302–304, May, 1957.
Macgregor, Frances Cooke: *Social Science in Nursing.* New York, Russell Sage Foundation, 1960.
Merton, Robert K.: *Social Theory and Social Structure.* Chicago, Free Press of Glencoe, 1957.
Montagu, M. F. Ashley: *The Direction of Human Development.* New York, Harper & Brothers, 1955.
Peplau, Hildegarde E.: *Interpersonal Relations in Nursing.* New York, G. P. Putnam's Sons, 1952.
Research staff, Washington University School of Nursing: "Progress Report in Personalization of Older Patients." Unpublished manuscript, 1959.
Weiss, Edoardo: *Principles of Psychodynamics.* New York, Grune & Stratton, Inc., 1950.
Weiss, James M. A. (ed.): *Nurses, Patients, and Social Systems.* Columbia, Mo., University of Missouri Press, 1968.

Suggestions for Further Reading

Aydelotte, Myrtle: "Issues of Professional Nursing." *Nursing Forum,* 7:73–85, No. 1, 1968.
Brown, Esther Lucile: *Newer Dimensions of Patient Care,* Part III. New York, Russell Sage Foundation, 1964.
Croley, M. Jay: "What Does a Psychiatric Nursing Specialist Do?" *Am. J. Nursing,* 62:72–74, February, 1962.
George, Frances L., and Kuehn, Ruth P.: *Patterns of Patient Care.* New York, Macmillan Co., 1955, pp. 166–175.
Hanson, R. C., and Beech, Mary Jane: "Communicating Health Arguments Across Cultures." *Nursing Res.,* 12:237–241, Fall, 1963.
Henderson, Virginia: "The Nature of Nursing. *Am. J. Nursing,* 64:62–68, August, 1964.
Hughes, Everett C., Hughes, Helen MacGill, and Deutscher, Irwin: *Twenty Thousand Nurses Tell Their Story.* Philadelphia, J. B. Lippincott Co., 1958, pp. 1–8, 47–61, 232–250, 268–277.
Johnson, Miriam M., and Martin, Harry W.: "A Sociological Analysis of the Nurse Role." *Am. J. Nursing,* 58:373–377, March, 1958.
Lambertsen, Eleanor C.: *Education for Nursing Leadership.* Philadelphia, J. B. Lippincott Co., 1958, pp. 45–55, 73–94, 105–107.
Little, Dolores: "The Nurse Specialist." *American Journal of Nursing,* 67:552–556, March, 1967.
McCabe, Gracia S.: "Cultural Influences on Patient Behavior." *Am. J. Nursing,* 60:1101–1104, August, 1960.
Macgregor, Frances Cooke: *Social Science in Nursing.* New York, Russell Sage Foundation, 1960, pp. 66–159.
Maloney, Elizabeth: "Does the Psychiatric Nurse Have Independent Functions?" *Am. J. Nursing,* 62:61–63, June, 1962.
Mead, Margaret: "Understanding Cultural Patterns." *Nursing Outlook,* 4:260–262, May, 1956.
Mead, Margaret: "Determinants of Health Beliefs and Behavior: III, Cultural Determinants." *Am. J. Pub. Health,* 51:1552–1554, October, 1961.
Moore, Marjorie A.: "Nursing: A Scientific Discipline?" *Nursing Forum,* 7:340–347, No. 4, 1968.
Paynich, Mary Louise: "Cultural Barriers to Nurse Communication." *Am. J. Nursing,* 64:87–90, February, 1964.
Rapaport, Lydia: "Motivation in the Struggle for Health." *Am. J. Nursing,* 57:1455–1457, November, 1957.
Saunders, Lyle: "Permanence and Change." *Am. J. Nursing,* 58:969–972, July, 1958.
Shuval, Judith F.: "Perceived Role Components of Nursing in Israel." *Am. Soc. Rev.,* 28:37–46, February, 1963.
Tuteur, Werner: "As You Enter Psychiatric Nursing." *Am. J. Nursing,* 56:72–74, January, 1956.

Chapter 2   Behavior

If our goal is the understanding of another person, it is useless to focus our attention upon one part or one aspect of his behavior. We must focus on the individual in his situation and see it as a whole, in detail and without distortion. In the light of our present knowledge, human behavior is a complicated phenomenon influenced by anatomy and physiology, biochemistry, psychology, and sociology all interacting in such a way that everything either is a part of or is in some way influenced by everything else.

The fact that people are more alike than they are different provides the opportunity for learning to better understand people and their needs. In order for man to survive, not only must he have various environments, with specific qualities available, but he must also maintain contact with these environments and through his total behavior carry on an interchange with them. We can illustrate this point in regard to the physiochemical environment. The human individual has to maintain a constant exchange with certain elements in the physiochemical environment around him, and if this supply is cut off his very existence is threatened. Closely related to this aspect is maintaining a constant exchange with certain elements in his internal physiochemical environment through such processes as metabolism and circulation.

Another necessary environment peculiar to man is the interpersonal, social or cultural environment. In contrast to plants and animals, people cannot live as human beings without maintaining contact with other people and without carrying on an interchange with them. As we shall see later, this interpersonal environment is extremely important in infancy, for without an interpersonal environment with certain qualities with which the infant has an adequate interchange, he will be unable to carry on the necessary interchange with his physiochemical environment and thus he will be unable to survive.

It seems plausible that many of the problems encountered in living are the result of experiences with an environment that either lacked the necessary qualities or with which, for some reason, the individual's behavior was ineffective in establishing and/or maintaining an adequate interchange. As we go on to elaborate certain aspects of human behavior, it will be helpful to remember that each aspect feeds into the whole interplay of forces which influences the individual's responses in any situation.

DEFINITION OF BEHAVIOR

The term *behavior* refers to the way in which an organism responds to a stimulus. Since we are primarily concerned with human organisms, our discussion will be limited to the behavior of people.

In considering behavior as action in response to a stimulus it may be helpful to explain the terms *stimulus* and *response*. By *stimulus* we mean that which incites certain changes within the individual, while *response* refers to action, both overt and covert, in relation to a given stimulus. The term *overt* refers to that which is readily discernible to the outside observer, whereas *covert* refers to that which must be inferred since it is not so readily observed. Just as there is an overt and a covert aspect of response, we find that the stimuli may originate in either the external or internal environment of the individual. For example, if the room temperature changes from warm to cold and one develops "goose flesh," he is responding to a stimulus, the change in room temperature, in the external environment. On the other hand, if one develops an increased body temperature, has a flushed face and feels warm, he is responding to a stimulus in his internal environment.

VARIETIES OF BEHAVIOR

For our purpose, three varieties of behavior will be considered: reflex action, goal-directed activity, and behavior as a response to frustration.

The first mentioned, reflex action, is the most simple type of activity and occurs automatically in response to a stimulus, such as is seen in the knee jerk when the patella region is tapped lightly with a percussion hammer.

The second type, goal-directed behavior, presupposes the existence of two conditions. First, there is always a need present within the individual or a change in his internal environment. Then there is a goal outside the individual or in his external environment which is capable of producing a change in the internal condition and thus satisfying the need. To illustrate, imagine an eight-month-old infant who is hungry and who is uncomfortable because of this change in his internal environment. This state of hunger will persist until he attains food, the goal, and ingests it. Then his internal condition will, in turn, change as his need is satisfied.

Behavior as a response to frustration, the third type of activity, is suggested by Maier[1] wherein a specific goal is not involved and a specific need is not satisfied. This may be clarified again by referring to the infant in the former illustration. Suppose that this infant has been hungry for two hours and has been increasingly loud in proclaiming his state of discomfort. Then, when his bottle of milk is brought to him, he responds by throwing it on the floor and spilling the milk. Consequently his goal of ingesting food is not reached and his hunger continues.

NEEDS

DEFINITION OF NEED

A need is an organismic condition which exists within the individual and which demands certain activity. A need evolves from a state of tension which disrupts the individual's equilibrium and produces a relative degree of discomfort which, in turn, propels him to do something about it in order to re-establish equilibrium.

SOURCES OF NEEDS

The need, then, is the basis of all "ongoing" behavior sequences, overt as well as covert, and it arises from three main sources. Most familiar are those such as hunger and thirst which arise as a direct result of metabolic processes. Then there are those which result direct-

---

[1]Norman Maier: *Frustration.* New York, McGraw-Hill Book Co., Inc., 1949, p. 161.

ly from a change in the individual's relationship with his external environment, such as a sudden drop in the temperature of the room. The third source is very common in evoking needs, although it is not often considered—that is, our symbolic behavior such as talking, reading or thinking. Who has not had the experience of suddenly finding himself ravenously hungry after hearing someone talk about a delicious meal that he has just eaten?

THE NEED-SATISFACTION SEQUENCE

The need-satisfaction sequence is characteristic of all goal-directed behavior and is a pattern established very early in life in relation to the biologic needs which are present at birth. At this time the infant has needs which can be satisfied only through his external environment, and as these needs are met his basic need-satisfaction pattern is established. On the basis of his interaction with the significant people in his environment, his need-satisfaction patterns are modified and elaborated. A very basic need-satisfaction sequence in relation to one of the so-called vital needs may be illustrated as follows: first, there exists within the organism a condition of disequilibrium, a physiologic tension state commonly recognized as thirst; this tension can be relieved only by an external object, in this instance, liquid, which becomes the goal. The tension state creates an urge toward activity which leads toward the goal. The activity always involves some neuromuscular act on the part of the individual experiencing the tension so that the goal is reached and the desire satisfied, thus relieving the tension which initiated the whole sequence. Therefore, when the individual recognizes this tension state as thirst, he begins action to obtain liquid, ingests the liquid, experiences satisfaction, and equilibrium is again re-established.

Then, there is the after-reaction to need-satisfaction which is called gratification. *Gratification* is usually defined as a pleasant expansive response following the satisfaction of a need. It may occur immediately following completion of the sequence, it may be delayed for some time, or it may not occur at all. Since gratification frequently becomes more important than the need-satisfaction to which it is a response, it is essential that we differentiate between satisfaction which is the termination of a need and the re-establishment of equilibrium, and gratification which is the after-reaction to the need-satisfaction sequence.

HIERARCHY OF NEEDS

There have been many attempts to enumerate and classify needs, but there has not been much clarification accomplished through these efforts because of so much duplication and overlapping. The authors have found that Maslow's concept of a hierarchy of needs is most practical and helpful in learning to understand the over-all content of behavior. Maslow[2] suggests the concept of five levels of needs ranging from the physiologic to those that represent a higher level of development. In his scheme, the first-level needs consist of the basic physiologic aspects such as hunger and thirst. The second level comprises the needs of safety—that is, of avoiding external dangers that might bring harm. The third level is the need for belongingness and love—that is, to be given love, warmth and affection by another person; the love needs involve both giving and receiving love. The need for esteem makes up the fourth level; it includes self-respect and self-esteem as well as the respect and esteem of others. With the satisfaction of these needs, one experiences feelings of self-confidence, strength and capability, whereas, if they are thwarted, one experiences feelings of inferiority, worthlessness and helplessness. The top or fifth level is the need for self-realization, that of being able to utilize one's potentialities to accomplish and achieve. As the infant develops and achieves satisfaction of his basic-level needs he is then freed to function on a higher level. On the other hand, if these more basic needs are not met adequately, then they claim priority, and activities on a higher level must be temporarily postponed.

CONFLICT

DEFINITION OF CONFLICT

Since conflict is such an important element of behavior, we can describe it as the opposition of two or more equally strong forces affecting the individual. Such interference may develop between such things as self-reactions, roles, attitudes and motives. If we are to describe conflict we will take into account several factors. First, there is a difference in the degree to which various individuals are susceptible to conflicts. Individuals differ widely in the ease with which they develop conflict and also in the nature and effectiveness of their response. This degree of susceptibility rests largely upon the biologic inheritance as well as the past experiences of the person. Second, we must consider the cultural norms or standards of the group of which the individual is a part. What does society condone and what does it prohibit? Third, there is the variety of competing reactions within the individual to

---

[2]A. H. Maslow: *Motivation and Personality.* New York, Harper & Brothers, 1954, pp. 80-92.

consider. These we sometimes refer to as ambivalent feelings, such as simultaneous feelings of love and hate for the same object. In addition, there may be incompatible reactions within a given society. These are sometimes similar to the ambivalent feelings of an individual. For example, a given society may condone the practice of cutthroat competition sometimes seen in modern industry but it may also sanction practicing the golden rule. We can readily see that cutthroat competition and the ideal upheld in the golden rule are incompatible. Conflict may also be described in terms of its consequences. Accompanying it is tension which may be either brief or prolonged, slight or severe. Another end result is the impoverishment of behavior or a reduction in activity responses. There is also a distortion of the ongoing pattern of behavior — that is, it tends to become warped in a certain direction or it becomes repetitive.

TYPES OF CONFLICT

Lewin[3] has contributed several concepts which may help us in understanding conflict. He describes three types of conflict.

In the first, the individual stands between two positive forces which attract him. For example, he is asked to go on a picnic with his family and also to play bridge with his companions. The two forces, the picnic and the bridge, both seem attractive to him and, therefore, these objects take on positive valences. The individual must decide which he will do, but in this type of conflict situation a decision is relatively easy as he selects one activity and excludes the other.

The second type of conflict situation is one in which there is a positive valence but a barrier exists between the individual and the positive attraction. As he tries to reach the goal, the barrier acquires a negative valence. The negative aspects of the barrier usually increase in strength and become stronger than the positive valence, and when this happens the individual retreats. To illustrate, let us picture a small child who sees some candy on the mantel. The candy seems attractive to him and is, therefore, said to have a positive valence; however, there is a chair in front of the mantel and several times he has fallen from this chair. The chair then becomes a negative factor and also serves as a barrier between the child and the candy. At first the child may make several attempts to climb up on the chair but then, as he remembers the times he fell, he withdraws temporarily, only to return again in a few minutes for another attempt. The duration of these withdrawal periods increases until finally he gives up.

---

[3]Kurt Lewin: *A Dynamic Theory of Personality.* New York, McGraw-Hill Book Co., Inc., 1935.

The third type of conflict situation occurs when the individual stands between two negative valences. For example, a child may be told to go to bed or he will be spanked. Since he does not wish to be spanked and also does not want to go to bed, he is repelled from both alternatives. We see him begin to vacillate and, as the pressures of these negative valences continue to build up, the child will attempt to escape from the situation by turning to fantasy or some other means of running away If a person is to have adequate experience in learning to cope effectively with various conflict situations, we have to assume that his environment provides ample opportunities for making a choice.

STRESS AND FRUSTRATION

EFFECTS OF STRESS

Stress and frustration are two related terms that we should clarify because of their many influences and implications on behavior in general. Stress occurs in a situation wherein pressures are felt by a person and these pressures, in turn, change his current behavior patterns. If the individual's behavior at the time he experiences the pressures is goal-directed, he will keep his goal in sight and perform in such a way that his need-satisfaction sequences will usually be completed even under a high degree of stress. On the other hand, if the stress becomes sufficiently great and reaches a point above the stress threshold of this individual, he may then experience frustration. When his tolerance level is reached and frustration occurs, his behavior will no longer be goal-directed and his need-satisfaction sequences will be either temporarily or permanently interrupted. In addition to these changes, there are many physiologic responses which may occur, such as an increase of tension, a change in pulse rate and respiration and an unpleasant feeling tone. The person who experiences frustration also usually feels that he is being punished by somebody, since he is being denied the satisfaction of his needs.

RESPONSES TO FRUSTRATION

Maier[4] suggests that there are four classes of responses which are thought to be characteristic of behavior induced by frustration. First is *fixation*, which he describes as a response which is strong or persistent

---

[4]Norman Maier: *Frustration.* New York, McGraw-Hill Book Co., Inc., 1949, pp. 77-82, 101-104, 107-109, 111-112.

and which cannot be changed by usual methods of retraining. He found that the response in progress at the time frustration occurred was the most likely one to be fixated. An individual with a fixated response would be expected to encounter difficulty in learning in a situation similar to the one which had proved frustrating. A very common example of a fixated response is a prejudice. The second response is that of *aggression,* which represents some form of attack and is, in general, destructive. *Regression* is the third specific response, and it may be visualized as the opposite of progression; that is, the individual goes backward rather than forward. He uses responses which were effective at an earlier age and had been discarded but which are again adopted in an attempt to cope with the existing situation. The fourth response to frustration may be one of apathy or *resignation,* which represents the act of giving up, of withdrawing and escaping from the reality situation. Characteristic of all these responses to frustration is the fact that they are not goal-directed but their purpose is achieved in the tension reduction that occurs.

ANXIETY

Another basic element of behavior is anxiety, which is a feeling state experienced when a person is in some way threatened or believes himself to be in danger. Anxiety has been defined as a state of dread or apprehension with respect to some anticipated danger. It seems to serve as a signal which alerts the individual to the possibility of excessive excitation, from within or without, that might upset his equilibrium and create a painful, unpleasurable state. As a warning, the anxiety acts as a stimulus to defensive action to handle the excitation. Anxiety, as such, consists of an unpleasant affect, felt as fearfulness, and concomitant physiologic signs which are interpreted as preparations for action, either flight or struggle. Although the actual danger remains unknown, the individual responds as though the threat came from the external environment and can only be dealt with by attacking it or running away from it. The unpleasant feeling tone is rather diffuse and persistent and gives rise to a feeling of helplessness. In our culture, anxiety seems to be directly related to the anticipation of a loss of esteem, either by oneself or by others. Whenever anything happens which threatens to disturb one's usual pattern of interacting with others, one tends to experience anxiety. It is generally agreed that the experiencing of anxiety is inevitable; therefore, the important thing is how the individual learns to cope with it.

Anxiety may be interpreted in many ways, depending upon the theoretical frame of reference one uses. There is what is sometimes called free-floating anxiety that produces a feeling of uneasiness, a feeling that something is wrong, a feeling of restlessness, which may provide the impetus to constructive physical activity if it remains below a certain level. On the other hand, any increase of anxiety above one's level of tolerance becomes a threat to one's psychological integrity, and regression ensues and defensive patterns become necessary. As the individual prepares to defend and protect himself, the extent of his awareness is always reduced or restricted so that he becomes oblivious to cues either from himself or from others that would illuminate the situation and help him to understand it and thereby learn to cope with it.

In situations in which one has had anxiety, one is unable to learn or to profit from his experiences because he cannot remember much of what has occurred, and most of his energy has had to be directed toward defensive activities in his attempt to alleviate the situation. Anxiety has a "contagious" quality and is readily communicated from one person to another; therefore, everyone in close proximity is soon contaminated and confusion and further disruptive interaction occurs.

BASIC ASSUMPTIONS IN REGARD TO BEHAVIOR WHICH HAVE IMPLICATIONS FOR NURSING

1. BEHAVIOR INCLUDES THE INDIVIDUAL'S TOTAL RESPONSE TO STIMULI. We have said previously that behavior is a response to a stimulus and that a stimulus may be from either the internal or external environment; therefore, we can conceive of total behavior as being incited from either inside or outside the body. For example, such vital functions as breathing and heart action are as much a part of our behavior as what we say and what we do. To illustrate further, increased respiration may be incited by a stimulus which calls for additional oxygen for the tissues, whereas a verbal response to a companion may be incited by a question which requires an answer. Both of these responses are incited by stimuli; therefore, both would be an example of behavior.

If we base our nursing care on the patient's total behavior, it will no longer be necessary to speak in terms of the old dichotomy, physical and mental, in regard to the care of an individual with a medical or a psychiatric problem.

2. THE BEHAVIOR MANIFESTED BY AN INDIVIDUAL IS GOVERNED BY HIS AVAILABLE ENERGY, WHICH IS ALWAYS WITHIN THE RANGE OF HIS MAXIMUM ENERGY POTENTIAL. Although the individual's maximum energy potential will remain fairly constant, the amount of energy

available to him at a given time may vary considerably. In this same respect, we find that the maximum energy potential varies from individual to individual. Therefore, the nurse cannot expect the same output from all individuals, nor can she expect the same degree from any one individual in all instances. As we shall see later, there are many factors which influence the amount of energy available to the individual in his day-to-day experiences.

3. ALL BEHAVIOR IS PURPOSEFUL. At first glance, it may appear that there will be many exceptions to this assumption; however, a close examination will reveal that there is always a purpose involved for the person behaving. Since this assumption is basic in learning to understand people, it is helpful to think in the following terms when we observe someone's overt action. What was he trying to accomplish? Was it in terms of maintaining something, gaining something or losing something? What did it mean to him? We also find that an individual's covert responses may be reviewed in the same manner. To illustrate, a germ may enter the blood stream, and the individual's response may be an increase in white blood cells. This response serves to combat the infection and is, therefore, purposeful to the individual.

4. ALL BEHAVIOR IS A RESPONSE TO CHANGED CONDITIONS IN THE INDIVIDUAL'S TOTAL ENVIRONMENT. This statement implies that all behavior has a cause even though it may be difficult to discover and even more difficult to understand once it is discovered. No response is thought to occur spontaneously without some stimulus to give it impetus.

5. THE RESPONSE OF AN INDIVIDUAL IN A SPECIFIC SITUATION IS THE BEST THAT HE IS CAPABLE OF MAKING AT THE GIVEN MOMENT. The acceptance of this assumption will make it easier for the nurse to accept the patient regardless of what his response may be. He may be responding as he does because of his low energy potential, because of his past experience in a similar situation or because of unknown factors. Nonetheless, it is a well-known fact that everyone utilizes all of his available potentialities to cope with his experiences.

6. WHAT AN INDIVIDUAL PERCEIVES AS HAPPENING TO HIM IS MORE INFLUENTIAL IN DETERMINING HIS BEHAVIOR THAN WHAT IS ACTUALLY HAPPENING TO HIM. We act and feel not according to what things are really like but according to our images of what they are like. In line with this assumption, the nurse may think that she is doing something helpful for the patient while he may perceive her action as something threatening; therefore, his response may be different from that which she anticipated.

7. THE PROVISION FOR THE SATISFACTION OF THE INDIVIDUAL'S EXISTING NEEDS WILL ALLOW FOR THE EMERGENCE OF MORE MATURE NEEDS. This statement implies that nursing care must be consistent

with the current level of the patient's needs, and, unless we can provide for his needs of the moment, we cannot expect him to make progress. In terms of this assumption, we can readily see why we meet with failure when we try to make the dependent, demanding patient more independent by ignoring his requests.

8. THERE IS INHERENT IN EVERY INDIVIDUAL A POTENTIAL FOR STRIVING FORWARD. This assumption expresses the hope that people, in general, are still capable of progressing as well as regressing. Furthermore, the movement must come from within the individual. There is nothing the nurse can do to the patient, but she can help him to mobilize these positive forces that will activate forward movement.

9. THERE IS BOTH AN OVERT AND A COVERT ASPECT OF EVERY BEHAVIORAL RESPONSE. Verbalizations, actions and other outward manifestations represent the overt aspect, with the simultaneously occurring thoughts, feelings and the general state of the individual representing the covert aspect of the response. If we consider only the overt manifestations of a person's behavior, we will have little real basis for understanding him because outwardly two persons can appear to be doing exactly the same thing, but their motives, feelings and other subjective experiences are quite different. Therefore, we can usually be accurate in saying what a person is looking at, but we cannot be certain what he sees. In the same way, we can readily say what someone is listening to, but we can never be sure what he hears.

10. THE INDIVIDUAL IN OUR CULTURE SATISFIES MOST OF HIS NEEDS THROUGH RELATIONSHIPS WITH OTHER INDIVIDUALS OR GROUPS OF INDIVIDUALS. From the moment of birth, each individual requires interaction with another person or persons if he is to survive, and this pattern of interaction continues to expand and become more elaborate as the individual grows.

Summary

An understanding of some of the basic concepts about behavior is a prerequisite for providing professional nursing care. If we can but grasp the concept of total behavior, then it will no longer be necessary for us to think in terms of the dichotomy, mental or physical. The concept of total behavior implies that the beating of the heart and the action of the stomach are just as important, and as much a part of the patient's behavior, as what he says and what he does. An attempt has been made to describe behavior in terms of both covert and overt aspects, as well as its stimuli from the environment, internal and external. Three varieties of behavior which the nurse may observe are reflex action, goal-directed activity, and behavior which is a response to frustration.

In order to understand behavior in relation to individual needs, it has been necessary to clarify the concept of needs, their sources, and the need-satisfaction sequence. Maslow's concept of hierarchy of needs may be helpful to the nurse in understanding the needs of her patients. Other basic concepts involved in understanding behavior are conflict, frustration and anxiety. Clarification of these aspects will help us in understanding the assumptions made about behavor which, as we shall see later, have many implications for nursing care.

Bibliography

Cameron, Norman: *The Psychology of Behavior Disorders.* Boston, Houghton Mifflin Co., 1947.
Dewey, Richard, and Humbler, W. J.: *The Development of Human Behavior.* New York, Macmillan Co., 1951.
French, Thomas M.: *The Integration of Behavior,* Vol. II. Chicago, University of Chicago Press, 1954.
Fromm, Erich: *Man for Himself.* New York, Rinehart & Co., 1947.
Frosch, John, ed.: *The Annual Survey of Psychoanalysis,* Vol. I. New York, International Universities Press, Inc., 1952.
Grinker, R. R., ed.: *Toward a Unified Theory of Human Behavior.* New York, Basic Books, Inc., 1956.
Lewin, Kurt: *A Dynamic Theory of Personality.* New York, McGraw-Hill Book Co., Inc., 1935.
Lidz, Theodore: *The Person.* New York, Basic Books, Inc., 1970.
Maier, Norman: *Frustration.* New York, McGraw-Hill Book Co., Inc., 1949.
Maslow, A. H.: *Motivation and Personality.* New York, Harper & Brothers, 1954.
Maslow, A. H., and Mittelmann, Bela: *Principles of Abnormal Psychology.* New York, Harper & Brothers, 1951.
Masserman, Jules H.: *Principles of Dynamic Psychiatry,* 2nd ed. Philadelphia, W. B. Saunders Co., 1961.
May, Rollo: *The Meaning of Anxiety.* New York, Ronald Press Co., 1950.
May, Rollo: *Man's Search for Himself.* New York, W. W. Norton & Co., Inc., 1953.
Montagu, Ashley: *On Being Human.* New York, Henry Schuman, Inc., Publishers, 1950.
Montagu, Ashley: *The Direction of Human Development.* New York, Harper & Brothers, 1955.
Mullahy, Patrick, ed.: *The Contributions of Harry Stack Sullivan.* New York, Hermitage House, Inc., 1952.
Saul, Leon: *Emotional Maturity,* 2nd ed., Philadelphia, J. B. Lippincott Co., 1960.
Stein, Maurice R., Vidich, Arthur J., and White, David Manning, eds.: *Identity and Anxiety.* Chicago, Free Press of Glencoe, 1960.
Sullivan, Harry Stack: *Clinical Studies in Psychiatry.* New York, W. W. Norton & Co., Inc., 1956.
Sullivan, Harry Stack: *Conceptions of Modern Psychiatry.* New York, W. W. Norton & Co., Inc., 1953.
Sullivan, Harry Stack: *The Interpersonal Theory of Psychiatry.* New York, W. W. Norton & Co., Inc., 1953.
Symonds, Percival M.: *The Dynamics of Human Adjustment.* New York, Appleton-Century-Crofts, Inc., 1946.

Suggestions for Further Reading

Anderson, Camilla M.: *Saints, Sinners, and Psychiatry.* Philadelphia, J. B. Lippincott Co., 1950, pp. 9-20, 41-58, 112-123, 151-177.
Bettelheim, Bruno: "To Nurse and to Nurture." *Nursing Forum, 1*:60-76, Summer, 1962.

Brill, Norman Q.: "The Importance of Understanding Yourself." *Am. J. Nursing,* *57*:1325-1326, 1957.

Engel, George L.: "Grief and Grieving." *Am. J. Nursing, 64*:93-98, 1964.

Farnsworth, Dana L.: "Mental Health, a Point of View." *Am. J. Nursing, 60*:688-691, 1960.

Godek, Isabelle: "Three Keys to Significant Behavior." *Am. J. Nursing, 59*:1564-1565, 1959.

Hammes, Helen J.: "Reflections on 'Intensive' Care." *Am. J. Nursing, 68*:389-390, 1968.

Hyde, Robert W., and Coggan, Norma E.: "When Nurses Have Guilt Feelings." *Am. J. Nursing, 58*:233-236, 1958.

Ingles, Thelma: "Case Study—The Worst Patient on the Floor." *Nursing Outlook,* *6*:99-100, 1958.

Ingles, Thelma: "Understanding the Nurse-Patient Relationship." *Nursing Outlook,* *9*:698-700, 1961.

Jourard, Sidney M.: "How Well Do You Know Your Patients?" *Am. J. Nursing,* *59*:1568-1571, 1959.

Maslow, A. H., and Mittelmann, Bela: *Principles of Abnormal Psychology.* New York, Harper & Brothers, 1951, pp. 45-49, 61-71.

Matheney, Ruth V., and Topalis, Mary: *Psychiatric Nursing.* 4th Ed., St. Louis, C. V. Mosby Co., 1965, pp. 69-75.

McCabe, Gracia S.: "Cultural Influences on Patient Behavior." *Am. J. Nursing,* *60*:1101-1104, 1960.

Nelson, Alice C.: "Why Won't Stevie Drink?" *Am. J. Nursing, 61*:44-48, 1961.

Rapaport, Lydia: "Motivation in the Struggle for Health." *Am. J. Nursing, 57*:1455-1457, 1957.

Thompson, Clara: "The Different Schools of Psychoanalysis." *Am. J. Nursing,* *57*:1304-1307, 1957.

Warters, Jane: *Achieving Maturity.* New York, McGraw-Hill Book Co., Inc., 1949, pp. 131-151.

Whiting, J. Frank: "Patients' Needs, Nurses' Needs, and the Healing Process." *Am. J. Nursing, 59*:661-665, 1959.

Chapter 3   Personality Structure and Characteristic Patterns of Adjustment

In order to analyze and better understand the complex behavior of the human organism, the schools of ego psychology describe personality topographically as consisting of three closely interrelated aspects that carry out various functions, some of which are conscious, others preconscious and still others unconscious; the id, the ego and the superego.

It must be noted, however, that the label which we attach to any one area or function of the individual denotes only a part of the total frame of reference. Each of these labels can then be utilized to better understand how an individual functions in specific situations. If one prefers other terms to describe the personality, one may focus on the self, the observing and criticizing functions of the self and the security operations which are called into play when anxiety threatens.

DEFINITION OF TERMS

THE ID

The id is thought to make up the total personality at birth. It is said to be primitive, which implies it has not been influenced by civilization or culture. The biologic traits are carried by the id, and it also contains the basic drives, impulses and desires. Furthermore, the id not only provides the source of life energy for the individual but is the one aspect of the personality in which the functions and processes are entirely unconscious. Since the id is primitive and promotes the demand for immediate satisfaction or release of tension and the avoidance of pain regardless of circumstances, the infant, who is all id, is said to function according to the pleasure principle.

THE EGO

Through his experiences with the external world, the infant's ego becomes differentiated as new functions become evident. The ego, which develops from the individual's inherent potentialities as a result of his interaction with his environment, is often referred to as that part of the personality that is in closest contact with reality. A part of this ego is the "self," or what is experienced as "I" and "me," as separate from everything that is "not me."

The ego has many functions, and its strength and stability are reflected in the way these functions are evidenced in the overt behavior of the individual. Many of the primary functions are in relation to reality, such as maintaining contact with reality and promoting the satisfaction of needs in accordance with the outside environment. It is through this function that the individual is able to evaluate reality situations and to become aware of both the advantages and dangers inherent in them. In this respect, the ego initiates warning signals when conflict and danger are imminent, so that more effective action will ensue.

In the same way, the ego functions in evaluating what goes on within the individual. Thus, the individual becomes aware of his primary impulses, desires and fears as well as his own standards and values. Then, in addition to these cognitive functions, the ego also influences overt action so that it is more in line with this awareness. In this way, too, the ego functions in determining which response, of all those possible in a given situation, is going to have priority from both a covert and an overt standpoint—that is, just how this individual will behave in a given situation.

Another important function of the ego is an integrative factor. It is this role that gives unity and coherence to overt behavior and helps to maintain "self-identity." In a similar fashion, the ego has the task of maintaining a "reasonable" equilibrium in the intrapersonal relationships or those between itself, the id and the superego.

THE SUPEREGO

The third aspect of the personality, the superego, is the last part to begin differentiation. It represents tradition or the demands of society and is developed through identification with the parent figures who enforce the prohibitions and taboos. Of primary concern are the moral issues of good and bad, right and wrong, and the superego functions as a restrictive force inhibiting certain behavior. Therefore, it is through the criticism of the superego that the individual experiences guilt. The superego functions in relation to both conscious and unconscious activities and throughout life is somewhat susceptible to change according to the influence of the persons significant to the individual.

Various functions and processes go on within the personality structure and are classified according to certain qualities and characteristics that they possess. First is the quality of consciousness, which is attributed to all of the thoughts, feelings, sensations and so forth of which we are aware at any given time. This conscious quality is transitory, and an idea which is labeled conscious can lose this quality and can also regain it a few minutes later. The second quality is that of unconsciousness, which is in some respects also transitory although not so much as the former. This quality is attributed to all thoughts, feelings, sensations and so forth that are not within the awareness at any given time.

This quality of unconsciousness has both a dynamic and a descriptive aspect. The descriptive aspect is sometimes called preconscious, and everything labeled with this quality is not within awareness at a given time but is capable of readily acquiring the quality of consciousness. Processes or ideas which are preconscious are also said to be latent. The dynamic aspect of this quality is in reference to that which is not within awareness at a given time and which cannot achieve the quality of consciousness by ordinary means. Processes possessing this quality are very powerful and can produce all the effects that ordinary ideas do without themselves becoming conscious, although these effects can become conscious as ideas.

The individual's so-called personality develops concomitantly with his general over-all development as he grows from a helpless infant governed by basic physiologic needs to an adult who functions as a biosocial unit.

As the individual develops and his ego becomes strong enough to exert more control over his behavior, he learns to utilize certain patterns when anxiety signals that danger is threatening. The patterns that are the most effective in relieving the increased tension are the ones that he tends to use again and again whenever anxiety is aroused and an adjustment is required.

ADJUSTMENT

The adjustment process is a fundamental pattern of behavior. The individual's adjustment can be said to be the characteristic manner in which he solves his main problems of life. In order to solve problems, however, the individual must perceive them; therefore, the manner in which he perceives and reacts to the problems which confront him will have a marked effect upon how he solves them. Since failure to adjust threatens the existence of the organism, we know how important adjustment in life really is. As conditions in the environment change, we can see people tending to vary their activities in response to these changes. They may solve their problems either by forming new responses, by changing the external environment or by modifying their needs. It is inherent in people to use their abilities as effectively as possible in an attempt to adjust to life. We need only to look around, however, to discover that some individuals seem to make a more satisfactory adjustment than others.

Efficiency in adjustment depends upon the ability of an individual to continue varying his responses until he achieves success in solving his problem or in his ability to change his image or perception of the problem to correspond with reality. We might say that the psychiatric patient has either lost or never developed his ability to vary his responses until he is successful. He retreats from reality because he has no available response to cope with the existing situation, and the response he makes may not solve his problem in a manner that is either satisfactory to him or acceptable to society.

PATTERNS OF ADJUSTMENT

REGRESSION

Regression is a process that is prominent throughout the spiral of development. After completing any given sequence of growth, we see the child again manifesting elements of behavior that were characteristic of his earlier behavior. This process may be implemented in relation to thinking, feeling, stages of development, ways of functioning and so forth throughout life. Through regression we return to patterns of activity that were effective earlier but have not been present in our current behavior (see the section "One to Three Years," in Chapter 4). Although regression is a vital part of our developmental sequence, it can have either a positive or a negative influence on everyday living as an adult. When reality becomes too frustrating, we may return to fantasy through regression rather than try to cope with the situation.

When we have an infection or some severe physiologic disturbance requiring bed rest, we may find that we feel like an infant — wanting to be cared for, to be treated tenderly, even though our overt behavior is that of an adult. When we become fatigued, we sometimes find that we cannot think as clearly as when we are refreshed. At these times, because of regression, we may revert to prelogical thinking and make connections on the basis of coincidence. Regression is a process whereby we can regenerate our energy and continue to function as an adult, but it is also a process that enables us to run from our responsibilities in reality and continue to function as a child. If one is functioning on an adult level, some degree of regression must occur before one of the following patterns is utilized.

COMPENSATION

Compensation is a pattern of adjustment, either conscious or unconscious, in which tension is relieved by overcoming or substituting for a weakness or lack that is either real or imagined. Before compensation takes place the individual must, first of all, have an awareness of his real or supposed defect. Compensation is concerned not only with freeing oneself from feelings of inadequacy but also with gaining approval from others. While the individual has a need to impress others favorably, he must also, if compensation is to be effective, maintain his self-respect.

Many feelings of inadequacy and weakness are alleviated by compensation; for example, the intelligent boy with poor hearing may overcome his feeling of lack by becoming a very skilled basketball player. In some instances the individual may actually overcome his handicap, as seen in the laryngectomy patient who learns to speak again by use of a special tube. The felt weakness may be turned into an asset, as when the tall thin girl becomes a fashion model. Compensation is also taking place when a strong characteristic of the individual becomes so prominent that it overshadows some weakness, as well as in many other situations.

This pattern of adjustment is said to have value when the substitute response brings with it increased gratification and makes it possible for the individual to be happy with himself as well as pleasing to others. Compensation may bring difficulty to the individual, however, if he is not able to achieve the substituted goal because he lacks certain abilities. For example, a child who cannot excel in sports and schoolwork may turn to playing the violin, but, if he does not have the talent or intelligence to master all the skills involved, he will be disappointed and experience once more a feeling of failure. The negative aspects of compensation can also be seen if the compensated activity becomes irksome to others or is actually antisocial in nature. Compensation is not constructive when it takes place in fantasy, with no acting out of the substitute response in real life.

CONVERSION

Conversion is a pattern which may be utilized when feelings and tensions rise far enough above the threshold of tolerance to become unbearable and no other means of discharge is immediately available. Conversion is said to be such a common pattern because of the general quality of the human body which makes it easy for any organ or function of an organ to be used to discharge excess tension.

In the process of conversion the excess tension is channeled through some organ or function and experienced as a somatic phenomenon. The individual feels relief because of the diminishing of the level of tension, and he can pinpoint, so he thinks, the source of his discomfort. He may say, "I feel bad because I have a headache," when realistically he has a headache because he feels bad. Each of us has his own favorite organ or system through which conversion takes place.

As we become aware of our patterns, we can retranslate the outcomes of the process from "body language" into the usual word language. For example, if an individual says, "I have a terrible headache, I feel like someone is beating me over the head," his simplest questions to himself could be "Is someone angry and directing it toward me?" or "Am I angry at myself and therefore beating myself over the head?" How many times have we heard someone say, "I've had it, I just can't take it anymore"? Such an individual might develop difficulty in swallowing or a loss of appetite, indicating that he is "full to the gills" or "fed up" with what ever is creating the intolerable stress in his situation.

DENIAL

Denial is a process that is utilized in an attempt to change some aspect of reality which is painful, anxiety-provoking or in some way threatening. Some believe that denial is used in relation to external stimuli in the same way that repression is used in relation to internal stimuli. Denial is a common pattern seen in early childhood and is employed when reality cannot be coped with and is "changed" through fantasy.

As a pattern in adult living, denial seems to be more and more common despite the fact that it creates havoc in one's interpersonal interactions, makes one more vulnerable to being hurt and really solves nothing. It may temporarily postpone anticipated pain, but it will inevitably lead to greater pain when the reality must be faced, accepted and coped with.

Dynamically, denial is utilized after the perception of something in the outside world that is painful. When energy is directed to block out the offending stimuli, one can remember clearly only that part of the situation which was not painful. Denial, if used extensively, can only lead to confusion because it reduces one's awareness of what is really going on. For example, many people are afraid of hostility and resort to denial whenever they are in a situation where hostility is expressed. Consequently they are not able to understand the situation, even in retrospect, and may feel guilty because they "must have done something." They may know generally that the interaction was unsatisfactory and disjunctive, but generalities do not lead to understanding; one must recognize the specifics of the interaction if one wants to understand.

DISPLACEMENT

The process of displacement has both a descriptive and a dynamic aspect. In a descriptive sense it involves an alteration in the arrangement of certain feelings, ideas or actions, resulting in a distortion of whatever elements are being dealt with. Sometimes a change of emphasis is involved: for example, in relating an experience, the insignificant details are emphasized and the important parts are touched upon lightly.

Dynamically, displacement involves both the discharge of energy and the phenomenon of substitution. Through this process, feelings that have been separated from the situation in which they were experienced (see "Isolation") and that have been repressed can be discharged in a reality situation without the person being aware of the source of his feelings. In other cases, feelings toward one object that have been suppressed can be discharged in a reality situation toward another object, but the person is immediately aware of what he has done. He may have just a flash of insight, but it is inevitable that he become aware because the experience has not undergone isolation. For example, something happens in class that makes a person very angry, but he cannot express it, so he takes care of it by suppression. When he arrives home he finds that his little brother has scattered the pages of an evolving term paper all over the house, so he proceeds to "blast" him, venting all of the anger that belonged in the previous situation. The angry person soon finds himself apologizing, because he knows that little brother's activity was not that catastrophic.

Displacement is also one means of resolving conflicts related to ambivalent feelings without resorting to more drastic measures. For example, a child has both positive and negative feelings about his father. As the intensity of these feelings increase, he may substitute the family dog as the target for his negative feelings and thus temporarily alleviate his conflict. Displacement is also one of the processes involved in the formation of symptoms. In the development of phobias, for example, fear of an external object is substituted for the fear of an unacceptable internal feeling or impulse.

FANTASY

Fantasy is a process normally prominent in early childhood whereby one attempts to cope with reality by imagination. It is primarily wish fulfillment and is based upon infantile experiences; thus it expresses the ways in which an infant perceives and misunderstands a frustrating reality. Fantasy involves primitive thinking in that pictures are used rather than words. It usually revolves around people since it is the child's interpersonal environment which proves most frustrating. A child may relive a painful experience in his imagination over and over again, each time substituting a different outcome. As the child struggles to establish his identity and to develop a sense of achievement and he constantly suffers minor defeats, he often thinks up elaborate situations in which he magically performs outstanding feats to provide himself with momentary reassurance.

The child inevitably attempts to provide for any unmet needs through fantasy. If he lacks playmates he creates an imaginary playmate to share his experiences. If his living experiences are not what he desires, he can through fantasy create a reality which is more pleasant. This process is very effective in childhood since it enables the child to keep functioning without becoming overwhelmed. After this time, however, fantasy which does not lead to action may become a real substitute for action, and to that degree it is pathological.

IDENTIFICATION

Identification is a process prominent in the so-called normal development of the infant and the child (see Chapter 4). It is a very early pattern of interaction with one's interpersonal environment and is a means of establishing one's identity. In early childhood the individual begins to imitate others, and through the process of reciprocal interaction he begins to be more like others. When identification is complete, we find that the individual has internalized the personal attributes and qualities of the people significant to him and that these qualities have become an actual part of him—so much so that he cannot distinguish them as apart from himself.

The teen-age boy may be said to identify with his favorite football star when he is seen with the same type of sport shirt and the same type of haircut. In this type of identification the teen-age boy may or may not have a close personal relationship with the individual; the football star may be someone the teen-ager only reads about or he may be someone that the teen-ager knows very well. We can readily see, then, that identification does not necessarily imply that there be close personal contact, but may result when the person identified with has desired personal attributes or qualities.

This process of identification normally occurs over and over again until after adolescence, when the individual's identity is firmly established. By means of this process one can derive satisfaction from sharing in the successes and failures of others, but this means that he experiences vicariously. To the degree that one is an autonomous person with the capacity for interdependent interaction, one will not resort to identification as a pattern of adjustment in day-to-day living. When we feel the lack of something that leaves our life incomplete, the need for identification is often stimulated. When we interact with someone who has unmet needs similar to our own, we also tend to identify. When we identify with someone we experience the same feelings simultaneously with him; for this reason we are not very objective about the situation, and confusion usually ensues.

INCORPORATION

Incorporation as a pattern of adjustment is utilized only when an individual has regressed to an infantile level in some area. It should be remembered that regression can occur in terms of feeling, thought or any other ego function and in relation to needs that have not been met, patterns of interaction with an "object" and so forth. Because of the many forms this regression may take, an individual can appear to be functioning on an adult level and at the same time be feeling very much like he did as an infant.

Incorporation as a defense is a process which seems to occur through a visual "taking in" of the individual who is the object of the incorporation. As implied in the foregoing statement, this pattern is a way of relating to the outside world. The person who is being related to in this manner seldom is aware, at the time, of what is happening in the interaction. He may, in retrospect, describe his experience as a feeling of being "gobbled up" or being "sucked into a drain"; "I felt exhausted, just as if I had been drained." As one becomes aware of this interaction in situations, he also may become aware of how he struggles to protect himself, and eventually he will be able to remain in such situations without being vulnerable to incorporative tendencies.

INSULATION

Insulation is a process through which we can protect ourselves from either internal or external stimuli, thus reducing the need to respond either to ourselves or to others. It is as if we erected a wall of asbestos between ourselves and the threatening stimuli. A person who is insulated internally will say that he has no particular feelings, that he feels nothing. This places him in quite a predicament, because he is unable to get any cues from himself to guide his action. If this condition continues for very long, he will inevitably have to implement his insulation to protect himself from external stimuli because of his increased vulnerability. With the completion of this process he manifests an attitude of cold indifference towards others.

The process of insulation can be very helpful in crisis situations, in which we must maintain our integrity and carry on as though nothing unusual had happened. If used beyond this point, however, the process is inevitably stifling to the person because he can only go through the motions of living. The superficial level of his existence makes life drab and monotonous.

ISOLATION

Isolation is a process in which we wall off certain ideas, attitudes or feelings, setting them apart from others: we set up little logic-tight compartments, strip all emotion from action, and separate emotional components from intellectual content. This pattern of behavior is often noticed when an individual tells of an experience very important to him but displays little feeling in the tone of his account. It is also seen, for example, in the teacher who advocates a democratic form of government but is unable to carry out these principles in her functions at school.

The concept of isolation is particularly useful, as we shall see later, in understanding the behavior of patients with schizophrenic or other pathologic conditions. This device has positive value in that it serves to keep the ego from being overwhelmed when one is just beginning to understand and to accept certain feelings that he had not recognized earlier. Isolation is also used in logical thinking, since objective thinking requires that we first isolate our feelings so that we can then analyze the facts.

PROJECTION

Projection is a process by which the individual attempts to get rid of his own undesirable thoughts and feelings by attributing them to others. Usually these disagreeable thoughts and feelings are those that the person himself holds in low regard, such as his hatreds, his moral delinquencies, his limitations and his inadequacies. In the state of fear, for example, there is an increased tendency to project suspicion, evil thoughts and designs onto others.[1] Frustration increases the tendency to project aggression.[2]

The expression of projection occurs in many forms. It is seen in the fantasy involved in art, literature and the theater. It occurs in exclusiveness, as illustrated by members of an organization who, having had difficulty themselves in being accepted for membership, wish to rigidly enforce entrance requirements for others. Righteous indignation and fault-finding with other people are also common forms. Phases of self-projection are observed in those who ascribe to another person various kinds of dishonesty or immorality and who are eager to help administer harsh punishment to those who have broken the rules. Projection represents a failure to permit recognition of unpleasant characteristics in oneself.

Just as we find that some people are more vulnerable to being projected upon, we find other people who are masters at projecting. Whether or not the increased frequency of projection is an outcome of our so called "paranoid society" is questionable; it would seem to be more of a product of the relative immaturity of the individuals who make up our society. The individual who uses projection frequently is at a disadvantage because it prevents him from looking at things (primarily himself and the way in which he interacts with others) as they really are, but the one who really suffers is the individual who is the target of the projection.

What does an individual experience who has been the recipient of someone's projection? Although the descriptions vary, all seem to have certain commonalities. First, there is a state of confusion created by having someone else's feelings superimposed upon one's own. If the individual is not too certain about what his own feelings are, he may tend to feel overwhelmed and helpless in the situation. If it has been hostility which has been projected upon him, he may find himself becoming very angry about something which previously had not posed a problem. Feelings are always exaggerated where projection is involved. On the other hand, the individual may begin to doubt his

---

[1] H. A. Murray, Jr.: "The Effect of Fear upon Estimates of the Maliciousness of Other Personalities." *J. Soc. Psychol.*, 4:310–329, 1933.

[2] E. H. Rodnick and S. G. Klebanoff: "Protective Reactions to Induced Frustrations as a Measure of Social Adjustment." *Psychol. Bull.*, 39:489, 1942.

motives, his intentions, or his identity when formerly he had been pretty clear about these things. One very frequently reported experience is a sudden, intense feeling of inadequacy by individuals who had functioned with a feeling of self-confidence and competency.

The sooner an individual can clarify through consensual validation — that is, by talking with someone who understands the dynamics of human behavior — the sooner he will be able to separate his own feelings from those which have been superimposed upon him and the sooner he will again be able to function as himself. The greater the degree of insight one has and the greater the awareness one has of one's own self and his ways of functioning, the less vulnerable one will be to the projections of others.

RATIONALIZATION

Rationalization is a justification or logical excuse made for an emotionally determined response which is unacceptable to the individual. In rationalization the individual admits the act by saying, "I did it because. . . ." The reason given, however, is not the real motive for his behavior but one that is face-saving. It seems that the individual almost momentarily recognizes the real motivation, but it threatens his security so much that he hastens to forget it and thus gives a reason that is acceptable to himself. Here the thinking serves to disguise the hidden motives of behavior and thus makes it possible to avoid facing the true ones. Rationalization differs from falsehood in that it is unconscious on the part of the individual. At the time, the individual really believes his reason, although he may become aware of the true motive in retrospect. The concept of rationalization seems to differ from that of projection in that it comes the closest to dealing consciously with unconscious material. In projection the individual would be apt to deny the act or feeling as well as the reason.

The types of justification in rationalization can be seen in many situations. For example, the individual may rationalize by saying, "It's all for the best." In another situation, he may feel somewhat bitter and remark, "It wasn't worth it anyway." He may also attempt to place the blame on circumstances or other persons by such excuses as "I didn't hear," or "I'm just getting over a cold." In other instances, the individual may give an argument of necessity. For example, the man purchases a new car that he cannot afford but justifies the fact to his friends by saying that his old one is too difficult for his wife to drive. Rationalization is also seen frequently in the postponement of disagreeable tasks. To illustrate, the student goes to a movie because, as he states it, "I need to be relaxed before I can start on my term paper."

We can usually tell when an individual is rationalizing, as he stumbles and halts in his attempt to find a reason. In discussing the topic of his action with him, he is apt to lose his temper if the adequacy of his reasons is questioned. Very often, too, one can see inconsistencies in the individual's thought or the principles involved.

Although commonly used by the average individual, rationalization serves to alleviate anxiety only momentarily and is always in danger of being toppled over by force of circumstance. By rationalization an individual can completely fool himself about the type of person he is and the motives which underlie his actions until something occurs that forces him to face things as they are. Although at times it may be considered a worthy method of meeting and accepting very difficult and disagreeable situations, rationalization in general is an unstable form of adjustment. An effective adjustment involves facing reality, which, of course, is circumvented in rationalization.

REACTION FORMATION

This process is discussed in the section "One to Three Years," in Chapter 4.

REPRESSION

In the dynamic process of repression, undesirable or traumatic thoughts, feelings and memories are kept below the level of awareness. Repressed material is usually not readily accessible to recall but may, by intensive therapy, be brought into awareness. It takes a constant exertion of energy to keep repressed material out of awareness. Consequently, less energy is available for constructive activities.

In addition to dynamic repression, there is passive repression. This is the process we use to dispose of all the irrelevant, immaterial details which impinge upon us every day. The energy is gradually withdrawn from this material, which then settles down and becomes a part of our memory; it is available when or if needed but does not necessarily interfere with our daily living. On the other hand, that which is dynamically repressed is continually striving for expression and distorting our overt behavior, in addition to requiring more and more energy to keep it out of awareness.

SUBLIMATION

Sublimation as a process in development is discussed in the section "Three to Six Years," in Chapter 4.

SUPPRESSION

Suppression is the process whereby we temporarily postpone the experiencing of certain feelings, ideas or action by intentionally keeping them out of awareness. In contrast to repression, that which is handled by the process of suppression can readily be recalled and, if necessary, dealt with by the use of other processes. For example, something happens in a working situation that we do not understand or cannot solve at the time, but we say to ourselves, "I just won't think about it now." The effectiveness of this process depends upon the significance of the idea or event, the intensity of the feeling, the period of time the delay must be maintained and the amount of available energy we have to devote to this process. The more highly charged the material, the more energy it requires to maintain the postponement, and, if other pressures arise, repression or some other process may be implemented.

Summary

From the topographical standpoint, the personality structure is said to consist of three interrelated aspects with certain characteristics and functions. The processes and functions that go on within this structure have been classified as conscious, preconscious and unconscious, depending upon the qualities and characteristics which they possess.

Although it is difficult to visualize a personality structure per se without relating it to the general development of the individual or his current patterns of behavior, we will acquire new meanings for these terms as we learn to relate them to the dynamics of the behavior of individuals in everyday life.

Adjustment as a process can be said to be the characteristic manner in which the individual solves his main problems of life. When an organism fails to adjust, its existence is threatened, and likewise the individual is threatened when he fails to cope with his problems. Efficiency in adjustment depends upon the ability of the individual to continue varying his responses until a successful solution of his problem is attained.

Learning to cope with a situation or adjusting successfully does not necessarily imply that the individual always brings about a change within himself or in his overt behavior. He may attempt to or actually bring about a change in his reality situation and thus be able to function more effectively.

The authors have attempted to outline some of the patterns used by the average individual in his adjustment process. All of us use variations of these patterns to some extent in our everyday life. We have a tendency to use, again and again, the patterns of adjustment that are most effective in relieving increased tension in periods of anxiety and frustration. The important point is not that we use these patterns in everyday living but to what degree we are keeping ourselves chained to our infantile feelings, reactions and anticipations—to what extent we have to blindfold ourselves or distort reality in order to maintain our feeling of capability in daily living.

Bibliography

Alexander, Franz, and Ross, Helen, eds.: *Dynamic Psychiatry*. Chicago, University of Chicago Press, 1952.

Breuer, Joseph, and Freud, Sigmund: *Studies on Hysteria*. New York, Basic Books, Inc., 1957.

Cameron, Norman: *The Psychology of Behavior Disorders*. Boston, Houghton Mifflin Co., 1947.

Caplan, Gerald, and Leboviei, Serge, eds.: *Adolescence*. New York, Basic Books, Inc., 1969.

Erikson, Erik H.: *Identity and the Life Cycle*. New York, International Universities Press, Inc., 1959.

Erikson, Erik H.: *Identity, Youth and Crisis*. New York, W. W. Norton & Co., 1968.

Erikson, Erik H.: *Insight and Responsibility*. New York, W. W. Norton & Co., 1964.

Federn, Paul: *Ego Psychology and the Psychoses*. New York, Basic Books, Inc., 1952.

Fenichel, Otto: *The Psychoanalytic Theory of Neurosis*. New York, W. W. Norton & Co., Inc., 1959.

Freud, Sigmund: *Beyond the Pleasure Principle*. London, International Psychoanalytic Press, 1922.

Freud, Sigmund: *Group Psychology and Analysis of the Ego*. London, International Psychoanalytic Press, 1922.

Freud, Sigmund: *New Introductory Lectures on Psychoanalysis*. New York, W. W. Norton & Co., Inc., 1933.

Freud, Sigmund: *The Problem of Anxiety*. New York, W. W. Norton & Co., Inc., 1936.

Freud, Sigmund: *Moses and Monotheism*. New York, Alfred A. Knopf, Inc., 1939.

Freud, Sigmund: The Ego and the Id. London, Hogarth Press, 1947.

Freud, Sigmund: *Three Contributions to the Theory of Sex*. New York, Nervous and Mental Disease Monographs, 1948.

Freud, Sigmund: *Outline of Psychoanalysis*. New York, W. W. Norton & Co., Inc., 1949.

Freud, Sigmund: "The Economic Problem in Masochism." In *Collected Papers. II*. London, Hogarth, Press, 1950, p. 255.

Freud, Sigmund: "Formulations Regarding the Two Principles in Mental Functioning." In *Collected Papers, IV*. London, Hogarth Press, 1950, p. 13.

Freud, Sigmund: "The Unconscious." In *Collected Papers, IV*. London, Hogarth Press, 1950, p. 98.

Gardener, Riley W., and Moriarity, Alice: *Personality Development at Preadolescence*. Seattle, University of Washington Press, 1968.

Gould, Rosalind: "Repression Experimentally Analyzed." *Character and Personality*, *10*:259-288, 1942.

Hartmann, Heinz: *Ego Psychology and the Problem of Adaptation*. New York, International Universities Press, Inc., 1958.

Mikesell, W. H., ed.: *Modern Abnormal Psychology*. New York, Philosophical Library, Inc., 1950.

Murray, H. A., Jr.: "The Effect of Fear upon Estimates of the Maliciousness of Other Personalities." *J. Soc. Psychol.*, *4*:310-329, 1933.

Rodnick, E. H., and Klebanoff, S. G.: "Protective Reactions to Induced Frustration as a Measure of Social Adjustment." *Psychol. Bull., 39*:489, 1942.

Schilder, Paul: *The Image and Appearance of the Human Body.* New York, International Universities Press, Inc., 1950.

Schilder, Paul: *Introduction to a Psychoanalytic Psychiatry.* New York, International Universities Press, Inc., 1951.

Solnit, Albert J., and Provence, Sally P., eds.: *Modern Perspectives in Child Development.* New York, International Universities Press, Inc., 1963.

Spitz, Rene A.: *A Genetic Field Theory of Ego Formation.* New York, International Universities Press, Inc., 1959.

Sullivan, Harry Stack: *Conceptions of Modern Psychiatry.* New York, W. W. Norton & Co., Inc., 1953.

Sullivan, Harry Stack: *The Interpersonal Theory of Psychiatry.* New York, W. W. Norton & Co., Inc., 1953.

Symonds, Percival M.: *The Dynamics of Human Adjustment.* New York, Appleton-Century-Crofts, Inc., 1946.

Weiss, Edoardo: *Principles of Psychodynamics.* New York, Grune & Stratton, Inc., 1950.

Wittenberg, Rudolph: *Postadolescence.* New York, Grune & Stratton, Inc., 1968.

Suggestions for Further Reading

Anderson, Camilla: *Emotional Hygiene.* 4th Ed., Philadelphia, J. B. Lippincott Co., 1948.

Brenner, Charles: *Elementary Textbooks of Psychoanalysis.* New York, Anchor Books, 1960.

Brown, J. F.: *The Psychodynamics of Abnormal Behavior.* New York, McGraw-Hill Book Co., Inc., 1940.

English, O. S., and Pearson, Gerald: *Emotional Problems of Living.* 3rd Ed., New York, W. W. Norton & Co., Inc., 1963.

Freud, Anna: *The Ego and the Mechanisms of Defense.* New York, International Universities Press, Inc., 1946.

Group for the Advancement of Psychiatry: *Normal Adolescence.* New York, Charles Scribner's Sons, 1968.

Maslow, A. H., and Mittelmann, Bela: *Principles of Abnormal Psychology.* New York, Harper & Brothers, 1951, pp. 87–99.

Warters, Jane: *Achieving Maturity.* New York, McGraw-Hill Book Co., Inc., 1949, pp. 1–28, 78–92, 93–212.

Chapter 4 Biosocial Development in Early Life

"It has been said that the history of mankind depicts a spiral progress; the course of events returns at increasing interval to the neighborhood of the starting point."[1] According to Sullivan, Burns demonstrates the rhythm of the development of Western civilization, tracing it from 800 B.C. through the twentieth century.[2]

Just as we see a spiral progress in the phylogenetic development of mankind, we also see such developmental patterns in the history of each individual. In the growth of the infant and young child, we see periods of marked disequilibrium alternating with periods of relative quiet and calm. Gesell calls this pattern of rhythms a spiral development. As development proceeds, we see that each recurrence in this spiral pattern marks a higher stage of maturity and a wider base for the expanding personality.

This pattern of spiral progress not only is characteristic of the development of the individual and the development of civilization but is also evident as the individual progresses in each new era of learning and in the very process of living as the adult continues to meet each new crisis as it arises.

---

[1] H. S. Sullivan: *Conceptions of Modern Psychiatry.* Washington, D.C., W. W. Norton & Co., Inc., 1953.

[2] *Ibid*, p. 47f.

BIRTH TO ONE YEAR

The first period of existence for the human organism, the fetal stage, is truly a period of preparation wherein an intricate action system develops along certain more or less predetermined lines. The drive toward growth and development generates various needs which are satisfied, and the fetus exists more or less as a parasite. After birth, the infant must make many major adjustments if he is to survive. While some of these are automatic occurrences within the organism, others require the active assistance of an adult.

The infant's gross structure develops according to a predetermined formula set up by heredity, but the details of both structure and function are left to evolve as the process of growth continues after birth through interaction with the environment. At first his needs are purely biologic, and he must develop adequate patterns of activity with a physiochemical environment with the required ingredients if he is to survive. For example, we have an infant with a defect in his respiratory apparatus that interferes with the activity necessary for oxygenating the blood. If the defect is not corrected, this infant will not be able to develop the pattern of activity necessary for maintaining an interchange with his physiochemical environment and will not be able to survive. On the other hand, there is the infant who has all that is necessary for an adequately functioning respiratory apparatus, but his physiochemical environment has very little oxygen and a high degree of carbon monoxide. This infant will not be able to survive either, unless there is a change in the quality of his environment.

The infant begins life in a state of complete helplessness and is dependent upon an adult who must recognize and satisfy the infant's needs. So right from the beginning the infant also requires an interpersonal environment with which he must learn to interact effectively if he is to develop into a biosocial adult. Just as the infant has to have an adequate physiochemical environment, he also has to have an adequate interpersonal environment.

The infant's initial interaction with adults is stimulated through his cry as he becomes restless and communicates his discomfort. When the adult responds and offers him the breast or the bottle, his need is satisfied after he ingests the food. Then as his tension is relieved, he goes to sleep until the need is again manifest, and this basic activity pattern is repeated. During the first weeks of life, the oral zone is the infant's primary means of relating to the outside world. The mouth serves a dual function, as a portal for the passage of food and as a pleasure organ through the stimulation gained from sucking and eating. The infant experiences everything in momentary states—that is, he is, as yet, unable to make any connections between his experiences.

Although we refer to his basic activity pattern as an evolving need-satisfaction sequence, he does not yet relate his cry to his state of discomfort or his ingestion of food to his state of comfort. He experiences in terms of either/or and all or none, and each experience is an isolated instance.

The oral activities, although prominent, are not the only experiences of this period. The infant receives tactile, olfactory and vestibular sensations during the feeding process that are essential for his development. He now needs the stimulation gained through being held, rocked, spoken to and played with, and a little later the auditory and visual sensations will become increasingly important. All these sensations become integrated into the feeding experience since the infant, in his passive receptive state, seems to absorb his environment.

Because the infant relates to his environment through empathy, he is a pretty accurate barometer in relation to the quality of his interpersonal environment. When his environment is quiet, relaxed and relatively free from tension and anxiety, the infant reflects these qualities. On the other hand, when his environment is chaotic and filled with tension, conflict and anxiety, the infant will reflect these qualities. These latter qualities when absorbed from his environment produce increased tension in the infant which not only interferes with his patterns of activity necessary to reduce the tensions of his biologic needs but produces a state of discomfort from which he cannot escape but which he attempts to cope with by withdrawing and by shutting out the painful stimuli. If this condition continues over a period of time, the infant's survival will be threatened. Such a situation can be alleviated only by removing the noxious ingredients from his environment, and this would involve the person or persons from whom the tension and anxiety emanate.

The infant's personality at birth and for the first few weeks of life consists primarily of rhythms and tensions, as yet unmodified by the outside world. At this time he is unable to distinguish between what is part of him and what is outside. As his needs are satisfied through interaction with a gentle mother figure, the world becomes the source through which he learns to satisfy his needs and to restore a state which is relatively tension free. The latter state is pleasurable and is possible only when the needs are satisfied and equilibrium or a tension-free state is again restored. This is a state which the infant seeks constantly as he functions according to the pleasure principle and is insistent in his demands for immediate satisfaction and relief from tension.

During this period, the infant's development is centered on his relationship with his mother, which is his first social experience. The mother's sensitivity to the infant's needs, and her ability to be consistent in providing for them, has a marked influence on the capacity which the child develops to relate to people throughout his life. The infant has a very great need for the love and attention of the mother, and as she unconditionally gives to the infant he develops a sense of security, a feeling that all his needs will be satisfied, a feeling that he is respected. Then, as the infant responds positively to the mother, she in turn is stimulated to give him more to further comfort and protect him, and, as a result, reciprocal action is established. Out of these experiences evolve both the need and the capacity for interpersonal intimacy throughout life.

It has been stated earlier that the details of both structure and function evolve through interaction with the environment as the process of growth continues after birth.

At first the infant is passive; he reacts to the stimuli impinging upon him but he cannot interact until there is some structure developed. During this early period, the foundation or core of his personality is being established. As he experiences certain activities which are vital to his survival, a transformation of energy occurs. Some of this energy is invested in the evolving personality structure which will eventually provide boundaries and culminate in a distinct entity, an individual, separate and apart from everything else in his world.

This period, when all of the infant's energy is invested in himself, is commonly called the period of primary narcissism. The warmth and love provided by the infant's significant figures seems to serve as a catalyst to stimulate the self-investment of energy which is so vital to his future development. The time when primary narcissism is at its peak is one of the times when an infant is the most appealing to adults. He seems filled to the brim with "good" feelings—in fact, he appears just about ready to overflow.

Because of the consistency, continuity and quality of his experiences with his mothering figure, the foundation for a basic sense of trust has been established. With the development of sufficient structure which has been invested with sufficient energy, we see the infant's mode change from one that was primarily passive to one that is primarily active.

The basic pattern of development evolves from the infant's relationship and interaction with his significant people, and although the pattern remains primarily the same throughout, the processes within the pattern change as development proceeds.

The need-satisfaction sequence mentioned previously seems to be the model for the developmental pattern. The infant experiences increased tension, which produces disequilibrium; this makes it imperative that some action occur to reduce the tension and reestablish equilibrium. Since another person must provide for the satisfaction of the infant's needs, the basic requirements for an interpersonal situation are established very early. With two people involved there must be a link or a bridge established between them to provide for the rendering of services and later for reciprocal activity.

We cannot say specifically how the mother relates to her infant because that is a function of the degree of her maturity. We can, however, describe the processes by which the infant relates to his mother.

Some of the processes which are vital in the early development of the individual are later resorted to as defense mechanisms or as manifestations of the individual's attempt to adjust or to cope with his reality. Their significance in development will be the present focus. The utilization as defenses or patterns of adjustment was elaborated on in the preceding chapter.

We have said that a certain degree of structure must be developed for the infant's actions to change from passivity to activity, and this implies that his beginning boundaries have been established. He is no longer an extension of his mother because his beginning boundaries separated them. He now attempts to get closer to his mother through the process of *incorporation,* which is modeled after orality and implies a taking in through the mouth and swallowing. He not only gobbles up his food but also gobbles up that part of his mother which is involved in meeting his needs. He is indiscriminate about what he takes in and readily spits out that which disagrees with him. During this time, the infant begins to make connections between his experiences. These connections, however, are based on coincidence rather than on logic. For example, if two occurrences happen in a relatively short period of time, there is an automatic relationship established between them. Sullivan refers to this kind of experience as "parataxic hook-ups."[3] This is more or less the mode of our experiencing from late infancy, throughout childhood, and for many of us, on into adulthood.

As the infant continues to grow and to interrelate his experiences, he begins to differentiate himself from the world around him. According to his experiences, he may find that when he cries and makes an effort to communicate his feeling of discomfort, he is soon rewarded by achieving a state of comfort. On the other hand, he may find that no one responds to his cry or that his state of discomfort is only exaggerated by his trying to communicate it. If the infant has adequate positive experiences in having his needs met, he begins to experience a feeling of capability and a certain potential for striving to achieve is mobilized within him. These experiences also help to form the core of

---

[3]H. S. Sullivan: *The Interpersonal Theory of Psychiatry.* New York, W. W. Norton & Co., Inc., 1953, pp. 83-84.

his later feeling of self-esteem and self-confidence. If the infant does not have adequate positive experiences in having his needs met, he will continue to feel helpless and will develop a deep inner longing which will become more and more insatiable.

With further experiences the infant becomes more aware and begins to recognize the people in his environment. If all is well in his relationship with his mother, he is learning to trust and to depend upon her. As the mother becomes more "significant" in relation to the infant's achieving states of comfort, he begins to imitate her or to relate to her through primary identification. Although he still enjoys the "game" of gobbling up and of being gobbled up, he now begins to mimic the people in his environment. This is his attempt to bridge the gap between himself and others—"I want to be like them."

Primary identification is a step higher than incorporation and is the process which involves the imitation of others. The process alone does not bring about any permanent change in the individual although he may temporarily experience what the other person is experiencing. Primary identification does lead to a closer relationship and greater investment of energy in the other person, which brings about *secondary identification*, a process by which one person becomes like another. The total process of identification is completed when that aspect of the other person, invested with energy, is internalized and made a part of the infant. This internalization is also called *introjection*, a process through which part of one person is taken into the personality of another.

With the completion of the identification process, there is a more or less permanent change brought about in the personality structure of the infant or child. He then relates to his significant people differently because his perception of them has changed and his needs are changing. This process of identification is repeated over and over again, if his relationships with his significant people are maintained, until development is more or less completed.

By the end of the first year of development, we find that the infant has made remarkable progress. There has been an elaborate development of his action system, and it is important for him to be free to exercise his new capacities. He can gain a sitting position unaided, crawl, stand alone and, usually, walk in an upright position. He is capable of activities that require relatively fine muscular coordination in both eating and playing. He still needs and enjoys social experiences to strengthen his self-identity, and he already responds positively to an appreciative audience and is apt to prolong his performance if there is adequate social give and take.

ONE TO THREE YEARS

The second phase of development, ages one to three years, has often been called the period of mastery of biologic skills and the acquisition of communicative language. If the infant has been successful in learning to live the role of the baby of the family and has survived this early period of development with optimum achievement, we now begin to see the differentiation of many sub-roles in his behavior. What these roles shall include and how they shall be played depend upon the biologic constitution of the child and upon the reactions of other persons toward his appearance and behavior. As a rule an infant is not perceived or reacted to by his parents as just their new baby, but he evokes a response which is a composite of many factors. How they feel about each other, whether or not the baby was really wanted, how they feel about "Uncle Joe," whose chin is just like that of the baby's and so forth.

During the early part of this period, the child usually manifests evidence of the beginning of many new lines of development that provide new ways of adaptation and also introduce new problems. Since the new experiences often seem quite threatening, the child tends to regress temporarily before he again moves forward, alternating periods of progression with periods of regression, thus developing in a spiral. *Regression* is a process of returning to earlier states or patterns after a higher level has been reached. This is the time when the reality principle first begins to influence the child's behavior. In contrast to the pleasure principle under which the child functioned previously, the reality principle involves the postponement of immediate satisfaction in order to gain greater satisfaction later through mastering the reality situation. Mother now feels that the time has come to "make" him into an acceptable member of the human race. So in many instances when he anticipates tenderness, he not only does not receive tenderness but gets disapproval, which only intensifies or aggravates the need for tenderness. From the period of childhood on, the characteristics of one's interpersonal situations are described by H. S. Sullivan in his theory of reciprocal emotions: "Integration in an interpersonal situation is a reciprocal process in which (1) complementary needs are resolved or aggravated; (2) reciprocal patterns of activity are developed or disintegrated; and (3) foresight of satisfaction, or rebuff, of similar needs is facilitated."[4]

---

[4]H. S. Sullivan: *The Interpersonal Theory of Psychiatry.* New York, W. W. Norton & Co., Inc., 1953, p. 198.

The child learns different reactions to his two parents, depending upon their expectations and reactions to him—for example, being mother's boy and father's boy. Then within each of these roles there is a further differentiation of good boy, bad boy and so on. Although the child is living out these social roles, he is unable to recognize, identify or analyze them. Consequently, in these interpersonal situations during childhood, multiple roles are structured that are successful in avoiding anxiety and punishment. According to Sullivan, these roles are organized to the degree that each one will be equally entitled to be called "I" later on.[5] It is the acting out of these roles structured in childhood that introduces an irrational element in the interpersonal situations of adults: "Me expects you to behave toward me like me expects you to behave."[6]

The child makes great strides in his muscular coordination, and all motor functions become more active and controlled. He alternately goes through periods when he is very active and unable to stay in one place very long, and periods when he is somewhat of a dawdler. As he learns to master fundamental motor skills, his life space grows, and, as the range of his activities increases, there is more opportunity for conflict to arise. As he develops each new ability, he has to have the opportunity to repeat these activities over and over again. He becomes more active, gets into more things and even becomes quite self-assertive at times. Stress very often develops during mealtime or when it is time to get dressed, when he insists on doing things for himself even though his results are upside down, backwards or inside out. As he exercises his new abilities, he experiences a sense of achievement, and it is natural for him to become angry with a mother who interferes and tries to regulate his activities. If the mother can accept his anger as a normal part of his development, it will not interfere with their relationship and he will learn that he sometimes has to defer to the wishes of others, that intervention in his activities is inevitable and reasonable, and he will be able to do so with a sense of achievement rather than with a sense of resentment and helplessness.

It is usually about the middle of this period, two or two and one-half years, that a child is able to withstand being separated from his mother without too much suffering. He now knows that when mother goes away, she will also come back. This change is manifested because by now he has internalized enough of his mother to maintain her as a constant "object," whereas previously his mother had to be present or nearby for him to feel secure.

One of the major tasks the culture imposes on the child during this

---

[5]Ibid, p. 209.
[6]Carol L. Brady, verbal communication.

period is that of learning sphincter control. In mastering this task, the child is likely to encounter many problems, the intensity of which depends a great deal upon the degree of security he has experienced during the previous period. His need for his mother's love is still very great, and it is often the greatest influence in encouraging him to accept the restrictions imposed in order not to lose his mother's love. His having to give up the pleasure principle in denying himself immediate satisfaction in soiling may give rise to ambivalent feelings—that is, the child feels love and hostility simultaneously toward the mother. The mother thus introduces a conflict in the child between the desire for her love and approval and the desire for immediate relief of tension. The child will be able to solve this conflict without too much difficulty if his relationship with his mother has been such that adequate love has been given to provide for the development of his ego. With the resolution of this conflict, the child accepts and internalizes the requests and prohibitions of his mother. After this occurs, the conflict is between the impulse to gain immediate satisfaction and the internalized restriction; and the sphincter behavior is now under the control of the ego, which is warned by anxiety of any threat that the impulse may break through.

During this time, the child is learning to be more discriminating in regard to all stimuli. At first he has only an immediate time concept, but by the end of this period he can make plans for the immediate future and also remember them. He builds up his concepts of property rights and learns that certain articles belong to certain people; however, at times he claims as many things as possible for his own without the slightest basis for his claim. Through all of these experiences he is learning a rudimentary form of sharing, establishing the roots for his later generosity and taking his first step toward interdependent social relationships. Then as he becomes increasingly more aware of and more responsive to his environment, he alternates between periods of shyness and periods of eagerness to go out into the world. He is also beginning to develop more elaborate patterns of verbal communication.

This period when so many biologic skills must be mastered is definitely a period when patterns related to self-control become fixed, and it is important that a framework of flexibility be provided within which these patterns may be learned. The important point is not that the child has to learn certain ways of behaving but that the relationship between him and his mother have a minimum of distortion. The child interprets his experiences according to the way he feels, and the way he feels depends partly upon his mother's reaction and the feeling she communicates to him.

During this time, more lines for his future character traits are established, and they will be influenced by many factors, such as his inheritance, constitution, potential and experiences in interacting with the world about him. Later creativeness and ability to relate intimately to others, to give, to be productive and to feel capable are some of the characteristics which have their origin in this period. The foundation for later reaction formations, which result in what are called reactive character traits, may also be developed at this time.

A *reaction formation* is a process used to alleviate unresolved conflicts involving feelings, attitudes, impulses and desires. Of two conflicting elements, the one that is more acceptable or desirable is usually strengthened or reinforced, while the other one disappears; a certain channel seems to be built for the expression of the reinforced element while strong emotional forces insure the repression of the one that must be kept hidden. The element which is allowed expression then becomes excessive or exaggerated. For example, the person for whom everything is just "too too" is basically a very hostile person who would be overtly very destructive without this reaction formation. In another instance, a person may be overly meticulous and may insist that everything be in a certain order whereas actually he would like to be very disorderly and messy. The overt manifestation of any behavior related to a reaction formation is rigid and cramped.

As the child experiences a feeling of acceptance and respect from the people in his day-to-day living, he begins further to structure the roles he will take in relation to them and to the world in general. He learns what their expectations are of him, and he in turn builds up his expectations of others. Although he readily learns to be alert to the cues from others with whom he interacts in terms of their facial expressions, feelings and gestures in relation to what he does, he also gets cues from himself from the way he is feeling and what he thinks is going on. When he is given the freedom to respond to his own cues as well as to the cues of others, he is learning to be himself. He will then have more opportunity to experiment, to vary his roles and to develop more spontaneity and skill in interacting with others.

The child also has to be given the opportunity to make choices, to make decisions, if he is going to learn to trust his own judgment and to develop into an autonomous person. The child who is constantly told what to do, how to do it, what to feel and what he needs will seldom find out who he really is, how he really feels or what he really wants. Instead he will develop an overpowering feeling of helplessness and inability to communicate and an inability to rely upon himself for cues to his reactions in interpersonal situations.

THREE TO SIX YEARS

The period from three to six years of age, commonly known as the oedipal phase or the latter part of childhood, is a time when a great many developments occur that produce changes in the child's overt behavior. First of all, there is a beginning physiologic development of the sex organs, with the accompanying increase in sensations that are a new source of pleasure. These sensations and the awareness of the differences in body structure may evoke considerable anxiety. Until this time children of both sexes have felt pretty much the same, but now they begin to feel differently and this change is reflected in their play. The little girl begins to play at keeping house, cooking, caring for her dolls, imitating her mother. She actually begins to feel like a girl, whereas the little boy shows more masculinity in his play activities. Activities of both begin as imitation because of the admiration each feels for the parent of the same sex, and this process later leads to secondary identification and introjection, which bring about further changes within the personality.

There is also an increase in curiosity about their own bodies, as well as the bodies of others, which results in their exploring themselves and others and also exhibiting themselves. This activity brings them into conflict with social barriers and taboos. Then, too, there is usually a change in the parents' attitude in permitting such activities; previously the child's tendency to display his body was considered cute. This change on the part of the parents usually provokes anxiety and confusion in the child. Accompanying these exploratory activities and increased curiosity is the gradual development of an awareness of sexual differences in the boy and the girl, which may also evoke great anxiety. Along this same line, the discovery that mother and father engage in some kind of secret activity arouses further curiosity and may produce anxiety in some children. At the same time, curiosity about pregnancy and birth usually arises and many misconceptions and phantasies evolve, depending upon the child's own development.

Until this time the child's relationship with his mother has dominated his activities, and even the father's role has been more or less that of a substitute mother. During this period, however, the child learns the differentiation of the male and female role with regard to both himself and the significant people in his environment. From this point on, the development of the boy and the girl differs.

The little boy begins to associate himself more with the masculine members of the family as identification with the father grows. Through part of this identification, he wishes to take the father's place and do what he does, and there is an intensification of his feeling for his mother as he becomes romantically devoted to her. He now sees his father as a rival for his mother's attention and affection. The little boy becomes possessive and protective of the mother. He imitates his father's behavior with her and likes to play games in which he assumes his father's role. Since he still wants to be loved by his father and he knows that his father is powerful because of his size, strength and dominant position, he may see the father more and more as a threatening figure. The boy may begin to fear this rival figure and to have many hostile feelings toward him that produce varying degrees of guilt. He may begin to idealize his father and to become more dependent upon him while trying to please him in every way. In this idealized image the father is usually seen as an asexual person and is internalized as that. Through this introjection of the father image, these sexual prohibitions become a part of the boy's personality and his superego is established. Then, by identifying with the father, the little boy learns to play the masculine role.

The girl has a difficult task to accomplish, since she must change her love object from mother to father. As she turns to her father, she may display much antagonism and hostility toward her mother. These feelings produce guilt, and she feels threatened in regard to the satisfaction of her dependent needs by the mother, toward whom she is quite ambivalent. Her conflict is between the desire to be in the mother role and be loved by the father, and the desire to be a child and be loved by mother. Both desires appear as threats which produce fears and anxieties during this period. Therefore, in order to resolve her conflict, the little girl sublimates her feelings by transferring some of them to other adult women significant to her and by playing at participating in their activities. She is then able to identify with her mother and to strengthen their relationship, which forms the basis for her later roles as a woman.

Sublimation is a process, prominent in childhood and in the latent or juvenile period of development, that creates more or less permanent changes in the structure of the personality. In contrast to reaction formation, which reinforces repression, sublimation cannot be used in relation to impulses, urges or drives that have been repressed because a free, unobstructed flow of energy is necessary. Through this process certain impulses or drives are discharged indirectly and their energy is utilized in varied constructive activities. Dynamically, a permanent channel is formed for the discharge of the impulse involved, so that when it arises, it gains expression through this channel without having to wait for the green light which is controlled by the ego.

During this early period, the overt manifestation of sublimation is a prototype of the more complete sublimation that will occur later on.

The interpersonal environment is very important in either facilitating or deterring the development of this process by providing models and alternative ways of solving conflicts. Many people believe that sublimation is the most effective of all the patterns used in adaptation, from the standpoints of both the individual and civilization.

This era in development is sometimes called the normal phobic period because of the many fears and anxieties which the child experiences. He frequently has nightmares and likes to hear stories about animals, witches and monsters that gobble up whatever or whomever is threatening the children in the story. In his play, we often see him assuming the role of ferocious animals, and this activity, sometimes called "identification with the aggressor," helps him to feel more adequate in coping with his own fears and anxieties.

SIX TO NINE YEARS

After the child has temporarily resolved the feelings related to the family triangle, the phase called the *juvenile* or *latency period* is possible. This period usually begins at the age of six and is marked by a repression of the child's sexual tendencies and the manifestation of the need for compeers or other persons of the same age and with similar interests. In contrast to the former period where sexual curiosity and interest were at their height, there now appears to be a desexualization of interest, with other objects and areas becoming the focus of attention.

With the energy made available through a resolution of the conflicts of the earlier periods, greater learning and intellectual growth become possible. The gratification during this period centers primarily on learning, building, accomplishing and collecting, which are all varied forms of achievement. The child's shift of attention to this type of activity is facilitated by his identification with his parents' nonsexual interests.

As the child's interest expands beyond the home, he is apt to appear somewhat casual in his contact with his siblings, parents and others in the immediate family circle. He begins to supplement his parents with new adults who become the objects of his identification: those in reality, teachers and group leaders; and those in fantasy, historical or television figures. Although he appears to want to escape completely from the domination of his home in his evident attempts to break away from his parents, his dependent needs remain very strong. Therefore, he still needs considerable encouragement and approval consistently to enable him to cope with stressful situations, and, even then, he is readily provoked into regressing to more infantile behavior.

Another major task of the child during this period is to fit into a group of his peers. This is the period when he is trying to locate his own place in the social world, and his choice of companions may sometimes be quite a trial to his parents. The gang, therefore, becomes one of his first experiences with independent social organization outside the home as he begins to associate more closely with his peers, usually those of the same sex. The child gains strength through identification with the group; but this process is possible for him only if he is able to lose part of his own identity as an individual and to gain satisfaction in his new identity as a part of the group. If he is insecure and lacks confidence in himself as a person, this new experience may be too threatening to him, and he will be unable to identify with the group. Children of this age have little sensitivity to the feelings of others and sometimes seem almost cruel in their interaction with their playmates.

The group formed during this time usually consists of members of the same sex, and part of their code is contempt and hostility for members of the opposite sex. This part of their code is thought to aid in the repression of some of their earlier sexual feelings toward the parent of the opposite sex. There is also a development of intense group loyalty that requires strict adherence to the rules and mores of the gang. The use of secret language and other symbols is quite common in these groups. These activities promote a feeling of strength and a feeling of independence.

Sometimes we find that girls do not form so closely knit, cohesive groups as boys do during this period. They are more likely to form close intimate relationships with individuals and tend to be more docile and overtly dependent than the boys. This behavior is an indication that they have been successful in identifying with a feminine mother. They are also more occupied with feminine activities like playing with dolls and keeping house.

The fantasy life during this period of development is rich and varied, although the degree of daydreaming will vary from child to child. While in reality all interest in the opposite sex is denied, a great part of their fantasy may be taken up with this interest. Another very common fantasy is the "conquering hero" theme, where the child places himself in a favorable role and accomplishes miraculous feats. In another, he imagines that he is not really the child of his own parents but has had some other origin. All of his conflicts may be re-enacted in his daydreams.

This period is often said to be the time of character formation. This is the time when the ego, busy with repressing and sublimating the sexual tendencies, adopts certain characteristic ways of coping with both internal and external stimuli. Some of the predominant tendencies of the earlier periods may again become evident and may even become exaggerated and integrated as character traits.

During the latter part of the previous phase of development, the part of the personality called the superego, which functions as an inhibiting factor, was established. During this period, the superego functions in a strict and unrelenting manner, readily producing anxiety and guilt for the slightest deviation from sanctioned behavior. Consequently, the child is apt to become compulsive and magical in both his play and work activities in his attempts to cope with the strict demands of his superego. Although this period of development is often called one of latency, we can see that it is one of tumult and conflict, with the promotion of constant reorganization.

This is the period in life when the child begins to develop many new patterns in his relationships with his peer group. Two of his outstanding needs at this time are having companions of the same age and interests as himself and being accepted by others. In his attempt to satisfy these needs he undergoes socialization and is graduated at the end of this period with an "orientation in living."[7]

Interaction with other children in his group helps the child to learn to live with other people. First, he has to learn to compete, which places him in opposition to or rivalry with others. Since the capacity for competition is valued in our culture, this tendency may become an exaggerated, troublesome pattern. He also has to learn to compromise — that is, to be willing to yield to others in order to reach an agreement. Another skill which he must develop is cooperation, to give and take, to be able to do things with others in such a way that everyone feels satisfied and worthwhile. Throughout this period the child learns to adapt himself to the demands of others. If he develops these abilities in situations wherein he can maintain some feeling of worth, achievement and esteem, he will have a solid basis for consolidating and refining his interpersonal skills on a higher level during the ensuing spirals of development and maturation.

NINE TO TWELVE YEARS

At about the age of nine years, the child begins to show both interest and concern for another person. His relationship with this other person, a member of the same sex, is different from any previous relationship. This relationship marks the beginning of the capacity for love which, in essence, is the capacity to care for and be as concerned about another person as one is about oneself.

----

[7]H. S. Sullivan: *The Interpersonal Theory of Psychiatry.* New York, W. W. Norton & Co., Inc., 1953, p. 243.

The child for the first time manifests a sensitivity to the feelings of others and what may happen to them He becomes concerned about what is important to them and what h can do to increase the'r w ll being. This relationship provides an opportunity for him to have an intimate exchange, a sense of closeness with another person. He and his chum have no need for pretenses and are free to discuss their most intimate feelings and thoughts about themselves, other people and anything that interests them. This type of interaction is called collaboration, with both persons sensitive to each other and working together toward some mutual achievement. From this opportunity to share his thoughts and feelings and to experience this sense of closeness, the child is able to change many of his infantile ideas about both himself and others and to increase his and his chum's sense of personal worth.

During this period, too, the child begins to manifest a new attitude toward his learning experiences. As other people and his interactions with them become more meaningful, a whole new world opens up for him, and he reaches out in his attempt to learn how to best prepare for what is to come.

TWELVE YEARS TO MATURITY

The period from the beginning of the activity of the sexual glands to the time when the individual is both sexually and socially mature is usually designated as the period of adolescence. During this time, the child grows rapidly and becomes fatigued quite readily. He is expending a tremendous amount of energy to maintain control of his intensified impulses and desires, and this, in turn, influences the degree of attention that he is able to give to his everyday activities.

In addition, he has an intense desire to be independent and to gain an emancipation from his parents, which leads to considerable overt hostility toward, and depreciation of, his parents. He may openly rebel against the wishes and prohibitions of the family. At the same time, he usually becomes more closely identified with his peer group and develops a strong feeling of loyalty toward the members. Sometimes he will verbally agree with the group, taking a stand against his parents since, at times, merely to agree with the parents makes him feel more dependent upon them.

Throughout adolescence both intense loyalty and jealousy are concomitant aspects of most friendships. Not only members of the peer group are objects for relationships at this time, but the youngster may become quite attached to an older person whom he idealizes. Although such relationships may be labeled homosexual, they really have a different basis, such as the youngster's need for dependent security which he is not able to fulfill with his parents because of his strong drive toward independence.

As he attempts to transfer his affection or object love to those other than his parents, the characteristics of his group begin to change gradually. The first evidence is usually when one member of the group admits or demonstrates an interest in a member of the opposite sex. The rest of the group are apt to consider this act as gross disloyalty and proceed to taunt and kid the nonconformer relentlessly. This kidding is rather characteristic of the adolescent group and seems to be one of their primary means of handling their anxieties.

The group often gathers for lengthy discussions of various abstract subjects, and the idealism manifested during these sessions is quite lofty. The subjects discussed and the ensuing arguments reflect the conflicts of the group; therefore, the periods serve as a thinking-through process preparatory for action and also as a means of avoiding certain actions until the group members are ready for them.

The adolescent's intrapersonal relationships are in a constant state of disequilibrium, and this turmoil is reflected in the extreme vacillations evident in his overt behavior as he rapidly swings from one extreme to the other. The intensity of his superego is seen in the rigid standards and prohibitions which he sets up for himself in his attempt to master his intensified impulses and desires as well as in his attempts to sever his dependence upon his parents. The reorganization of his ego is of primary importance as he attempts to establish himself as an adult. He functions according to the pleasure principle at one moment and at the next is very realistic. He tries to be an adult but regresses rapidly when he finds it too difficult. His fantasy life tends to be rich and varied as he tries out his solutions to his many conflicts, although he usually faces reality readily again as he continues his attempts to grow toward maturity.

MATURITY

Not all individuals who achieve adulthood from a chronological standpoint simultaneously achieve maturity. The achievement of maturity is hindered in some individuals because they apparently lack the essential inherent capacity, while others have experienced too much trauma during the early years of their development. The results may be evidenced in defects ranging from those which involve only a part of the personality to those which involve the total personality.

In the material that follows, an attempt will be made to enumerate various patterns of behavior that are believed to be characteristic of the mature person, and there will of necessity be some overlapping in the concepts.

First of all, we anticipate that this person has arrived at a working philosophy of life which gives meaning to his efforts and stability to his actions. This philosophy will be a realistic code of values which structures his general plan of life. In other words, he will live his philosophy. If he understands and accepts certain beliefs, principles and values, they, in turn, will determine his action. The core of his values may be religious, aesthetic or scientific but it provides a certain amount of unity and consistency to his life.

Second, we anticipate that this individual will be tolerant. A tolerant person is not one who merely "puts up with" something or endures it. In contrast to this, a tolerant person is accepting, both of himself and of others. Since he has learned to accept himself, he is also able to accept others for what they are.

The third characteristic we anticipate is that he will be self-objective. The mature person has become an object to himself and is able to see himself as he is with all his assets and liabilities. Although he understands his limitations, he does not necessarily passively accept them, but his level of aspiration is fairly realistic. He functions with a minimum of self-deception and participates vigorously in activities which have value for him. Since he is able to take himself and his capacities for granted he also manifests a self-confident attitude.

The mature individual will also be capable of giving as well as receiving. He usually thinks more of what he can give rather than what he can get from an experience. He does not view giving as an obligation, but he gives spontaneously and spends his energies on aims outside of himself. He is able to collaborate since he does not always have to play the role of giver, but he can also accept affection, compliments and other things without feeling guilty and having almost impulsively to give something in return. So we anticipate a person who is able to give a great deal but one who is also able to enjoy receiving.

A fifth characteristic of this mature person is that he has developed the ability to establish an effective heterosexual love relationship—that is, he has the capacity both to love and be loved and will want to share with another individual as well as to receive. He is also able to give without expecting an equal return, as is essential with children. He is able to enjoy nonsexual interests as well as sexual interests with his mate, and their roles, masculine and feminine, are complementary.

In addition, we could anticipate that he has to some degree developed his capacity for self-realization. He will be both creative and productive and utilize his available energy to this end. He is able to use his own talents, skills and powers within the structure of his own realistic set of values. Furthermore, he will be able to seek and to find

fulfillment of his needs for both satisfaction and security without interfering with the needs of others.

We expect also that this individual has learned how to master his
environment in ways which are primarily realistic. He gains pleasure
from planning, organizing, overcoming difficulties in his work, assuming his responsibilities and doing well with a job. He has found
outlets for expressing his aggression whereby it is not destructive to
others, although in instances of attack he is successful in handling his
aggression effectively. Furthermore, this person experiences a minimum of irrational anxiety. He will not always have a feeling of impending doom but can well display anxiety if external conditions warrant
it.

All these characteristics may be anticipated in the mature individual to some degree, although the degree to which they are manifest
may vary considerably since the concept of maturity itself is relative. In
view of these characteristics of maturity, what changes can we expect to
have taken place in the various aspects of the personality of the person
who is relatively mature?

The first aspect, the id, will be basically the same, but the relationship between it and the other factors in the personality structure will be
different. The ego is the dominant factor in the personality, showing a
great deal of adaptability in its liaison role between the id, the superego
and external reality. The individual's ego is able to cope with old
anxieties when there are similarities between current and former problems; and although functioning within the framework of reality, the
individual can now permit greater satisfactions without experiencing
the anxiety and guilt formerly associated with them. In addition, this
person, because of his mature ego, is able to tolerate considerable stress
before revealing any degree of disorganization or decompensation. On
the other hand, the superego also reveals many changes in its functions. Although it still functions in the role of a critic, it will more or
less give appropriate warnings rather than punish as it did in childhood. The individual, of course, experiences guilt if the reality situation
warrants it, but this guilt is primarily conscious with a minimum of
unconscious guilt.

The patterns which each mature person utilizes in adjusting to
external reality are the same as for anyone else, since all adults are
more or less a product of their childhood. He is not, however, obligated to use any one of his old patterns if they prove inadequate, but
he is free to explore new possibilities.

Summary

We have described the infant as being born with a certain heritage,
endowment and potential that will develop if certain experiences are

possible. All infants have common basic needs both physiologic and interpersonal that must be provided for if they are to survive. In spite of their similarities to other human beings, each infant is a separate, unique entity and will develop at his own pace. To some degree, it appears that man is a product of his culture; however, he has an inherent capacity to learn and, therefore, to change, not only himself but also his environment.

We see the infant begin his journey in life in a state of passive dependency with specific needs which, if satisfied, lead to the development of a solid foundation for all later experience. As he goes through each spiral of development and has adequate opportunity to utilize each new ability as it evolves, we see him gaining a greater sense of self-identity and capability. By the time he is ready to go to school, he is in many respects somewhat of a finished product in the limited world centered in his home and family. His next learning experiences are focused upon learning to live with people who are pretty much like himself, as his world extends to encompass the school community and other related horizons. We see him developing various interpersonal skills in his play and in his work, and if he simultaneously experiences a feeling of self-esteem and worth he will be able to refine these skills as he continues to grow and to develop.

Gradually we see a new pattern of behavior evolving as the child begins to reveal a sensitivity to the feelings of others and begins to show concern about what happens to others. This new interest in and concern about people is the beginning of the capacity for love, which sets the stage for a new type of relationship. He is now able to experience a sense of closeness with another person and to have an intimate exchange of what were previously "private" thoughts and feelings. These experiences open the door to a whole new vista of learning, and we see him begin to reach out in order to be better prepared for future life.

As he moves upward through the spiral of development, we see him reach the level of maturity, which is characterized by a high degree of adaptability to stress. This person is one who is able to use the energy he does not need for survival for productive, creative activities. In this generous productive state the individual also requires security, and we see him gaining this internal peace when he can adjust his internal needs in a flexible way to the changing external and internal conditions.

We see the child develop in a progression-regression sequence from dependence through independence to interdependence or maturity, which is not a static state but one in which the individual continues to grow, to expand and to reach out.

Bibliography

Alexander, Franz, and Ross, Helen, eds.: *Dynamic Psychiatry*. Chicago, University of Chicago Press, 1952.

Cameron, Norman: *The Psychology of Behavior Disorders*. Boston, Houghton Mifflin Co., 1947.

Caplan, Gerald, and Lebovici, Serge, eds.: *Adolescence*. New York, Basic Books, Inc., 1969.

Erikson, Erik H.: *Identity and the Life Cycle* New York, International Universities Press, Inc., 1959.

Federn, Paul: *Ego Psychology and the Psychoses*. New York, Basic Books, Inc., 1952.

Fenichel, Otto: *The Psychoanalytic Theory of Neurosis*. New York, W. W. Norton & Co., Inc., 1945.

Freud, Sigmund: *Beyond the Pleasure Principle*. London, International Psychoanalytic Press, 1922.

Freud, Sigmund: *The Ego and the Id*. London, Hogarth Press, 1947.

Freud, Sigmund: *New Introductory Lectures on Psychoanalysis*. New York, W. W. Norton & Co., Inc., 1933.

Freud, Sigmund: *Outline of Psychoanalysis*. New York, W. W. Norton & Co., Inc., 1949.

Freud, Sigmund: *The Problem of Anxiety*. New York, W. W. Norton & Co., Inc., 1936.

Freud, Sigmund: *Three Contributions to the Theory of Sex*. New York, Nervous and Mental Disease Monographs, 1948.

Freud, Sigmund: *Moses and Monotheism*. New York, Alfred A. Knopf, Inc., 1939.

Freud, Sigmund: *Group Psychology and Analysis of the Ego*. London, International Psychoanalytic Press, 1922.

Freud, Sigmund: "On the Transformation of Instincts with Special Reference to Anal Erotism." In: *Collected Papers, II*. London, Hogarth Press, 1950, p. 164.

Freud, Sigmund: "The Infantile Genital Organization of the Libido." In· *Collected Papers, II*. London, Hogarth Press, 1950, p. 244.

Freud, Sigmund: "The Passing of the Oedipus-Complex." In: *Collected Papers, II*. London, Hogarth Press, 1950, p. 269.

Freud, Sigmund: "On Narcissism: An Introduction." In: *Collected Papers, IV*. London, Hogarth Press, 1950, p. 30.

Frosch, John, ed.: *The Annual Survey of Psychoanalysis*, Vol. I New York, International Universities Press, Inc , 1952

Gardener, Riley W., and Moriarity. Alice· *Personality Development at Preadolescence*. Seattle, University of Washington Press, 1968

Gesell, A., and Ilg, F. L.: *Infant and Child in the Culture of Today*. New York, Harper & Brothers, 1942.

Hartmann, Heinz: *Ego Psychology and the Problem of Adaptation*. New York, International Universities Press, Inc., 1958

Josselyn, Irene: *Psychosocial Development of Children*. New York, Family Service Association of America, 1948.

Lewin, Kurt: *A Dynamic Theory of Personality*. New York, McGraw-Hill Book Co., Inc., 1940.

Piaget, Jean: *The Origins of Intelligence in Children*. New York, International Universities Press, Inc., 1952.

Piaget, Jean: *The Construction of Reality in the Child*. New York, Basic Books, Inc., 1954.

Schilder, Paul: *The Image and Appearance of the Human Body*. New York, International Universities Press, Inc., 1950.

Silverberg, William: *Childhood Experience and Personal Destiny*. New York, Springer Publishing Co., Inc., 1952.

Spitz, Rene A.: *A Genetic Field Theory of Ego Formation*. New York, International Universities Press, Inc., 1959.

Sullivan, Harry Stack: *Conceptions of Modern Psychiatry*. New York, W. W. Norton & Co., Inc., 1953.

Sullivan, Harry Stack: *The Interpersonal Theory of Psychiatry.* New York, W. W. Norton & Co., Inc., 1953.
Wittenberg, Rudolph: *Postadolescence.* New York, Grune & Stratton, Inc., 1968.

Suggestions for Further Reading

Adams, Margaret M.: "Appraisal of a Newborn Infant." *Am. J. Nursing, 55*:1336-1337, 1955.
Badgeley, Elizabeth Wadleigh: "Making Friends with Children." *Am. J. Nursing, 57*·1558-1560, 1957.
Bettelheim, Bruno: *Dialogues with Mothers.* Glencoe, Ill. Free Press of Glencoe, 1962.
Cameron, Norman: *The Psychology of Behavior Disorders.* Boston, Houghton Mifflin Co., 1947, pp. 89-102.
English, O. S., and Pearson, Gerald: *Emotional Problems of Living.* New York, W. W. Norton & Co., Inc., 1945.
Erikson, E. H.: *Childhood and Society.* 2nd Ed., W. W. Norton & Co., Inc., 1964.
Erikson, E. H.: *Insight and Responsibility.* New York, W. W. Norton & Co., Inc., 1964, pp. 111-157.
Gesell, A., and Ilg, F. L.: *Infant and Child in the Culture of Today.* New York, Harper & Brothers, 1942.
Group for the Advancement of Psychiatry: *Normal Adolescence.* New York, Charles Scribner's Sons, 1968.
Jersild, Arthur T.. *The Psychology of Adolescence.* New York, Macmillan Co., 1963, pp. 177-226, 393-409.
Maslow, A. H., and Mittelmann, Bela: *Principles of Abnormal Psychology.* New York, Harper & Brothers, 1951, pp. 125-152.
Peplau, Hildegarde E.: "Anxiety in the Mother-Infant Relationship." *Nursing World, 134*:12, 33, 1960.
Warters, Jane: *Achieving Maturity.* New York, McGraw-Hill Book Co., Inc., 1949, pp. 93-140.

Chapter 5   Biosocial Orientation in Later Life

THE MIDDLE PERIOD OF LIFE

The period of middle age is said by some to begin at the climacteric, but for our purposes we will refer to the middle years as that period in family life where there are again but two figures, the mother and father, who, because of their shared experiences in the joys, anxieties and responsibilities of rearing a family, are now very different persons. They have perhaps struggled financially and have shared much, including sexual pleasures, joy with the addition of each child, anxiety over childhood illnesses, and disappointments. Their children have come of age, been emancipated from the home, and have begun families of their own. These years of experiences have made the couple wiser, their judgment keener, but also have brought a gradual decline of physical power and agility.

There is also the middle-aged person who has never married or whose marriage has been terminated by divorce or death. The student with an interest in the single person approaching old age will find this topic discussed in several of the references at the end of the chapter.

Changes begin to occur in the physical appearance of the middle-aged person. The hair tends to gray, and men may begin to grow bald. Usually there is a gain in weight, especially around the "middle," and wrinkles in the skin begin to make their appearance. The sense organs do not seem so keen. high tones are not so easily heard, and eyeglasses become a necessity. Sensations of pain are not usually so acute, and taste is not so discriminating. Tremors of the muscles are sometimes noticeable, and rest periods are more frequent. Sometimes there is anxiety and fear that sexual life will disappear. Rebellion may occur, especially in the male, since he has been the provider and the power symbol in the family. He may now want to prove that he is as "good as ever" and may take on extramarital sexual interests.

Since our culture does not seem so tolerant of the aged as some, those in middle life often try to hide their signs of aging. Although aging is said to begin at conception, the middle years seem to bring keener cognizance of it. Thus, we see the middle-aged man wearing a girdle and a toupee and riding around in a convertible. We see the aging woman tinting her hair, buying all sorts of skin preservatives and the like. Some people, threatened by such things as the loss of agilities, laugh, are witty and poke fun at their stress. Perhaps this is why there are so many jokes concerned with the middle-aged man attempting to prove his physical power.

Illness during this phase of life takes a longer period in running its course, and many diseases become chronic. In women, the menopause may bring with it symptoms of tension, depression and vague somatic conditions. Children have left home, and it may be difficult for the parents, especially the mother, to make an adjustment. While there is often financial gain because there are fewer to support, and because the chief provider has acquired a stable position in his occupation or profession, this is often not enough to make up for the loss of affectionate bonds. Although interests are more narrow, they also change. Interests are less adventurous, and are usually of such a nature that less physical efficiency is required. When one's interest in outside affairs has fallen off, there is a tendency to focus on oneself, and there is more concern with functions of the body. While this interest in the body may be valuable in that serious diseases may be detected earlier, it may also be over-used.

During this phase, there is often a tendency to look back, and to realize that many hopes and ambitions of one's life will never be fulfilled. The male usually realizes that he has gone about as far as he will go in his job. When grandchildren appear on the scene, they are a constant reminder that one is growing older. Although most people of this age derive much wholesome pleasure from the grandchildren, there are others who try to relive the period when their own children were small and therefore tend to "take over." This pattern may be seen in the widow whose interests have become too narrow, and who becomes quite meddlesome in the households of her children.

The more flexible person, with healthy patterns of adjustment in early life, will more readily adapt to his new status in life during the middle years. The better he adjusts to this period, the easier it will be to adjust to retirement. Some individuals, however, need a great deal of understanding and help in finding new outlets. The right kind of help in living a normal life, and the early detection and correction of health problems, will make the period of retirement and old age a happier one.

The period of middle age is often more difficult for the female than the male. The cessation of the menses, and the loss of the children from the home frequently cause a sudden realization that she is getting older. The male, on the other hand, does not become quite so cognizant of this fact until he retires. By the time he retires, his wife has often made many of the necessary adjustments. It is fortunate, indeed, that these stressful periods do not occur to both husband and wife at the same time.

While it is desirable that preparation for the later years go on all through life, it is perhaps during the middle-age period that there is the greatest readiness on the part of the individual for such preparation.

THE OLDER PERSON

Because of the increasing proportion of older persons in our society, the gradual decline in agility of the older person, the increasing cost of chronic and disabling illnesses in a culture that places high values on the production of material goods, and for other reasons, older people seem to threaten our social order. Although the pessimistic attitude of our culture toward older people is not always justified, as we shall explain later, the urgency for understanding and for constructive action is mounting.

POPULATION CHANGES

Let us examine first some of the population changes in regard to age in our country. Our country's population of those in the age group 65 and over is on the rise; it is five times larger than this same group in 1900. For 1985 the projected number of persons over 65 years of age in this country is 25 million if one assumes that there will be no major changes in the rate of mortality.[1]

---

[1]Matilda White Riley and Anne Foner: *Aging and Society.* Vol. I: *An Inventory of Research Findings.* New York Russell Sage Foundation, 1968, pp. 16-17.

The interrelationships of the factors of fertility, mortality and immigration have contributed to the increase in numbers and proportion of older persons. With new advances in medicine, there has been a decline in mortality rates of older persons, so that the life span of the individual has increased. Since immigrants tend to be younger, restrictions on immigration to the United States have also had a great influence on the population structure.

Our elder population also differs from the general population. In the older age group there are more women than men, and a little over half these women are widowed. About one-fifth of older people are in living arrangements apart from their relatives.[2] The older people are further characterized by the fact that they are predominantly a group with only grade school education.

Within the United States the greatest concentration of older persons is in the New England and Great Plains states. The low percentage of older people in the southern states results from the high birth rate in that area. Even though the lowest proportion of older people is in the south, the greatest *increase* in the proportion of older persons occurred between 1940 and 1950 in states with milder climates, such as Arizona, California, Florida and Nevada. It is predicted that "by the year 2000, even assuming no unusual progress in cutting down the death rate, we can expect to have an aged population of more than 27 million persons. This would represent approximately 1 in 8 of our total population."[3]

The increase in the proportion of older persons not only is characteristic of this country but is a trend also in the world population structure. Persons 60 years and over constitute about seven per cent of all the earth's inhabitants.[4] The rapid population change has many social implications that will both directly and indirectly affect the practices of nursing in other countries, as well as the United States.

THE SOCIAL IMPLICATIONS OF AN AGING POPULATION

Since older people are considered more conservative, and will make up an increasingly large proportion of the population, it is anticipated that there may be reluctance in implementing needed measures for social, economic and political change. Older people use differ-

---

[2]Philip M. Hauser and Ethel Shanas: "Trends in the Aging Population." In Cowdry's *Care of the Geriatric Patient.* St. Louis, C. V. Mosby Co., 1968, pp. 968–973.

[3]U.S. Department of Health, Education, and Welfare. Report No. 20 prepared by Agnes W. Brewster, and Dorothy McCamman: *Health Costs of the Aged.* Washington, D.C., U.S. Government Printing Office, 1956, p. 2.

[4]New York State Joint Legislative Committee on Problems of the Aging. *Making the Years Count.* Legislative Document No. 32, 1955, p. 4.

ent goods and materials than younger people, and some influence would be exerted on the type of materials produced to meet the changes in the consumer's market.

Because of the increasing proportion of older people, employment practices and retirement plans of the future may favor the older person. Considering the number of children dependent upon others coupled with the number of oldsters dependent upon others, there will be a small percentage of workers in our society, and they will have to provide for an increasing number of persons.

> If we don't do something about using the disabled, and chronically ill, and the older age group, by 1980, for every able-bodied worker in America there will be 1 person physically handicapped, chronically ill, or age 65 or over to be supported.[5]

At the present there is considerable discrimination against the employment of the older worker, although in the research of industrial psychologists it has been noted that the older worker tends to stress accuracy over speed, and that certain manual skills are maintained. Older industries, such as clothing manufacturing, tend to utilize the skills of older workers more than the newer industries, such as aircraft construction.

In the future, since there will be a smaller percentage in the younger age group suffering from acute disease, it is expected that more time will be available to health workers for concentration on the health problems of older persons. There is already an increased demand for education in the problems of older persons. Perhaps because of our cultural attitudes toward the aged, the various health professions and occupations seem to have been slow in accepting gerontology.

It has been as recently as 1942 and 1945 that the American Geriatrics Society and the Gerontological Society respectively were founded.

CULTURAL ATTITUDES TOWARD THE AGED

The older person, like those in other age groups, wants to feel loved and needed, and wants to maintain his social status in society; however, as he becomes older, it becomes increasingly difficult for him to make significant contributions to the economy. While some opportunities to gain respect are present in all societies, so, too, is neglect found in all cultures.

---

[5]Howard A. Rusk: "Rehabilitation: Nature and Magnitude of the Problem." In U.S. Senate Committee on Labor and Public Welfare, Selected Documents — Volume V: *Public and Private Services for Older People: Rehabilitation, Housing and Living Arrangements, Education and Community Services.* Washington, D.C., U.S. Government Printing Office, 1957, p. 12.

Simmons indicates that in primitive cultures the aged seemed to have more prestige in climates which were mild, in tribes that had a permanent residence, in areas where there was an abundant food supply, and in those societies that viewed life after death as attractive. In certain primitive Eskimo communities, the aged who could no longer care for themselves were killed outright or abandoned, but in other societies prestige increased with advancing years. The Incas and Aztecs were known to have organized assistance for the aged and disabled.[6]

The literature of the Greeks indicates favoritism of youth and lamentation of old age. Sparta and ancient Athens, on the other hand, valued the wisdom and judgment of the aged.

In ancient China, old age was treated with reverence and respect. Because the old were considered wise, when they spoke, the young listened. The philosophic attitude toward a calm, tranquil life in which one has time to reflect on the finer things in life is favorable to, and even respectful of, the advancing years.

In contrast, our country, in general, manifests an attitude of indifference and neglect toward the aged. There are exceptions, as in some rural areas where the aged may be an asset to the family. Modern disease control has added years to the life span of man but has contributed little to make this period more enjoyable. In crowded industrial sections where space is precious, the aged are in the way and are treated with a general indifference and neglect. The old are removed from the homes of their families, tucked away and soon forgotten in a variety of institutions offering shelter and custodial care. In many such institutions the aged man or woman is ignored and treated as an inanimate object. He is cut off from his former social system, and surrounded by others who are unable to treat the dignity of being human with love and respect. With more knowledge and understanding of the older person, the nurse is able to act in such a manner that old people can enjoy being a part of a social system in which they feel wanted because they can contribute in some fashion.

In one way or another, the old man must embrace the world with an impulse of love. Rigidity, aridity, hardness exclude the possibility of love. On the other hand, love may endure in all its splendor and vitality if a certain inner activity and versatility be preserved; therein we have an essential precondition of all inner growth and further development.[7]

---

[6]Leo W. Simmons: *The Role of the Aged in Primitive Society.* New Haven, Yale University Press, 1945, p. 240.

[7]A. L. Vischer: *Old Age: Its Compensations and Rewards.* London, George Allen and Unwin, Ltd., 1947, p. 194.

CHANGES IN ANATOMICAL STRUCTURES AND PROCESSES

Vischer states that "senescence begins when the phenomena of atrophy predominate, become more emphatic and are externally perceptible."[8] The older person's skin becomes wrinkled, thin and dry, with brown pigmentation. The hair becomes gray and thin and the nails tend to thicken. The senses of seeing, hearing and touch are impaired. Farsightedness is especially common, and the visual field is narrowed. The inability to distinguish colors has also been noted. In general, there seems to be a gradual dysfunctioning of visual structures. There is also a gradual decline in hearing, especially the acuity for high tones. Taste, too, becomes blunted, which makes eating less interesting for most people.

In advancing age there seems to be brittleness and shrinking of the bony structures, but little change is noted in tendons and ligaments. The skeletal muscles lose strength, and motor activity is slowed down markedly. The teeth, if present, seem to grow more yellow; if they have been replaced by ill-fitted dentures, they may be very annoying to both the older person and others. Although there are some changes in the brain, such as deposits of waste matter, and minute areas of softening, these do not always correlate with the degree of intellectual functioning. Another interesting aspect in relation to the aged is that the two sexes begin to look more alike, with voice and facial appearances more similar.

The size of the heart tends to increase with advancing age; the valves tend to become more rigid; and the blood pressure, especially the systolic, tends to increase. The chest wall is less elastic, and the capacity of the lung tissues to ventilate the pulmonary blood is lessened. On the other hand, the smooth muscle organs such as the stomach and intestines are least affected by age.

The homeostatic mechanism of the body seems able to take care of normal demands, but there are changes in its reserve ability to meet the unusual demands of pathologic conditions. In general, there is slower repair of tissue, and the individual is slower in recovering from illnesses. All of us are aging every day, and it is not a process peculiar to the older person.

Cavan, Burgess, Havighurst and Goldhamer[9] summarize the physical criteria of old age as follows:

1. Gradual tissue desiccation
2. Gradual retardation of cell division, capacity of cell growth, and tissue repair

---

[8]*Ibid.*, p. 23.

[9]Ruth Shonle Cavan, Ernest W. Burgess, Robert J. Havighurst, and Herbert Goldhamer: *Personal Adjustment in Old Age.* Chicago, Science Research Associates, Inc., 1949, pp. 2-3.

3. Gradual retardation in the rate of tissue oxidation (lowering of the basal metabolic rate)
4. Cellular atrophy, degeneration, increased cell pigmentation and fatty infiltration
5. Gradual decrease in tissue elasticity, and degenerative changes in the elastic connective tissue
6. Decreased speed, strength and endurance of skeletal neuromuscular reactions
7. Decreased strength of skeletal muscle
8. Progressive degeneration and atrophy of the nervous system, impaired vision, hearing, attention, memory and mental endurance

It should be emphasized that aging does not occur in all parts of the body at the same time nor at the same rate.

CHANGES IN SOCIAL ROLE AND POSITION

Sarbin has defined role as a "patterned sequence of learned actions or deeds performed by a person in an interaction situation."[10] Thus, one person in the interaction may be playing the role of teacher and another person in the interaction may be in the role of student. The teacher, however, may have many other roles in life. She may also be a mother, a volunteer worker in the hospital and a grandmother. The student, too, may have the role of paper boy, Boy Scout and family sibling. In a position or status, "the person learns (a) to expect or anticipate certain actions from other persons and (b) that others have expectations of him."[11] The child, for example, expects to be fed, bathed and loved, and the mother, in contrast, is expected to provide food, protection and gentleness. "The organized actions of the person, directed toward fulfilling these role expectations, comprise the role."[12] Although role and position or status are interdependent on one another, they are not the same thing. Often in nursing the word role is used merely to describe the duties of the nurse on the job, as, for example, the instructor might ask, "What is the nurse's role in giving medications?" Here the instructor is usually asking the student to enumerate a list of duties or steps in the procedure for the administration of medicines. Although social scientists have several definitions of the word *role*, it usually means more than a mere description of one's duties. "Whatever agreement has been attained in the use of the term *role*, centers around the organized *actions* of a person coordinate with a given status or position."[13]

---

[10]Theodore Sarbin: "Role Theory." In Gardner Lindzey, ed.: *Handbook of Social Psychology*, Vol. I. Cambridge, Mass., Addison-Wesley Publishing Company, Inc., 1954, p. 225.
    [11]*Ibid.*
    [12]*Ibid.*
    [13]*Ibid.*

The aging process involves many changes, and one is an important change in role and status. The older person usually has a lower status than the middle-aged person; however, a few gain in status, as, for example, a capable attorney who becomes a judge in his later years. An unfavorable change in role and status is stress producing in the older person.

During the middle-age period, it was the mother who had a marked change in role—that is, she gave up her role as mother, and emancipated her children. Her next role was that of grandmother, but no longer did she have full say about her children's care, and it became necessary, if she was to remain happy, to find new interests. The father, during the middle years, did not need to find so many new interests because he had his job and often was at the stage of greatest achievement in his career. Retirement, on the other hand, leaves considerable time, and the male must then take on different activities. If the marriage has not been a particularly pleasant one, this additional time with the spouse will be even more disagreeable than before retirement.

It has been noted that our culture does not ascribe much prestige to the aged. This is exemplified by our compulsory retirement practices at the age of 65. With the increased cost in living and the increased cost of medical care, the aged person living on a small pension often must move to a lower-income dwelling. The expectations that a culture has toward a group has marked influence on its role and position. Expectations of the aged group as depicted by television and motion pictures is also believed to influence the roles of older persons. Television seems less discriminating toward the aged than motion pictures. The above examples are but a few of the facets of our social life that indicate a change of expectation of the behavior of older people.

There is a decrease in role activity with age, with older women exceeding older men in continuing in their established roles. However, older married men and women living together are highest in role activity.

Often the older person has a heightened interest in religion and becomes a more active participant in church work. The church accepts the aged, and does much to make life happier and fuller for them. In fact, it is one of the few places that do not discriminate toward the aged. In church, the older person is always welcome and needed.

CHANGES IN PSYCHOLOGIC ADJUSTMENTS

Because of the physical and mental changes, and a change in role and status, old age seems to have more periods of crisis than any other period of life. Preparation for, and acceptance of, some of these changes will make the transition from middle life to later life much easier for the individual. In general, the way an individual meets a crisis is determined to a large extent by the patterns of behavior that he has used in earlier life. However, there also seem to be other characteristics common to later life. Partly because of changes in the body which influence the concept of the self, the older person may tend to direct his hostility toward himself, and therefore may be subject to feelings of depression and loneliness. On the other hand, resentment over the way his family or society has treated him may be directed toward younger people with whom the older person lives.

The inability of the older person to see or hear well may bring on feelings of suspicion. If he feels unwanted, he may resort to telling stories about his earlier achievements. In order to conserve energy, he may tend to eliminate stimuli from his environment; thus, if it is an effort to hear, he may "tune out" trivial conversations.

The older person, like people of all ages, wishes emotional security, esteem, recognition, physical comfort, new experiences and the like; however, some of these desires increase in old age and some, such as the desire for sexual expression, decrease in some but increase in other cases.

The desires, aspirations and demands of the older person seem to have become better defined through the years, and his expectations in relation to these have become more specific. The older person also experiences a disruption of his habit patterns. When he is retired, his old habits are no longer applicable, and he is forced to find new ones. Forming these new habits may be quite difficult, especially if they are in conflict with old, long-established ones. It also takes more time for the older person to learn the new habits required of him: therefore, it is important to give the older person time to respond in a significant manner.

The number of individuals with whom the older person interacts is likely to decrease because his friends of the same age begin to die, and because he cannot get around as well as he formerly did. In general, the older person's orientation to time seems to contract. The past and present seem to flow together, with fewer plans made for the future. The minute acts and annoyances of daily living, therefore, may appear greater to him.

Some older people become interested in preserving culture, and become more inspired by great works of art, literature, philosophy and religion. Such interests open new avenues to the aged. In some cultures the aged learn new tasks very quickly. It is thought by many that old people can learn quite readily if properly motivated. The older person tends to be more accurate in what he learns than the younger person. Judgment, too, is often not impaired. In fact, because of the older person's previous experience, judgment is often enhanced. If one continues to learn and to exercise judgment, it is believed that these attributes are less apt to become rusty from disuse.

Another characteristic of older people is that they are apt to become quite rigid and fixed in their daily routines. It has been suggested that this may be closely related to the fact that older persons do not wish time to pass but want everything to stay as it is.

Sometimes older people tend to hoard useless objects, and to become careless in their personal habits. If interest is maintained in other events, however, they tend to have more motivation to keep up their appearance.

The older individual may harbor many fears, especially the fear of pain and helplessness if he becomes disabled. Although he may also have a tendency to center his thoughts on bodily processes, he may not always mention these because he thinks it may cause others concern. He may also be greatly disturbed by his faulty memory.

In general, whatever personality traits characterize the individual earlier in life seem exaggerated in later years. Thus, if the individual was stingy in early life he will probably be miserly in old age, and if he was generous in his early years, he tends to be even more so as he grows older.

It should be pointed out that, even though an older person may become more dependent in old age, he is not like a child. His body is different from a child's; his personality, because of his many and varied experiences, is not like that of a child. Society should not treat him as it treats children. Both youth and the aged have their separate roles in society. In fact, one wonders how the aged, meeting the many stressful situations confronting them, manage to make so many adjustments. There is much hope for people who can make some adjustment to so many stressful situations.

Summary

The middle-aged person and the older person have been discussed from a social, cultural, biologic and psychologic point of view.

We prefer to think of the middle period of life as that period in family life when there are again but two figures, although it is said by some to begin at the menopause. This is not to say that single or widowed people do not experience middle age.

Population changes indicate a rise in the age group 65 and over. The social implications of such a population trend indicate a need for social, economic and political change in the future.

Cultural attitudes toward the aged vary from culture to culture and from time to time. In traditional China old age was treated with reverence and respect. In our country today the aged are, in general, viewed with indifference.

The physiologic changes that accompany old age have been described within the chapter. However, it should again be emphasized that aging does not occur in all parts of the body at the same time nor is the rate of aging the same in all parts of the body.

The aging process also leads to changes in role and status. We see that changes in role occur at different periods for men and for women. During the middle period it is the mother who gives up her role of childbearing, while in later years it is the man whose role changes at retirement.

Some of the changes in patterns of behavior that accompany the aging process are brought on by the physical changes and the changes in role and status already mentioned. Thus, the inability to see or hear well may bring about feelings of suspicion. Because of retirement, the number of persons with whom one interacts may become limited.

In general, the more flexible the person was in his early life, the better he will be able to meet and solve problems in later life.

Bibliography

Agate, John N., Ed.: *Medicine in Old Age.* Philadelphia, J. B. Lippincott Co., 1965.

Anderson, John E., ed.: *Psychological Aspects of Aging.* Washington, D.C., American Psychological Association, Inc., 1956.

Cavan, Ruth Shonle, Burgess, Ernest W., Havighurst, Robert J., and Goldhamer, Herbert: *Personal Adjustment in Old Age.* Chicago, Science Research Associates, Inc., 1949.

Committee on Labor and Public Welfare, United States Senate: *Studies of the Aged and Aging: Guide to Significant Publications.* Selected Documents—Volume VII. Washington, D.C., U.S. Government Printing Office, 1956.

Committee on Labor and Public Welfare, United States Senate: *Studies of the Aged and Aging: Public and Private Services for Older People.* Selected Documents—Volume V. Washington, D.C., U.S. Government Printing Office, 1957.

Cowdry, E. V., ed.: *The Care of the Geriatric Patient.* St. Louis, C. V. Mosby Co., 1968.

Cumming, Elaine, and Henry, Wm. E.: *Growing Old.* New York, Basic Books, Inc., 1961.

Dubl'n, Louis I.: *Statistical and Social Implications in the Problem of Our Aging Population.* University of Pennsylvania Bicentennial Conference (pamphlet, n.d.).

Gilbert, Jeanne: *Understanding Old Age.* New York, Ronald Press Co., 1952.

Greenleigh, Lawrence F.: *Changing Psychological Concepts of Aging.* U.S. Department of Health, Education and Welfare. Public Health Service, National Institutes of Health (mimeographed), 1953.

Howell, Trevor H.: "George Cheyne's Essay on Health and Long Life," *Gerontologist,* 9:226–228, Autumn, 1969. Part I.

Illing, Hans A.: "Environment and Aging." *J. Am. Geriatrics Soc.,* 6:405–410, May, 1958.

Kleemeier, Robert W., ed.: *Aging and Leisure.* New York, Oxford University Press, 1961.

Lansing, Albert I., ed.: *Cowdry's Problems of Aging,* 3rd ed. Baltimore, Williams & Wilkins Co., 1952.

Lemkau, Paul V.: *Mental Hygiene in Public Health,* 2nd ed. New York, McGraw-Hill Book Co., Inc., 1955.

McConnell, John W.: "The Impact of Aging on the Economy." *J. Gerontol.,* Supplement No. 2, 13:42–47, 1958.

Neugarten, Bernice L., ed.: *Middle Age and Aging.* Chicago, University of Chicago Press, 1968.

Podolsky, Edward: "Changing Attitudes on Growing Older." *J. Am. Geriatrics Soc.,* 6:352-354, April, 1958.

Pollak, Otto: *Social Adjustment in Old Age.* New York, Social Science Research Council, 1948.

Riley, Matilda White, and Foner, Anne: *Aging and Society.* Vol. I: *An Inventory of Research Findings.* New York, Russell Sage Foundation, 1968.

Rose, Arnold M., and Peterson, Warren A., eds.: *Older People and Their Social Role.* Philadelphia, F. A. Davis Co., 1965.

Simmons, Leo W.: *The Role of the Aged in Primitive Society.* New Haven, Yale University Press, 1945.

Tibbitts, Clark: "The Impact of Aging on Social Institutions." *J. Gerontol.,* Supplement No. 2, *13*:48-52, 1957.

U.S. Department of Health, Education, and Welfare. Social Securities Administration: "Health Costs of the Aged." (Prepared by Brewster, Agnes W., and McCamman, Dorothy.) Report No. 20, Washington, D.C., U.S. Government Printing Office, May, 1956.

Vischer, A. L.: *Old Age: Its Compensations and Rewards.* London, George Allen and Unwin, Ltd., 1947.

Suggestions for Further Reading

Brill, Naomi: "Basic Knowledge for Work with the Aging." *Gerontologist, 9*:197-203, Autumn, 1969. Part I.

Burgess, Ernest W.: "Family Structure and Relationships." In Ernest W. Burgess, ed.: *Aging in Western Societies.* Chicago, University of Chicago Press, 1961, pp. 271-298.

Busse, Ewald W., Barnes, Robert H., Silverman, Albert J., Thaler, Margaret, and Frost, Laurance L.: "Studies of the Process of Aging. X: The Strengths and Weaknesses of Psychic Functioning in the Aged." *Am. J. Psychiat., III*:896-901, June, 1955.

Cohen, Elias S.: "Cultural Attitudes Toward Aging and Their Implications for Public Planning." *J. Am. Geriatrics Soc., 8*:337-343, May, 1960.

Cumming, Elaine, and Herry, William E.: *Growing Old.* New York, Basic Books, Inc., 1961.

Donahue, Wilma: "Psychologic Aspects in the Management of the Geriatric Patient." In E. V. Cowdry, ed.: *The Care of the Geriatric Patient.* St. Louis, C. V. Mosby Co., 1958, pp. 27-38.

Engel, George L.: *Psychological Development in Health and Disease.* Philadelphia, W. B. Saunders Co., 1962, pp. 195-196.

Friedmann, Eugene A.: "The Impact of Aging on the Social Structure." In Clark Tibbitts, ed.: *Handbook of Social Gerontology.* Chicago, University of Chicago Press, 1961, pp. 120-144.

Gilbert, Jeanne: *Understanding Old Age.* New York, Ronald Press Co., 1952, pp. 3-173.

Hall, Bernard H.: "The Mental Health of Senior Citizens." *Nursing Outlook, 4*:206-208, April, 1956.

Hauser, Philip M., and Vargas, Raul: "Population Structure and Trends." In Ernest W. Burgess, ed.: *Aging in Western Societies.* Chicago, University of Chicago Press, 1961, pp. 29-53.

Lansing, Albert I.: "General Biology of Senescence." In James E. Birren, ed.: *Handbook of Aging and the Individual.* Chicago, University of Chicago Press, 1960, pp. 119-135.

Neugarten, Bernice L., et al.: *Personality in Middle and Late Life.* New York, Atherton Press, 1964.

President's Council on Aging: *The Older American.* Washington, D.C., U.S. Government Printing Office, 1963.

Riegel, Klaus F.: Personality Theory and Aging. In James E. Birren, ed.: *Handbook of Aging and the Individual.* Chicago, University of Chicago Press, 1960, pp. 797-851.

Rodstein, Manuel: "The Aging Process and Disease." *Nursing Outlook, 12*:43–46, November, 1964.

Rose, Charles L.: "Social Factors in Longevity." *Gerontologist, 4*:27–37, March, 1964.

Shock, Nathan W.: "Age with a Future." *Gerontologist, 8*·147–152, Autumn, 1968. Part I.

Shrut, Samuel D.: "Attitudes Toward Old Age and Death." *Ment. Hyg., 42*:259–266, April, 1958.

Tibbitts, Clark: "Social Change, Aging and Public Health Nursing." *Nursing Outlook, 6*:144–147, March, 1958.

Vischer, A. L.: *Old Age; Its Compensations and Rewards.* London, George Allen and Unwin, Ltd., 1947.

Wolff, Kurt: *The Biological, Sociological and Psychological Aspects of Aging.* Springfield, Ill., Charles C Thomas, Publisher, 1959.

Chapter 6   Observational Skills

Everyone observes the behavior of other people, whether this observation be intentional or incidental. The cause or purpose of this widespread practice has been attributed to many factors. It has often been said that idle curiosity is the primary motive for observing other people; however, it has also been suggested that perhaps a basic desire to understand others is inherent in everyone. Regardless of what we accept as the basic cause or purpose of this tendency, we find that the nurse, in general, is no exception. In addition, the nurse has usually been taught to watch her patient carefully for signs and symptoms that indicate certain disease conditions and complications. The nurse in psychiatry, however, soon finds that she requires a further refinement of these skills of observation because her subject of study is the patient and all aspects of his interaction with his environment. Some of these reactions may be overt and readily discernible while others, often the most important, are safely hidden from the casual observer. The following material discusses the observation and the recording of behavioral data as a function of the nurse.

DEFINITION OF OBSERVATION

Observation is an active process requiring that we be alert to all the stimuli that are impinging upon us. This process implies that we use all our sense organs, depending of course, upon the stimuli present. That is to say, when we are observing we touch the substance, smell the odor, taste the food, hear the sound and see all that is visible. Observation is one method of collecting data. It is sometimes considered as a search in order to discover something unknown, such as the details of Mrs. A.'s reaction when she loses at bridge. For the nurse, observation is the chief method of collecting data in regard to her patient's behavior.

Observation consists of many skills that are developed through persistent and guided practice. The skill of observation is not peculiar to the nursing profession alone since we find that the tool is utilized by many groups. The navigator observes the course of his ship just as the bacteriologist observes the microorganism and the politician observes his growth or decline in popularity.

We can summarize, then, by saying that observation is a method of collecting data in order to discover something unknown. It is also an active process, and a skill that requires the use of all our sense organs.

THE PROCESS OF OBSERVATION

What takes place when we observe something? The process seems to happen so automatically that seldom are we aware that it is not an instantaneous occurrence. For further clarification let us try to analyze the process of observation to determine what occurs when we observe.

First, there is a *stimulus*. Then, assuming that we have an individual with the necessary physiologic prerequisites, sense organs and an intact nervous system, this stimulus gives rise to the second step, a *sensation,* which is merely the stimulation of a sense organ. Third, we give meaning to this sensation in terms of our past experience, and this meaning we call *perception*. If the sensory experience is new or unfamiliar, however, we are apt to have difficulty perceiving it and we may be unable to organize this incoming data so that it has meaning for us.

The fourth step, *a focusing of attention*, occurs as we perceive and attempt to make the stimulus more clear and distinct. The third and fourth steps are so closely related that any fluctuation in one aspect is bound to influence the other. The accuracy that we develop in perceiving is to a great extent dependent upon our ability to focus our attention on the particular phase of our total environment that is under observation at the time.

When we pay closer attention, the fifth factor, that of *interest,* enters in, and we tend to become interested in what we perceive. As our interest is aroused, the last step in the process occurs, and we tend to *limit the field,* to concentrate more closely on whatever we are observing and to exclude irrelevant stimuli.

As we can see, the individual does not observe automatically like a machine, with certain stimuli being fed in and certain stereotyped results being produced. Any observation that a specific individual may make will be influenced not only by his past experiences and his total condition at the time but also by the skills that he possesses.

CHARACTERISTICS OF GOOD OBSERVATION

Good observation is *purposeful*. Such a purpose may be general or it may be specific, but it is not just aimless looking around. For example, the nurse may be observing and trying to communicate with a newly admitted patient for the purpose of collecting as much detailed data as possible about the patient in order to discover what may evoke the one little spark of interest in his new environment. This type of observation is fairly general and somewhat nonstructured in that the nurse is not focusing her attention on any one aspect of the patient's behavior. On the other hand, the nurse may observe the patient for very specific reasons. For example, it may be important for a nurse to observe the patient's reaction to his interview with the psychiatrist or to watch his specific reactions following electrotherapy. In this instance, the nurse is focusing her attention upon certain aspects of the patient's behavior for very definite reasons. In many instances the nurse may observe the same patient for both general and specific reasons; but regardless of whether the purpose is general or specific, it should always exist.

Secondly, good observation is *planned*. That is, the nurse does not merely "drop in" on a situation at any time she happens to be passing by but arranges her work so that she can spend the major part of her time with her patients. It is important that the nurse make some general plans for the duration and number of observations that are necessary for the effective care of her patients. Some thought should also be given to the interval between observations. This last aspect is important not only for the nurse to be assured of the patient's welfare or to have something to write on the chart, but also to obtain a fairly adequate sampling of observational data throughout the patient's stay in the hospital.

Objectiveness is also a characteristic of good observation. By objectiveness we do not mean a cold emotional detachment, as though we were observing a slide under a microscope; we mean rather truth in what one observes. Only experience can teach us this. However, we can sometimes improve our objectiveness by comparing our observations with those of others and discussing them in conferences so as to see how our data are similar or different from the observations of others.

Objectiveness in observation does not apply only to observing the patient and his surroundings; it also refers to objectiveness in the intentional observation of oneself.

THE NURSE AS AN OBSERVER

As an observer the nurse has three functions: the spectator, the participant and the introspectionist. Sometimes it appears as though the experienced nurse were performing all three functions simultaneously, but actually she may skillfully oscillate from one activity to another in certain situations.

As a *spectator* the nurse seems to "look on" the situation with a minimum of interaction with others. However, in this activity she may act somewhat as a catalyst to bring about desired reactions in others without actually participating actively in the situation. Through her very presence in the hospital environment she may act as a stabilizing influence even though she is merely looking on. It is somewhat analogous to the situation in which the child feels safe playing in the back yard because he knows that his mother is in the house and will occasionally look out the window. In the hospital we have seen the night nurse acting as spectator when she sits in the doorway of a room because a patient feels apprehensive and has requested her support. In other situations the nurse as a spectator may keep out of the range of vision of her patients so that she may learn of their interaction when they are apparently unaware of her immediate presence. The nurse as a spectator may also be exemplified in many other circumstances. When the nurse cares for a patient during an insulin therapy coma she again acts as a spectator and a catalyst with a minimum of interaction with the patient during the coma phase. In this situation, the patient is unconscious and the nurse is assisting in bringing about the desired physiologic reactions. In other instances the nurse may observe the static environment as a spectator. She may notice that the room is too dark or too cold for the comfort of the patient, or she may check the ward resuscitator to assure herself of its effectiveness.

We have said that a minimum of immediate interaction occurs between the nurse and the patient in that the nurse is not participating with the patient at a given moment. This idea, however, does not imply that the nurse herself is not active. The primary intention of the nurse is directed toward acting as a catalyst to "set off" an interaction rather than to become a primary part of the interaction.

The terms catalyst and spectator also imply a factor of distance. We do not mean that the nurse is rigid or emotionally cold and, therefore, goes about without feelings of her own. Since the nurse is human we realize that she, too, has feelings and will express them in the spectator role, chiefly by her attitude. The distance factor merely means that the nurse is not *primarily engaged* in the interaction which she has "set off." The nurse may perform this activity not only in caring for patients but also in her relations with patients' relatives and her co-workers. The head nurse on a psychiatric unit is often seen to do this as she creates the nonspecific emotional atmosphere on the ward that is so essential as a medium for the therapeutic care of her patients.

As a *participant observer* the nurse is actively engaged in the inter-action with her patient or some other person. This can be seen when the nurse is participating in activities with a specific patient or group of patients. The nurse carries out such a function when she interacts with the patient during an interview or conversation or some nursing tech-nique that she is performing. Unlike the nurse as a spectator, the participant observer function is one in which the nurse shares more with the patient. While she is participating she is also observing. How the nurse participates will be further clarified in another chapter.

As an *introspectionist* the nurse observes herself. That is to say, she is able to recognize and understand her own reactions to others and her own reactions to herself. When you ask yourself, "Why does the patient in room 203 irritate me?" or "How was I instrumental in helping Mrs. J. to become less dependent upon me?" you are playing the role of the introspectionist. The skillful nurse frequently observes herself when she has elicited some behavior in a patient that she did not anticipate. Perhaps Mrs. B. answers the nurse's request to take some medicine in a very sarcastic manner. The nurse may then ask herself, "Was there something in my manner that brought about this reaction in Mrs. B.?" or "How do I feel about administering this type of medication?"

We can now see that the nurse may perform all three observational activities in a given set of circumstances but not at a given instant. For example, the nurse will undoubtedly interact with the electrotherapy patient in a participant manner before the patient eases into coma. During this period the nurse may momentarily observe herself. During the patient's coma phase the nurse may act as a spectator and may also do some reflective thinking in regard to self-observation. The skill that the nurse develops in observation will undoubtedly depend on her ability to observe and understand herself.

FACTORS THAT HINDER THE DEVELOPMENT OF SKILL IN OBSERVATION

There are many factors that are apt to function detrimentally in the nurse's attempt to refine her skills in observing behavior. The most obvious of these, of course, is a defect in the sense organs or other areas of the nervous system. It is a well-known fact, however, that some people who are unable to receive any visual stimuli have, in spite of this handicap, become very keen observers of human nature. Since it is doubtful that the nurse would be handicapped to this degree, she should at least have the potentials for developing skills in this area.

Another factor, not quite so obvious, is the erroneous idea that most of us have about our ability to observe. It is unusual to find a person who is either aware or will admit that he is not always alert or observant of what is going on about him. As a rule, it is difficult to develop any further skill or to acquire any greater understanding of a subject until we become aware of the level of skill or understanding already possessed. We first have to discover our weaknesses if we are to become skillful, and this discovery at the most may only deflate our ego temporarily.

We are also handicapped by the state of passivity that has probably enveloped each of us at some time or other. As we go about our daily activities, we tend to get into a rut to the degree that we take everything for granted. We seldom stop to think about the why or wherefore of anything and just drift placidly along in our ignorance, actually oblivious to three-fourths of what is going on about us. We need to wake up and again become an active and constructive part of our environment if we would be good observers.

A fourth important factor that will impede one's progress is limited knowledge and experience with the type of subject being observed. As was brought out previously, accuracy in perception requires at least familiarity with the particular kind of stimuli involved if they are going to have any meaning for us.

The last factor to be mentioned here, although there may be many more, is a lack of motivation to develop skills in observation. As we all know, there can be little actual learning in any subject unless there is a desire to learn. After fully overcoming the previously mentioned barriers, however, the individual usually does not encounter a problem in motivation but thoroughly enjoys his growing awareness and alertness to the world about him.

WHY THE NURSE OBSERVES PSYCHIATRIC PATIENTS

A rather close bond exists between human beings when they share their feelings and experiences with one another. Because the nurse spends considerable time with her patients, it is only natural that she share *certain* common experiences with them. It is for this reason that the nurse is often able to furnish valuable data that no other worker has the opportunity to discover. The nurse, therefore, can contribute much to the total care of the patient if she can communicate to others what she has observed in her relationships with the patient. To the psychiatrist her observations offer considerable data that may substantiate the diagnosis and the treatment plan. She is also helpful in furnishing other members of the psychiatric team with information that will enable them to carry out their roles in the care of the patient more effectively.

An extremely important reason for the nurse to observe the patient is that she may anticipate his behavior and thereby prevent the patient from injuring himself or others. Close observation helps the nurse to understand the patient better and, therefore, facilitates a better relationship with him. The nurse's observations also offer many implications for planning comprehensive nursing care and evaluating such care. In addition, the nurse gains considerable insight into her own behavior by self-observation. Such an understanding not only will improve her nursing care but will also help her to achieve maturity and to assume her functions as a nurse more readily.

RECORDING OBSERVATIONS

To record means to write down, to give a true account or description of a circumstance or incident. We can examine this concept more closely if we are aware of what constitutes good recording.

ATTRIBUTES OF GOOD RECORDING

The use of psychiatric terminology is discouraged in objective recording. The notes should be written in common, everyday descriptive language, since it is much more important to relate exactly what the patient did or what he said than to know only what was characteristic of his actions. The person reading the notes will then be able to interpret what has been recorded and decide for himself whether or not certain behavior trends are evident. Just as psychiatric terms have different meanings for many of us, we find that some ordinary English words may also portray somewhat different concepts to each of the persons reading the notes, although sometimes not to the same degree. A more accurate communication of observations is possible, therefore, with a minimum use of psychiatric terminology and an emphasis upon descriptive terms.

Personal opinion and interpretation are minimized in good recording. A report should exclude expressions of the writer's approval or disapproval of occurrences, persons or objects that he is describing. An objective report, then, keeps the amount of personal feeling portrayed to a minimum. Therefore, we have constantly to be on guard against the use of "loaded words." These words are those charged with the emotion of the writer, which may arouse negative feelings in the reader. One reporter might use the following expressions:

A bunch of fools who are suckers enough to fall for Senator Smith's ideas met last evening in that rickety firetrap that disfigures the south edge of town.[1]

We very readily recognize this reporter's feelings about this incident through the number of "loaded words" he includes. On the other hand, another reporter might give the following account of the same incident:

Between seventy-five and one hundred people were present last evening to hear an address by Senator Smith at the Evergreen Gardens near the south side of town.[1]

This report of the incident, in contrast to the other, depicts an objective record of the occurrence.

Another attribute of good recording is that the data are *recorded as soon as possible* after the incident has been observed. After we have observed a number of occurrences during the day we sometimes forget very important details or are unable to recall just exactly how or when they occurred. The nurse should arrange her work to enable her to record her observations at intervals throughout the day. Such an arrangement may also provide for better patient care, since all of the nurses will not be confined to the office at the end of the day to record their notes.

Therefore, when we record observations of behavioral data as descriptive details of the interaction that took place and include a minimum of personal interpretation and feeling, we will be apt to communicate a true account of what actually occurred.

Summary

We have attempted to formulate a concept of observation by emphasizing that it is a skill, an active process, and a method of collecting data for the purpose of discovering something unknown about the subject of study. In analyzing this process we find that it is a sequence of events which seem to occur automatically and simultaneously. The skill in observation is facilitated by a knowledge of the process involved,

---

[1]S. I. Hayakawa: "Reporting What We See and Hear." In Leslie L. Hanawalt and Emilie A. Newcomb, eds.: *Writing from Observation.* New York, Harcourt, Brace and Co., 1942, p. 439.

an understanding of the roles the nurse may play, and an awareness of the constituents of good observation as well as the factors that may impede progress in the development of this skill. For the effective communication of observation to others in the hospital setting, skill as a recorder should also be developed. Therefore, the attributes of good recording have also been discussed in the foregoing material.

Bibliography

Festinger, Leon, and Katz, Daniel: *Research Methods in the Behavioral Sciences.* New York, Holt, Rinehart and Winston, 1953.

Gee, Wilson: *Social Science Research Methods.* New York, Appleton-Century-Crofts, Inc., 1950.

Good, Carter C., and Scates, D. E.: *The Methods of Research.* New York, D. Appleton-Century Co., 1954.

Hanawalt, Leslie L., and Newcomb, Emilie A., eds.: *Writing from Observation.* New York, Harcourt, Brace and Co., 1942.

Hayakawa, S. I.: "Reporting What We See and Hear." In Hanawalt and Newcomb, *op. cit.*, p. 439.

Masserman, Jules H.: *Principles of Dynamic Psychiatry,* 2nd ed., Philadelphia, W. B. Saunders Co., 1961.

Reik, Theodor: *Listening with the Third Ear.* New York, Grove Press, Inc., 1956.

Selltiz, Claire, et al.: *Research Methods in Social Relations.* New York, Holt, Rinehart and Winston, 1962.

Sullivan, Harry Stack: *Conceptions of Modern Psychiatry.* New York, W. W. Norton & Co., 1953.

Van Dalen, Deobold, B., and Meyer, Wm. J.: *Understanding Educational Research.* New York, McGraw-Hill, Inc., 1962.

Suggestions for Further Reading

Becker, H. S., and Geer, B.: "Participant Observation: The Analysis of Qualitative Field Data." *In* Adams, R. N. and Preiss, J. J., eds.: *Human Organization Research.* Homewood, Ill., Dorsey Press, 1960, pp. 267-289.

Berthiaume, Aileen B.: "Observing Is More than Watching." *Nursing Outlook, 5:*290-293, May, 1957.

MacGregor, Frances Cooke: *Social Sciences in Nursing.* New York, Russell Sage Foundation, 1960, pp. 181-202.

Pearsall, Marion: "Participant Observation as Role and Method in Behavioral Research." *Nursing Research, 14:*37-42, Winter, 1965.

Weber, Marilyn: "The R.N. as Observer in Psychiatric Research." *Nursing World, 131:*7-8, June, 1957.

Chapter 7   Communication Skills

THE IMPORTANCE OF COMMUNICATION

It has been postulated that every individual has an inherent need to communicate. Communication with self and with others enables people to relate to one another, and this relationship, in turn, serves as a channel which provides for and enhances further communication. Communication involves sharing with another what is primarily one's own and implies a reciprocal action. We exchange views, express our inner thoughts and feelings, by both verbal and nonverbal means.

MISUNDERSTANDINGS

When we think of the many uses we make of words, it is not surprising that there are so many misunderstandings. The meaning of a word depends upon the experiences and the motives of the person who uses it. Every individual has a personal collection of associations related to the circumstances wherein this word and its meaning were added to his collection. Another factor is that the meanings of words change for each of us as we continue to grow. This is the reason we seem to gain new meanings that increase our understanding each time we reread something.

We use words in our attempts to communicate; we also use words in our attempts to not communicate. We use words to control others, to strike out, to express love, to express hostility, to hide behind, to create confusion and just for the enjoyment of the motor activity involved. We talk ourselves into and out of things and situations. In our attempts to bridge interhuman space, we use words. In many respects we have collected these words without ever understanding the reality to which they refer.

Man has always tended to hide everything he could not understand behind a name or a word of some kind. For without a name, this "something" or whatever it is arouses fear—our old fear of the unknown! Look at the way we react when we have a "pain." We want this pain to have a name, a diagnosis; then we usually feel better, regardless of what it is.

More and more we function under the delusion that naming something is synonymous with understanding it. This has become our magic formula: I know it; I give it a name; therefore I have mastered it. So whoever knows the name has power, or so he feels! Through words and names, many things have become more obscure rather than more clear.

DISCUSSION

It has been said that the road to genuine understanding is by way of becoming clear about one's confusion instead of concealing it or having it covered up by verbal symbols. If we function under the assumption that everyone means the same thing when he uses certain words, we find that very little communication takes place. This assumption is probably why the discussion method has so often fallen into ill repute. We enter a discussion to clarify a problem or situation, and after a couple of hours we often find that not only have we not found a solution to the problem but that the issues are more cloudy than when we began. Undoubtedly a great many words were exchanged and probably a great many feelings (See *Interaction*, Chapter 8), but it is very clear that the lines of communication were not open.

It may have been an instance of "Your feelings are so loud, I can't hear a thing you're saying." In the verbal expression of everyday life, the deeper levels of communication are too often ignored. We often express just the opposite of what we feel; we swallow our deeper feelings and try to forget them—even though they may frequently give us indigestion.

Discussion is a process wherein we critically examine our own ideas, opinions, feelings and attitudes about something, as well as the ideas and insights of others. By sharing in the experience of others, communication takes place. It is only through deep and genuine discussion that vague ideas condense into clear thoughts. We often hear people say that they are hesitant to express themselves, to say what they believe and to act accordingly, for fear that they will offend others. This, of course, is a false belief because if one's motives are positive such action can only encourage others to do the same, making it possible for authentic communication to ensue. It is when we pretend to have convictions and sound off with a lot of glib generalities, which inevitably evaporate on closer scrutiny, that people are offended and rightfully so.

ACKNOWLEDGING COMMUNICATIONS

That which is communicated may be thought of as signals that evoke a certain response in the recipient, and their communication may be intentional or unintentional. What was formerly thought to be a criterion for successful communication is no longer considered applicable to the communication between people. According to Ruesch,[1] we can better determine the success of a communicative act in relation to the reduction of tension experienced by the sender. This reduction of tension is believed to be closely related to the kind of acknowledgment and the degree of understanding that the recipient of the signals gives the sender. We have all been in situations wherein we experienced pleasure from the release of tension following a successful communication, as contrasted with the persistent and increased tension we have experienced when our attempts to communicate have failed.

When a person says something, his anticipations may vary from expecting that he will be either understood or misunderstood or that his message will be distorted; consequently, with this orientation he directs his attention toward the recipient's response. Acknowledgment, as seen by Ruesch, is a response which shows that the recipient of a message accepts the content. So, in person-to-person contacts, we see people trying to secure acknowledgment of their communications.

Ruesch elaborates upon four possible forms of acknowledgment that have been identified in the process of communication. The first form involves understanding and requires a benevolent attitude on the part of the recipient, who responds in such a way that the sender knows that his message has been received and really understood and, as a consequence, experiences a sense of well-being. In the second form of acknowledgment, the recipient responds in such way that the

---

[1]Jurgen Ruesch: *Disturbed Communication.* New York, W. W. Norton & Co., Inc., 1957, pp. 34-55.

sender knows that his message has been received but that it has not been understood, although the recipient communicates an attitude of readiness to listen further, of wanting to understand. In this interaction, when the sender gets the signal that this person wants to listen and will try to understand his communications, he experiences satisfaction almost to the same degree that he would have had his message been understood. A third form of response involves mutual agreement, wherein the recipient of the message discovers and signals to the sender that he is in complete accord with the content, that he sees it the same way. Both the sender and the recipient experience pleasure from reaching an agreement, although this is thought to be different from the pleasure experienced in being understood. The fourth possible response involves mutual disagreement, wherein acknowledgment may be varied. First of all, the recipient may not give any acknowledgment that the message had been received and may get up and leave. On the other hand, he may respond with hostility or decide that an agreement cannot be reached, and the communication process disintegrates in the ensuing battle. Phases of understanding, lack of understanding, agreement and disagreement are believed to occur in the process of any healthy, potentially successful communication, but when disagreement and misunderstanding become the end goals, the process becomes pathologic.

There are many devious ways of acknowledging a person's statement that not only will prove quite stressful but will also distort the message that is being sent. One very common experience is trying to communicate with someone who, in his eagerness to give acknowledgment, always tries to complete your statements before you can even get them verbalized. One cannot have a pleasurable, successful communication with a person who responds in this manner. Another quite different response, which is probably more destructive, is the tangential one. In making a tangential response, we ignore the intention of the sender and reply to some incidental aspect of the situation. In this kind of response the content of the message is totally disregarded and a new message is initiated.

Since everyone wants to be understood, we realize how very important our responses are to the communications of others. It will be helpful to study our own patterns of communication and become alert to the kinds of acknowledgment we give and the reaction of others to these responses. This achievement gives us a sound basis for learning to communicate meaningfully with people.

In our interaction and communication with others, people seek for consistency in feelings, verbal expression and action, and if it is not manifest in our interpersonal situations, confusion usually results. The quality of our interaction with others has a direct influence on the

effectiveness of our communication. We tend to integrate situations —
that is, initiate and carry through — according to our basic orientation
toward life and toward the world in general: "loving" people who have
a positive outlook on life, who feel secure in their identity and who
have progressed to the level of interdependent relations tend to integrate situations that are warm, friendly and conducive to continuing
interaction and communication, whereas "hateful" or "malevolent"
people who have a negative outlook on life, who are not quite sure who
they are, who are hindered by infantile dependency strings or who are
still fighting for their independence tend to integrate situations which
are cold or alternately "hot," "cold," and "sticky" and conducive to
disjunctive interaction and a lack of communication.

FORMS OF COMMUNICATION

For practical purposes, communication will be divided into the
verbal and nonverbal aspects, although we seldom have one without
the other.

VERBAL COMMUNICATION

By verbal communication, either written or oral, we mean that
which involves the use of words for the purpose of conveying and
clarifying one's ideas, thoughts or feelings to others. Unless the person
or persons to whom we are trying to impart the context comprehends
the communication, the process is incomplete. For example, the head
nurse told the staff to be permissive with a particular patient but to
watch him closely. Thinking that the staff understood her directions,
the head nurse was surprised to learn that someone had allowed the
patient to go home to visit his mother when he had asked for permis-
sion. When she inquired about the incident, the response was, "Well,
you said to be permissive." It was then obvious that the communication
had not been successful.

Another important aspect of verbal communication is that which is
written. The following is an example of an observation that was recorded in order to communicate information to the physician:

Mr. M. came into the sunroom fully dressed in sport clothes. He stood for
a minute in the center of the room with a pained expression on his face . . .
eyebrows drawn together and the corners of his mouth turned down,
lips parted and breathing through them so that his respiration was audible to
those in the room. He was rubbing his back with his left hand and holding a
lighted cigarette in his right hand. Talked very loudly, "Oh, my back, oh, my
back!"

He stopped moaning long enough to say "Hello" to a student nurse who came into the room and said, "Good morning, Mr. M."

He sat down in a straight-back chair, still rubbing his back with his left hand, then looked about the room. He got up, all the time rubbing his back . . . "I've never hurt so much before!"

He walked as if in pain, crouched down, and took two or three steps to a leather chair. He sat down carefully and slowly in a slouching position, clinging to the arms of the chair and supporting his weight with both hands.

"Oh, it's terrible!"

"Oh, is it that terrible, Mr. M.?" said a student nurse as she smiled at him. He looked at her and did not reply. He then sat up straighter so that his entire back rested against the chair. Exhaling heavily, he bent over slightly and rubbed his back again.

"They must have done something to it on my first treatment . . . it didn't hurt before I had them. The doc said something about another x-ray of it." He pulled a pack of cigarettes out of his pocket, put one in his mouth and lit it. Then he crossed his knees and sat looking straight ahead, puffing so heavily on the cigarette that sparks flew from it.

By referring to the criteria for "good" recording near the end of Chapter 6, it can readily be seen that the sample just given meets the criteria, and an accurate description of this patient's activity at a given time is available for communication to the physician. Often we find that written communication requires further elaboration orally, and the physician may desire to discuss it with the persons concerned in order to clarify the incident.

NONVERBAL COMMUNICATION

Nonverbal communication includes the attitudes, feelings and thoughts that we convey either intentionally or unintentionally through such media as our posture, gestures, facial expression, vocal tone and inflections.

This type of communication is probably one of the most powerful tools available when used under the conscious direction of the individual. In this instance, the term powerful means the degree of influence inherent in the process. In any situation where two or more persons interact, this nonverbal communication is inevitable. It may, therefore, be readily seen that a negative influence may result just as easily as a positive one. For example: Miss K., a professional nurse with very definite standards in regard to the indiscriminate use of alcoholic beverages, found that she was to care for Mr. S., a chronic alcoholic admitted the previous evening. Miss K. considered herself a liberal, nonprejudiced individual and was not conscious of her true feelings in this respect. She assisted Mr. S. with his routine morning care as she thought she would care for any other patient. However, after breakfast Mr. S. asked, to her surprise, "Why do you dislike me so? Have I offended you in any way?" Although she tried to reassure him that she liked him, his first impression prevailed.

In this instance, the nurse's disapproval of the patient's behavior was communicated to him without her being aware of it. As is illustrated here, it is very difficult to mask one's true feelings about a given idea or action, and it is practically impossible when the individual is not conscious of them himself. Since it is a natural tendency for people to disapprove of the behavior of others that is contrary to their own personal standards, the approval or disapproval of the actions of others is one of the easiest to communicate. The nurse should constantly be alert to this fact.

Usually we find that the proximity of the two persons involved enhances the readiness of the communication, as brought out in the example. Mr. S. might not have become aware of the nurse's feeling about him so early in his hospitalization if he had not had direct contact with her. On the other hand, it is also believed that the more intense the feeling, the less direct the contact need be for communication to take place.

As has been implied by the inevitability of this type of communication, it is such a natural process that we often ignore it or are not even aware that it has taken place. We may find that patients do not always respond so directly as Mr. S. did to the communication of feelings. Nevertheless, we know that they are aware of the atmosphere that is created, whether it be pleasant or unpleasant, accepting or critical.

In interpersonal situations, feelings and gestures seem to have a mandatory function. They not only direct the other person's behavior but they also prolong and sustain certain reactions and disrupt others. That which we communicate to others on this nonverbal level is an extension of our attitudes, and it is this communication that has so much influence in evoking response in others. This feeling tone that we communicate to others and they communicate to us is an important factor in appraising the friendliness of people. It may be one of friendliness and warmth, one of coldness and hostility, one of primarily increased tension, or one of "nothingness," depending upon the amount or degree of protective covering the person wears. Have you ever had the experience of interacting with someone from whom you received no feeling tone? These experiences are puzzling because we lack the data that give meaning to what is going on. It is like a song without a musical score, that becomes something entirely different when we add the music.

Another clue in appraising the friendliness of people is the physical distance that they maintain between themselves and others. We desire intimate contact with people with whom we are familiar and comfortable, so we bridge the distance between us and come close to these persons. On the other hand, we desire to keep people with whom we feel strange and uncomfortable at a distance, so we stay away from them and keep them as remote as possible.

Verbal and nonverbal communication usually occur at the same time, and it is often difficult to separate them when observing an actual situation. It may be helpful now to consider some of the communication tools in more detail.

TOOLS OF COMMUNICATION

ADVICE

The giving of advice is fairly simple and popular, but it is not very effective as a therapeutic tool. Advice presupposes that one individual is not capable of directing his own activity—therefore, the two individuals are on different planes. The person giving advice selects the goals and directs the other person toward these goals. Advice, if accepted and acted upon, fosters dependence. The person who seeks advice seldom really desires it, and it may serve as a springboard for projecting the blame for failure in the future. Advice may be helpful in alleviating acute anxiety, but even here it is purely supportive and the relief is only temporary. The nurse, therefore, will rarely encounter a situation in which this method is indicated.

PERSUASION

Persuasion is seldom advocated for the nurse. It is more direct than suggestion and more coercive. It also has a pleading or argumentative quality which usually is not conducive to effective nurse-patient relationships.

RECORDING

Recording is another very important communication skill in nursing. For a detailed discussion of recording, see page 85.

APPROACH

Usually, when we think of approach, we think of coming nearer to something or of reducing the spatial distance between two objects, but in nursing the term often refers to the planning or thinking that is done prior to any action that is taken. The topic will be considered only in general terms here and will be discussed in more detail in Part III.

Let us briefly consider the two types of approach, the verbal and the physical. The *verbal approach* is the most common and occurs whenever the nurse makes contact with the patient by use of the spoken word, such as when she greets her patients or when she explains what is to be done before a plan of treatment is administered. Seldom do we find an instance where the verbal approach is not indicated, and, even though a patient seems to be unaware of what is going on, he will often respond if the nurse takes the initiative through the verbal approach.

One of the most important aspects of the verbal approach to patients is the nonverbal communication that inevitably accompanies it. The tone of the nurse's voice, her inflection and her general manner as she makes this contact influence the patient's response to her.

The *physical approach* is any direct contact the nurse makes with the patient by means of touch. It is sometimes used as an emergency measure. For example, if the nurse suddenly comes upon a patient who is harming himself or others, it may be necessary to make a physical approach; but the need for such approaches can be minimized if close observation is maintained.

Should an instance arise in which it is necessary to control the patient's activity by physical means, a verbal approach used simultaneously usually makes the contact more effective. If the nurse makes no attempt to communicate her intentions to the patient, he is apt to misinterpret the nurse's action and require more stringent methods of control.

While there are some patients who respond better to a purely verbal approach, there are other patients whose response is enhanced by a simultaneous tactual stimulation. For example, certain elderly patients feel much more secure if the nurse takes their arm or hand as she speaks to them, particularly if she wishes them to rise from a sitting position. There are other patients who may respond better to the combined method of approach, but this will be dealt with in more detail as we discuss the care of patients with specific problems.

FACTORS TO CONSIDER IN DETERMINING THE PLAN OF APPROACH. The first factor to consider is the nurse herself. The nurse should examine her own attitude toward the patient and determine whether it is positive or negative—that is, is she attracted toward the patient or is her first impulse one of avoidance? A positive attitude is essential for creating an atmosphere of acceptance. While it may not be possible to have a positive attitude toward all patients, a knowledge of her attitude will aid the nurse in determining the plan of approach.

Closely related to this attitude of acceptance is the factor of tolerance. By tolerance we do not mean that the nurse should merely tolerate the patient's behavior, nor should she necessarily approve it. Tolerance implies a noncritical, noncondemnatory attitude on the part of the nurse, regardless of the patient's overt behavior.

Another factor which the nurse will consider is her interest in the patient. Is she caring for the patient merely because he is assigned to her, or does she have a genuine interest in helping him to regain his health?

The next factor to be considered is the patient. An approach based upon an understanding of the patient and his problems is most apt to bring the desired results. The nurse should be able to anticipate the patient's reaction fairly accurately if she has this understanding. One important question for the nurse to consider is how is the patient apt to interpret the situation? Will the patient interpret her actions as helpful, or will he feel threatened? Then, what level of approach will be necessary to communicate her intentions to the patient? Is he one who readily comprehends the spoken word, or will it be necessary to reinforce the spoken word with a tactual approach?

The nurse then determines her purpose in approaching a particular patient. In considering the purpose we usually think in terms of both the immediate and long-term goals for the patient. Whereas the immediate goal for approaching the patient may be to help the patient to dress, a long-term goal may be to help the patient to become more independent and capable of making his own decisions. Therefore, both the immediate and long-term goals have to be considered within the framework of the over-all plan for therapy.

IMPORTANCE OF APPROACH.   Approach has always been given an important place in psychiatric nursing, probably because the first impressions gained by the patient influence his immediate and over-all adjustment to the hospital situation. Just as the first approach made to the patient as he enters the hospital is often important in influencing his reactions throughout his hospitalization, so may the first approach to a patient on a given morning set the pace for his reactions throughout the day.

Planning the approach usually fosters more consistency in providing therapeutic care for patients. In many situations where the staff is team oriented, the physician prescribes the approach or attitude that is to direct the personnel in the care of a given patient. For example, the physician may indicate that the staff should be actively friendly toward a certain patient. On the other hand, a matter-of-fact approach may be more appropriate. These more specific prescriptions of attitudes have been thought to be very helpful in aiding the staff to be more consistent in their contacts with patients. However, it is essential that there be a clarification of terminology to ensure a minimum of discrepancy in the meaning of the terms to everyone concerned. Assuming roles and acting "as if" we were a certain person or were feeling a certain way is not considered very effective in promoting growth except in very structured situations, such as in psychodrama or in role playing. But even in these situations, one has to really experience the role to achieve any insight or understanding.

SUGGESTION

Suggestion as a tool of communication includes both encouragement and reassurance and, if used effectively, can be a powerful tool in helping the patient to change his behavior. First, the nurse utilizes this method by being an example of an effective biosocial person. As we know, a demonstration is helpful whether we are learning new skills or refining old ones. It is sometimes helpful to encourage the patient and to comment on any progress, no matter how small: for example, "You're feeling better," or, "You're improving." We do this in the hope that it will strengthen the patient's motivation in that direction. Suggestion is also helpful in getting patients to participate in, or to refrain from, ward routines and certain activities. For example, a patient may wish to clean out her closet at 5 P.M. The nurse might say, "Why not wait until after dinner when you'll have more time?"

Suggestion should always be positive; the nurse's selection of words is most important. For example, it would be more appropriate to say, "How about playing shuffleboard?" rather than, "You wouldn't like to play shuffleboard, would you?"

Another important way in which a nurse uses suggestion is through her nonverbal activity. This is especially true with certain patients who seek constant reassurance and who are apprehensive. How the nurse acts and the attitudes she communicates with this type of patient will be far more effective than any verbal communication she may attempt. By these nonverbal cues, the nurse can give the patient the reassurance that he is not being "laughed at" or criticized. Another way in which the nurse may provide reassurance for the patient is by her neutral response when the patient says or does something that frightens or embarrasses him. In most instances, situations that are labeled "reassuring the patient" are in reality situations "reassuring the nurse." True assurance comes from within and the nurse may facilitate this by helping the patient gain a new perspective on a problem or by helping him learn new ways of coping. The use of suggestion is further illustrated in the social milieu or therapeutic environment which is created in the hospital. Discussion of this aspect is found in Chapter 21.

LISTENING

It has been said that listening to someone is the most precious gift we can bestow. Listening is another skill involved in communication, and the role of the nurse as a listener cannot be overemphasized. Developing skill as a listener is one of the most difficult tasks confronting a nurse in psychiatry. This difficulty evolves primarily from two factors, nursing tradition and the nurse herself. The student nurse is usually taught that the "good' nurse keeps busy doing things for people. The emphasis has long been upon the use of material objects and procedures that require a manipulation of these objects. In the role of a listener, the nurse is, to all appearances, passive and very definitely lacks material objects to manipulate. The nurse herself often feels that she is not doing anything constructive and is wasting time. Consequently, she is apt to feel guilty because of her previous orientation. Therefore, prior to developing any degree of skill as a listener, the nurse must become aware of her own feelings when she is placed in this role. If such situations are anxiety provoking, she must develop some means of handling her anxiety other than through manipulating material objects.

In the role of a listener the nurse simultaneously plays another role—that of the participant observer—which clearly defines how active her function really is. The nurse's role as a listener may be planned or it may be incidental. Since the nurse does not always know what role the patient will ascribe to her, she should be very flexible. Not only is the listening role very time consuming but it requires great patience on the part of the nurse, since we tend to feel ill at ease when periods of silence occur in our contact with others. Our first impulse is to fill in these gaps by a comment or a question, but we can function best by learning to wait and, as is often said, to show respect for periods of silence. It may be that the patient is reluctant to go on, or it may be that he does not know just how to express what he wants to say. If his train of thought is interrupted, the opportunity may not again arise for him to express this particular thought. As long as the patient feels pretty much at ease, it is often most helpful if the nurse refrains from comments. On the other hand, if the patient is obviously becoming more tense and shows signs of embarrassment, a pertinent remark or question by the nurse may enable him to continue talking.

The role of the nurse as a listener is inevitably tied up with the use of conversation as a means of communication. Therefore, the listening role is further elaborated as we discuss the nurse's use of this method. It is a well-established fact that the more immediate the opportunity for discussing a disturbing experience, the more effective is the relief provided through talking about it. Whether or not patients will be encouraged to talk will depend upon the directions given by the individual therapist. Only if the nurse is aware of the plan of therapy and how far the patient has progressed in his therapy will she be able to function as a positive factor in cooperating with the physician and others concerned with the patient's welfare.

In summary, we might say that a good listener is interested in what is being said and shows this interest through his posture and attention and other nonverbal cues rather than frequently interrupting to tell what he might have done in a similar circumstance. Since a complete absence of response may be interpreted as a lack of interest, the nurse may make brief relevant remarks to indicate that she knows what has been said. As the nurse becomes more sensitive to the feelings of others, she will be able to determine more readily when to remain silent and when to comment. A good listener is one who concentrates on what is being said and the feeling that is being communicated rather than on what he is going to say when the opportunity arises.

CONVERSING WITH PATIENTS

Although conversation is usually considered a game of social contact in which there is a mutual exchange of ideas, the nurse utilizes identical skills in working therapeutically with patients. In addition, the experienced nurse in cooperation with other team members uses both interviewing and psychotherapeutic techniques to carry out her role as a positive agent in the hospital environment. Since there is reciprocal action, it is implied that the nurse talks "with" rather than "to" patients. Conversation is considered a little more than just talk. It is more sustained, has more continuity, and there is supposedly some connection between the verbalizations of those participating. When we have a conversation with "genuine" participation by those involved, we are verging on communication, which requires a sharing of experiences related to the topic at hand.

SPONTANEOUS CONVERSATION. In spontaneous conversation, the aim may be varied. The nurse may be attempting to get acquainted with the patient or the patient with the nurse. It may offer a brief interlude of social interaction for the patient and help him to feel more a part of the situation. An opportunity for the patient to practice various social skills may be provided by incidental conversation. Much can also be accomplished through alleviating some of the inevitable monotony experienced in the usual hospital situation by occasionally stopping in to "pass the time of day." In certain instances it may be beneficial merely to divert the patient's attention from his current thoughts or problems by keeping him engaged in conversation. For example, a patient who is undergoing intensive individual psychotherapy may suddenly begin to talk of his intense dislike for his wife. The nurse, knowing that this was one of his basic problems unacceptable to him previously, may wish to divert his attention and save his communication for his conference with his doctor later in the day. However, she should be reasonably sure she is only postponing the communication and not stifling it completely.

The same rules for any social discourse apply in talking with patients. The essence of these rules is that one is courteous and offers ample opportunities for the patient to participate.

Helpful hints. During their initial experience, some nurses find it easier to converse with an individual patient, whereas others find it easier to converse with a group of patients. The nurse usually becomes aware of the phenomena when she analyzes her feelings in both situations. She can usually become more skillful if she begins where she feels most at ease and then gradually broadens her contacts to include both the group and the individual.

In initiating conversation with both groups and individuals, the nurse may find it helpful just to start talking about some commonplace topic that is not apt to provoke intense feelings, either negative or positive. A few of the topics that may be suitable in initiating such a conversation would be the weather, food, an event that is to take place in the near future, comments on something that is observable from the window and so forth. To become a good conversationalist requires both effort and practice just as in acquiring any other skill. It is sometimes helpful to catalog intentionally in your memory small bits of information as you browse through the newspapers or books so that you can relate them to patients if the occasion arises. The main difference between diversional conversation with patients and conversation with friends is that one does not relate details of one's personal life to patients.

THERAPEUTIC CONVERSATION. There are of necessity certain requirements in a situation if the use of this method is going to be plausible. First, the persons involved should be in relatively close proximity. Second, an approach is necessary to initiate the discourse. This may be on the part of either the nurse or the patient. Third, there must be a common means of exchange—that is, both persons must speak and understand the language or other symbols used. Fourth, there should be a feeling of freedom or trust on the part of both persons. "Real" communication requires an intimacy with the person with whom one is trying to converse.

The nurse carries on spontaneous conversation with all patients, but those she converses with therapeutically are a select group. In order to function in this manner, the nurse must be fairly sensitive to the feeling tones in the situation and she must be fairly valid in her interpretation of what occurs. In contrast to the speaking acquaintance which the nurse has with all patients, her relationship with these select patients is on a different level. For characteristics of the various types of relationships, see Chapter 8.

This type of relationship presupposes that the nurse has an understanding of the patient and his problem and also assumes that she has a basic understanding of the dynamics of human behavior. All nurses may not be able to use conversation as a therapeutic tool without special preparation and additional experience. When the nurse does function in this manner, she may do so in cooperation with the physician and other members of the team. On the other hand, she may find that she is the only other person in the situation and that she provides the kinds of interaction and communication experiences that are helpful to patients.

Although the conversation may be initiated by the nurse, the course of the conversation is dictated by the patient. In one respect the nurse serves as a sounding board for his thoughts, ideas and feelings. The nurse avoids the use of direct and leading questions, and it may be helpful to use statements in the beginning that cannot be answered by "yes" or "no." The verbal activity of the nurse is at a minimum, with the patient doing most of the talking. The nurse encourages the patient to talk by her nonverbal activity, such as nodding or various other gestures. If verbal activity becomes necessary, sometimes just a word such as "well" or "really" will enable the patient to continue. Another method of encouraging patients to continue talking is to repeat their last thought or word expressed. Of course, one must be fairly certain of how the patient really does feel. The patient can usually be encouraged to elaborate or clarify by using such phrases as "Can you give me an example of that?"

In this type of conversation the nurse's attention is primarily on the feelings that are being expressed or the latent meaning of the patient's expression rather than on the verbalized content as such.

Summary

When we communicate we share ideas in a reciprocal relationship. For the purposes of clarity, communication is discussed as verbal and nonverbal. By verbal communication, either written or oral, we mean that which involves the use of words for the purpose of conveying and clarifying one's ideas, thoughts and feelings to others. Verbal communication takes place only if it is comprehended by those for whom it is intended. Nonverbal communication, on the other hand, refers to the attitudes and feelings that we convey to others either intentionally or unintentionally through such media as our posture, facial expression and voices.

Methods of communication have been discussed in more detail. The nurse utilizes these tools as she works with patients. The types of approach, the physical and verbal, and the importance of each have been discussed, as well as the factors which the nurse considers in determining her plan of approach. Other communicative tools frequently employed by the nurse have been examined and special emphasis given to therapeutic conversation as it may be utilized in nursing situations.

Bibliography

Axline, Virginia: *Play Therapy.* Boston, Houghton Mifflin Co., 1947.

Bird, Brian: *Talking with Patients.* Philadelphia, J. B. Lippincott Co., 1955.

Brown, Roger: *Words and Things.* Chicago, Free Press of Glencoe, 1958.

Fromm, Erich: *Man for Himself.* New York, Rinehart & Co., 1947.

Fromm-Reichmann, Frieda: *Principles of Intensive Psychotherapy.* Chicago, University of Chicago Press, 1950.

Hayakawa, S. I.: *Language in Thought and Action,* 2nd Ed., New York, Harcourt, Brace and Co., 1964.

Hoch, Paul H., and Zubin, Joseph, eds.: *Psychopathology of Communication.* New York, Grune & Stratton, Inc., 1958.

Lewin, Kurt: *Dynamic Theory of Personality.* New York, McGraw-Hill Book Co., Inc., 1935.

Meerloo, Joost, A. M.: *Conversation and Communication,* revised Ed., New York, International al Universities Press, Inc., 1958.

Reik, Theodor: *Listening with the Third Ear.* New York, Grove Press Inc., 1956.

Ruesch, Jurgen: *Disturbed Communication.* New York, W. W. Norton & Co., Inc., 1957.

Ruesch, Jurgen, and Bateson, Gregory: *Communication—The Social Matrix of Psychiatry.* New York, W. W. Norton & Co., Inc., 1951.

Sullivan, Harry Stack: *Conceptions of Modern Psychiatry.* New York, W. W. Norton & Co., Inc., 1953.

Suggestions for Further Reading

Becker, Ruth Sulzmann: "Interpersonal Relations—in the Basic Program." *Am. J. Nursing,* 55:952-955, 1955.

Bird, Brian: "Psychological Aspects of Preoperative and Postoperative Care." *Am. J. Nursing,* 55:685-687, 1955.

Bojar, Samuel: "The Psychotherapeutic Function of the General Hospital Nurse." *Nursing Outlook,* 6:151-153, 1958.

Davidson, Henry A.: "Nonverbal Communication in a Hospital Setting." *Perspectives in Psychiatric Care,* 1:12-17, 1963.

Davis, Anne J.: "The Skills of Communication." *Am. J. Nursing,* 63:66-70, 1963.

Doan, Edith H.: "Making Communications Effective." *Nursing Outlook,* 2:420-422, 1954.

"Dr. Whatsisname": "Can Nurses Work with Individuals?" *Ment. Hosp.* 11:13, 1960.

Fernandez, Theresa M.: "How to Deal with Overt Aggression." *Am. J. Nursing,* 59:658-660, 1959.

Flynn, Gertrude E.: "The Nurse's Role: Interference or Intervention." *Perspectives in Psychiatric Care,* 7:170-176, 1969.

Fries, Olive H., and McLellan, Mary Lou: "Helping Patients Get Well." *Nursing Outlook*, 7:654-655, 1959.

Gregory, Elizabeth M.: "How to Help a Patient During an Emotional Crisis." *Nursing World*, 132:8-11, 1958.

Hart, Betty L., and Rohweder, Anne W.: "Support in Nursing." *Am. J. Nursing*, 59:1398-1401, 1959.

Hayter, Jean: "Reassure the Patient." *Nursing World*, 134:21-32, 1960.

Hewitt, Helen E., and Pesznecker, Betty L.: "Blocks to Communicating with Patients." *Am. J. Nursing*, 64:101-103, 1964.

Hibarger, Victoria E., Blanchard, William H., and Glogow, Eli: "Nurses Use the Group Process." *Am. J. Nursing*, 55:334-336, 1955.

Jackson, Joan K.: "Communication Is Important." *Am. J. Nursing*, 59:90-93, 1959.

Knowles, Lois N.: "How Can We Reassure Patients?" *Am. J. Nursing*, 59:834-835, 1959.

Marshall, Margaret A.: "Hopelessness." *Nursing World*, 133:30-31, 1959.

Merrill, Doris P.: "Self Knowledge: Aid to Better Nursing." *Nursing World*, 133:22-24, 1959.

Newman, Margaret A.: "Identifying and Meeting Needs in Short-Span Nurse-Patient Relationships." *Nursing Forum*, 5:76-86, 1966.

Norris, Catherine M.: "The Nurse and the Crying Patient." *Am. J. Nursing*, 57:323-327, 1957.

Pendall, Rudolph J.: "Speaking with People." *Nursing Outlook*, 2:96-97, 1954.

Peplau, Hildegarde E.: "Talking with Patients." *Am. J. Nursing*, 60:964-966, 1960.

Peto, Marjorie: "Communicating with Little Children." *Am. J. Nursing*, 57:602-603, 1957.

Robinson, Alice M.: "Communicating with Our Patients." *Nursing World*, 132:6-9, 1958.

Rohweder, Anne W., and Hart, Betty L.: "How Attitudes Are Taught and Caught." *Am. J. Nursing*, 60:806-809, 1960.

Schwartz, Doris: "Uncooperative Patients." *"Am. J. Nursing*, 58:75-77, 1958.

Speroff, B. J.: "Empathy Is Important in Nursing." *Nursing Outlook*, 4:326-327, 1956.

Stoneberg, Carla Johnson: "Communication through Art on a Psychiatric Ward." *Perspectives in Psychiatric Care*, 2:12-22, 1964.

Van Kaam, Adrian L.: "The Nurse in the Patient's World." *Am. J. Nursing*, 59:1708-1710, 1959.

Webb, Carolyn: "Communicating in Pediatrics." *Am. J. Nursing*, 60:194-195, 1960.

Chapter 8 Nurse-Patient Interaction

Interaction and communication are two of the most important aspects of human relations. As with other low-visibility functions in nursing, as well as in living, it is quality rather than quantity that is so important.

In this period of civilization, which has been labeled the "Age of Anxiety," we find more and more people running around like caged squirrels, hunting for something, plunging into activities, but always coming out feeling that something is missing. Now more than ever before, we hear people who are always in the midst of other people speak of being lonely. This feeling of loneliness and emptiness, then, can be added to the increasing list of unfulfilled "insatiable longings" (see Chapter 19). This experience, described by so many, is similar to anxiety in that we do not have anxiety, we are anxious—it strikes at the very core of our being.

Poets have described this experience of anxiety as "the fear of freedom." It seems paradoxic that we should have great fear of something that not one of us would hesitate to say is one of our inherent rights. We often delude ourselves with the words "we are free," "we believe in freedom," "we will fight for freedom." Yet when the pressures rise, we run from our responsibility, we refuse to take a stand, we become mired in a state of indecision. Last but not least, in our scurry to find a haven, we run from ourselves. Until we can be frank with ourselves, we cannot expect or even hope to have genuine interaction with another person.

How many times have we been told or have we told others: "We must be genuine." "We must have sincere interest in our patients." "We must respect them as individuals." "We must establish good interpersonal relations." "We must become skillful in therapeutic use of self." Many of these terms have become clichés that are hollow and empty, and we tend to use them to disguise both our ignorance and misunderstanding.

DEFINITION OF TERMS

According to Webster, *interact* means "to act upon each other," while interaction is defined as "mutual or reciprocal action or influence." The term *responsible* means "being liable to respond, to give a response," whereas *responsibility* refers to "the quality of being responsible." The word *genuine* means "proceeding from a reputed source, authentic, real in contrast to being false or artificial."

What do the meanings of all these words tell us? Intellectually, at least, we know that people want to interact with a "real" person—not a "cold" or "indifferent" person but someone who will respond. Life is not a state, it is a movement in the spiral of living. Nowhere in nature is life fixed; it is more a vibration-like succession of waves. Similarly, real personal contact or interaction is not a state but a momentary condition that must be continuously rediscovered.

As Meerloo sees it, people behave like armored cars, pushing each other around. They are sometimes both deaf and mute when others try to interact with them; they are afraid to get involved. We can, by offering material rewards or punishments, train people to behave in more socially acceptable ways. At least, we say, they are able to function again and it is not as time-consuming. However, it is believed that people change and become persons only through "real" interaction with other "real" persons. It is through this kind of interaction that we find out who we are, how we are, and what we truly believe; otherwise, we become more like robots who function "as if" they are really living, or we join the ranks of armored cars to push each other around.[1]

THE INTERPERSONAL ENVIRONMENT

In Chapter 2, Behavior, we mentioned that man requires various environments with specific qualities if he is to survive; also that he has

---

[1]Joost A. M. Meerloo: *Conversation and Communication.* New York, International University Press, Inc., 1952, p. 191.

to maintain contact with these environments and through his total behavior carry on an adequate interchange with them. Since one of the necessary environments peculiar to man is the interpersonal environment, the process of interacting with other people becomes a characteristic pattern of human behavior early in life. These patterns of interaction from infancy and childhood become the pattern of interpersonal relationships that characterize the living of each individual.

Throughout the life span of man we see him learning different patterns of interaction and different ways of relating to various environments. The infant establishes and maintains contact with his environment through the process of empathy. Just as he gobbles up his formula and anything else that comes within reach of his mouth, he literally gobbles up the tensions, the feelings and the pervading atmosphere in his immediate surroundings. If he has a warm, calm, comfortable environment, we anticipate that he will feel warm, calm and comfortable. On the other hand, if his environment is cold, tense and painful, we anticipate that he will feel cold, tense and painful.

As the infant grows, his way of relating to his environment begins to change, and he not only continues to absorb what is in his environment but also begins to imitate those persons with whom he interacts most. This change in his pattern of interaction strengthens his relationship with the people significant to him, and he now relates to his environment through the process of primary identification. All of these experiences contribute to the growth and development of the infant until, finally, we see manifestations that indicate that again his pattern of relating to his environment has changed and the predominant process is one of secondary identification. After this change has taken place, the child is not merely imitating his significant people but is beginning to act and feel the same way they do. Therefore, at certain times, we see the child appearing as a miniature replica of his significant people. Throughout development from infancy to maturity, we see the individual repeat this sequence of interacting with his interpersonal environment until he has his identity firmly established and is potentially an independent, unique entity.

Somewhere in this process of growing up, the individual appears to lose the early pattern of relating to his environment through the process of empathy. After the individual is secure in his new identity, we see a new pattern of interaction evolving, a new way of maintaining contact and interchange with the interpersonal environment. This new process of relating and interacting seems to have some elements of each of the individual's former patterns of relating but it, too, is called a process of empathy. In contrast to the earlier patterns of interaction, this more mature process enables the individual to maintain his own integrity while interacting with others and to sense or "feel" a situation without either getting his own feelings merged with the situation or absorbing the existing feelings.

When an individual has developed some understanding of himself, his needs, feelings, strengths and vulnerabilities, and is alert as to how he feels in a particular interaction, he will, in retrospect, be able to recognize the way he related to the person or persons involved in the interaction. As a rule, if he has related through empathy, he will have a fairly clear picture of what has occurred in the interaction and how and what the other person or persons were feeling, and he will be able to validate this experience in reality. On the other hand, if he has related through identification, he will be feeling differently than he was before the interaction began and will probably be somewhat confused, depending upon what occurred in the interaction and the degree and quality of the change in his general feeling state.

When a person begins to concentrate on his patterns of interaction and is intent on improving his interpersonal skills, he usually finds that the process of identification is characteristic of his interpersonal relations. Whenever this individual is in a situation wherein pronounced needs are manifested or intense feelings are expressed, he becomes extremely uncomfortable because he begins to experience similar feelings and/or needs. In some respects, this individual is somewhat at the mercy of his interpersonal environment, although inevitably he will fight back or strike out at whomever he feels is responsible for his uncomfortable state.

According to Sullivan, "The traits which characterize interpersonal situations in which one is integrated describe what one is."[2] If we really want to understand the way we interact with others, we have to study the day-to-day situations in which we find ourselves and find out who we are.

Not only do we find out who we are but we can also find out who the other persons with whom we interact really are. Are we interacting like an infant with some of our "ghosts from the past?" Do we expect the same from the person we interact with as we did from some important person in our past life—our mother, father or sibling? See Chapter 4 (the section, "Birth to One Year") for an elaboration of "parataxic hook-ups" and "me-you" patterns.

We have to look at our motives in our interpersonal situations. What do we anticipate? What do we want from the other person? Do we want his approval? Disapproval? Do we want him to feel obligated, appreciative, guilty? Do we want him to agree with us? To disagree? To argue? To fight? If this is what we "want," then this is usually what we

[2]Harry Stack Sullivan: *Conceptions of Modern Psychiatry.* Washington, D.C., William Alanson White Psychiatric Foundation, 1947, p. 123.

get. We more or less force people to support our infantile "neurotic" patterns of interaction. If they fall into our trap and react the way we "want" them to, it is further proof of our infantile belief that we are right, and the infantile part of us rejoices while the adult part of us is dissatisfied. What happens if the other person does not get enmeshed in our web and respond as we "wish?" What if he responds genuinely and realistically according to what he feels and believes? Then the infantile part of us becomes very angry and destructive, while the adult part of us feels guilty. We then tend to take care of our guilt by telling ourselves, "I am not angry. He is angry at me. He does not like me." It is much easier to be the victim than the person who is aware of his responsibilities and actions and is able to assume responsibility for them.

We have said that interpersonal interaction always occurs in an interpersonal situation; in fact, it makes up the situation, which exists for the purpose of satisfying the needs of those involved. The outcome of the activity of the persons involved can either be a reduction of their tension or an increase of their tension—that is, their needs may be either satisfied or aggravated (see page 49, Theory of Reciprocal Emotions).

When we feel dissatisfied, tense or in any other way uncomfortable after any interaction, it is time to look at the situation and try to analyze what has occurred. We need the details of what went on—the actions, reactions and feelings of those involved—to reconstruct the situation if we are really to understand. Since we tend to see and to hear only that which helps to maintain our self-esteem and our "picture" of ourselves functioning as we think we should, it is very helpful to review our interaction with someone else, provided that he is an autonomous, responsible adult who really knows who he is. This is one of the anticipated outcomes of an effective supervisory process. This kind of interaction is also what we refer to as positive, "healthy" interaction, which inevitably results in a therapeutic change.

We tend to think of a one-to-one relationship as involving two persons who are interacting in day-to-day living situations, but when we remember that each person may bring a varied number of his "ghosts from the past" into the situation, it is no wonder that so much of our interaction is clouded, negative and dissatisfying. This is one reason we have to become knowledgeable and skillful in our one-to-one interaction before we can possibly interact therapeutically with a group of persons. As has often been said, "Without human contact we die, and with human contact we sometimes become very weary."

A concept which has proven helpful in learning to analyze and understand interpersonal situations is that of "poles of interaction." Each individual has a pole of interaction on which the behavior reflecting his self-concept and self-esteem is evident. This behavior may range from a feeling of inferiority at the bottom of the pole, to a feeling of superiority at the top of the pole, with a feeling of adequacy and competence at the middle of the pole. Since "it takes two to tango," we always have two poles of interaction when two people are interacting; and the position of each individual on his pole can be plotted if we have the details of the interaction, including the feelings of the persons involved.

In constructive interaction, ideally, each individual functions within a range about the middle of his respective pole. Assuming that neither person is threatened and that each enters the situation feeling fairly comfortable and competent, a collaborative effort will ensue.

What happens if the foregoing description fits one person in the situation, but the other person is at the top of his pole, with a pseudo feeling of superiority because he feels threatened or because, for some reason, that is his usual pattern of interacting with others? In this type of interaction, the condescending attitude of the latter would communicate his superior position on his pole. If the other person is able to remain secure and evaluate the situation for what it is, he will be able to shrug it off and not be affected adversely. On the other hand, if he is shaken by this negative feeling tone, he may have to use one of his defensive patterns. For example, after perceiving the negative attitude, he may resort to denial (see Chapter 3) to block his awareness of the disturbing element. Similar to an ostrich with his head in the sand, he would no longer have the data necessary to evaluate the situation realistically, and would render himself more vulnerable to the attacks which would inevitably follow in such an interpersonal situation.

In learning to become more sensitive to what goes on in interpersonal situations, it is important to become aware of how one feels at the moment at which he becomes involved. Since there is a limit to our span of awareness or to our scope of awareness at any given time, we first have to focus on what is going on within us and then gradually broaden our view. First, self-awareness increases, then we can focus on the other person in the interaction, and gradually we can include the total interpersonal situation. This may seem like a time-consuming process, but in comparison with the amount of time each and every one of us fritters away in less constructive efforts, it amounts to very little. During the process of becoming more sensitive and expanding one's awareness in interpersonal situations, one tends to become overly sensitive; however, this condition gradually stabilizes. It is comparable to the swing of the pendulum from one extreme to the other, which can be observed in any change and which finally ceases near the center.

RELATIONSHIPS

When a person has experiences in positive interaction with another person, a more durable interpersonal situation evolves, which we call a relationship. Relationships with people are sometimes defined as a state of being mutually or reciprocally interested. Since reciprocal means to alternate or to act interchangeably, the whole process of relationship implies the interaction of two or more persons or things in which changes continuously occur. In nursing we also speak of rapport, which refers to a harmonious relationship in which there is mutual interest and respect. In other words, the nurse and patient find a common ground and respond to one another.

MOTIVES IN RELATIONSHIPS

A motive may be thought of as that which incites action. The motive also provides the urge to begin or continue a certain course of action. The actual motivation of behavior is a very complicated subject, but it will be well to remember that motives may be either conscious or unconscious—that is, the individual may be aware of why he is acting in a certain way, or, on the other hand, he may be completely unaware of the cause of his behavior. Therefore, we would expect the same to hold true for the nurse in her relationships with patients. For the sake of convenience we may classify the motives which underlie the nurse-patient relationship into two groups, those that are positive and those that are negative. The positive motive, which is essential for any therapeutic nurse-patient relationship, is a sincere interest in the patient and a genuine desire to help him. In spite of the importance of the positive motive, we often find that negative motives are common in nurse-patient interaction. The nurse may be merely *curious* about the patient. Although a degree of curiosity is usually essential for any learning, curiosity alone is not sufficient in establishing the desired relationship. The nurse may become so scientific that she may forget she is working with another human being and consider him an inanimate object of scientific interest. In her contact with patients the nurse may also be *testing the strength of her own personality*. She does this by exerting pressure upon the patient to act the way she wants him to act. Then, if she succeeds in getting him to perform accordingly, she is inflated because it indicates to her that her personality is stronger than that of the patient.

Another very common negative motive is an attempt to *minimize or justify the existence of one's own conflicts* through working with patients.

The nurse may do this by manifesting an attitude of superiority in feeling that "the patient is so much worse off than I am." Another motive is promoting *personal gain* irrespective of the patient's welfare through using "tricks" or skills indiscriminately. For example, if the nurse is caring for a very difficult patient who refuses to eat and who wants to go home, she may promise him that he may go home immediately providing he eats all of his meal. If the nurse knows that going home immediately is impossible for the patient and is merely making this promise because she wants to impress others with her skill, she is using her influence indiscriminately and not for the welfare of the patient.

In addition, the nurse may be *acting out her own conflicts* in relationships with patients. Let us consider the case of a young nurse who is still struggling to free herself from her mother, who persists in dominating her life. She has received an invitation to a formal dinner dance and has her heart set on a black net gown for the occasion. While shopping for the dress, her mother insists that a demure dotted swiss dress will be more appropriate. Consequently, she goes to the dance attired in the white dotted swiss. She feels that her evening is a "flop" because she does not make the impression that she had anticipated. She somehow feels that her mother is to blame for ruining her evening and feels rather resentful, although she does not openly express any of these feelings. The next morning, she does not feel much like going on duty and finds that many little things annoy her. One of her patients is even more demanding that day; after the nurse cares for her, she tells the nurse that she has not applied the dressing correctly and that it will probably fall off before the morning is over. The nurse responds with open hostility and sarcastically tells the patient that she knows what she is doing. From then on in her contact with the patient that day she will not give an inch and will not fill even the patient's logical requests. It is easy to see in this situation that the nurse is acting out her conflicts about being dominated by her mother in her relationship with this patient.

A final negative motive that we shall consider is that of *caring for the patient merely because the doctor, head nurse or instructor says that she should.* This does not necessarily involve the desire to follow orders nor does it imply that the nurse does not do as directed by the doctor or others, but if this is the primary motive in caring for the patient, an effective relationship will be impossible.

Usually there is one basic motive that is predominant over all the others and provides the underlying theme for the individual's actions. However, in certain situations subordinate motives may become dominant at various stages of nurse-patient interaction. Even though one's relationships with others are usually characterized by positive motives, anyone is apt to find that negative motives are responsible for her actions in certain situations.

ATTITUDES OF THE NURSE IN HER
RELATIONSHIPS

An attitude is a feeling tone which forms the background for our reactions to certain persons, places or objects, supporting and/or limiting the response. When certain patients are repulsive to us, we are apt to communicate this attitude, nonverbally and unintentionally, in caring for them. The patient is usually cognizant of our attitude toward him although we may not yet be aware of it. Attitudes cannot be observed directly but can best be inferred on the basis of the action and the feeling tone communicated. Perhaps we jerk the sheet a little suddenly when we make his bed or frown when we greet him. We can readily see that we will have considerable difficulty in developing rapport with this patient.

It is quite easy to say that "one must correct his attitude," but often we can change our overt actions only momentarily and our true feelings remain the same. First of all, it is necessary for us to become aware of our true feelings and to discover when and under what circumstances we feel this way. Sometimes just becoming aware will help us to change the attitude if it is not associated with strong feelings. A greater understanding of the patient and his needs may also help. At times just understanding the facts and talking them over with our instructor or another experienced nurse will help us to comprehend the situation more clearly. In other instances we may wish to discuss the problem with a psychiatrist. It is only natural that we will be attracted toward some patients more than others but, as we become aware of our attitudes, we can develop more skill in establishing effective interpersonal relationships. In many instances we will find that our attitude is such that we can readily develop rapport with patients with whom we are working.

PHASES IN AN EFFECTIVE NURSE-PATIENT
RELATIONSHIP

The first phase of the nurse-patient relationship is the period in which the nurse and patient more or less get acquainted with each other—a period of orientation. We can assume that the nurse will have had only a few contacts with the patient, with little opportunity to observe him, and, therefore, will have only a minimum of actual knowledge about him. Usually the nurse will have to take the initiative and be responsible for promoting and furthering the interaction. Even then the patient may not be too responsive to the overtures at this time and may require a longer period for testing. During this period the nurse's contact with the patient may be almost entirely structured by the ward routines and the immediate nursing measures required by this patient. Whether or not the relationship remains on this level or develops further will be influenced by several factors. The motive of the nurse in this relationship is probably one of the most important factors. If she has a genuine desire to help this patient and her actions communicate this feeling, the basis for a further relationship may be established. On the other hand, if the patient's needs are such that a more intensive relationship is not indicated at this time, or his problems are much more complex than this particular nurse is able to cope with, the relationship will probably remain at this level. The patient may also project a different role upon the nurse. This, too, will influence the course of the relationship, which will then be outlined in the over-all plan of therapy as indicated by the psychiatric team. If the over-all tone of the nurse-patient interaction has been primarily positive and sufficient time is available for further interaction, the next phase of the relationship will be possible. During this period there is apt to be considerable anxiety experienced by both the nurse and the patient. Also, there is apt to be a denial of this anxiety by various overreactions and a drive toward self-preservation.

The second phase of the nurse-patient relationship is initiated with a fairly well-established feeling of trust on the part of the patient. The patient now assumes a little more initiative in maintaining the relationship and looks forward to his contact with the nurse. The patient begins to identify with the nurse and is apt to manifest considerable interest in her as a person. Here, too, the patient is apt to do further testing of the nurse and may tend to feel rejected at the slightest opportunity. He may also relate things to the nurse in a very obvious attempt to shock her, because he still may not be certain that he is unconditionally accepted. A good bit of his activity may be to impress the nurse, and he is apt to do a great many things that he knows will please her. If both the nurse and the patient weather this phase of the relationship, the third phase usually becomes evident.

The patient is definitely dependent upon the nurse in *the third phase* and does considerable acting out of his problems in his relationship with her. It is important to remember that the nurse should not "make" the patient dependent on her. If one person is "made" to feel dependent on another, it is to satisfy the need of the second person; it is only a repetition of childhood experiences wherein the second person was made to feel helpless and ineffectual. Interaction of this sort is manipulative and destructive. On the other hand, if this person has dependency longings, he requires interaction that will enable him to learn to trust another person; thus he can learn it is safe to be dependent and his dependency needs can be fulfilled. As these needs are met, the need for independence will evolve and the patient will be on the road to achieving interdependence. This is the period in which the nurse uses all of her interpretative, communicative and other interpersonal skills in helping the patient to work through his problems. The patient is more expressive verbally, and the nurse will serve as a sounding board for him to clarify both his feelings and his thoughts. There is usually an increased mutual sensitivity to the feelings in all periods of contact. Although the patient may identify with the nurse, the nurse does not identify with the patient. The nurse emphathizes or "feels into" the situation but does not "feel with" the patient or situation.

The last phase of the nurse-patient relationship begins when the patient has worked out his problems to the extent that he no longer requires this intensive support, and it may be spontaneously indicated by the patient or by the termination of the period of hospitalization. If the relationship is to be resolved for any reason other than a spontaneous indication by the patient, some preparation will be necessary. If the nurse must leave and the patient's dependent needs are still quite marked, there should be some attempt made to transfer this relationship to someone else, and the patient should be prepared for this change several days in advance.

TYPES OF RELATIONSHIPS

INTERPERSONAL RELATIONSHIPS.   These involve the individual and his *external* environment, or that part of the environment outside the living organism. The individual may interact with one or more persons or he may react to the inanimate objects in his social milieu. We shall assume that an interpersonal relationship is interaction which requires that at least one of the persons involved be real. We have implied, by this statement, that people sometimes interact with an imaginary environment. Since the individual may perceive his external environment to be different than it really is, he tends to respond to it as he sees it. For example, a patient may believe that Miss R., the nurse, is trying to poison him when she brings his medication. Even though Miss R. has poured the correct dosage of the prescribed medicine, the patient may still not take it. Here we can see that the patient is reacting to poison, an imaginary object in his environment. We can also see that the object was not totally imaginary. There is a medication, but the patient has misinterpreted this stimulus as a poison. In this situation both the nurse and the patient are real figures in the interaction.

On the other hand, Mr. B. may be observed to talk considerably when no one else is in his room. When the nurse enters, Mr. B. states that he is talking to his friend, Jim. Since it is known that Mr. B. does not have a real friend named Jim, we know that he must have an imaginary friend with whom he interacts.

Individuals also interact with other persons in the environment who are real as well as to objects that are real. Under these circumstances, reality is perceived as it exists with a minimum of misinterpretation.

There are several characteristic patterns which commonly predominate in nurse-patient relationships and which are apt to develop in any group of people who are in proximity with one another. The first of these is the *domination-submission pattern* and is evident when one person is habitually submissive to another who wields power over him. In this instance the submissive person has a need to be dominated and controlled by someone else.

A second common pattern is the *parasitic relationship* in which the patient becomes totally dependent upon the nurse and any occurrence may be interpreted as a threat to his existence. This type of relationship may be fostered between the patient with very strong dependency longings and the nurse with a very strong or intense need to be a mother figure.

A third kind of interpersonal relationship is the *supportive* type wherein the patient is able to cope with everyday experiences with the support of another person. The supportive relationship is one of the most helpful in usual nurse-patient situations.

INTRAPERSONAL RELATIONSHIPS. Another broad area of relationships that is of concern to us is intrapersonal interaction. This type of relationship refers to the individual and his *internal* environment or that environment within the living organism. This statement implies that the individual's anatomy and physiology are a part of his internal environment. The functioning together of the body's organs to maintain life is an example of intrapersonal relationships. As was seen in Chapter 4, there is a part of the interpersonal environment that is internalized. As this part of the environment becomes internalized, it then becomes a part of the individual. For example, as the child develops and interacts with peers and adults, he gains a concept of himself. This concept is built up through his years of experience in terms of how significant adults reacted to him and how he, in turn, reacted to them. This concept of himself is just as much a part of his internal environment as his heart action or his inhaling and exhaling. For a more detailed discussion see "Birth to One Year," in Chapter 4.

As we shall see later, conflict situations may arise between the individual and either his internal or his external environment.

AREAS OF RELATIONSHIPS

The nurse interacts not only with patients but also with her co-workers, her family and her friends in the community. She has both professional and nonprofessional relationships in her home, the hospital and the community. All these experiences affect her and her future relationships with others.

Summary

The need to have interaction with genuine autonomous persons was discussed in terms of its scarcity and its significance. The characteristics of human interaction were highlighted from birth on—we see the infant develop into a biosocial adult. More emphasis has been given to understanding what goes on in our own interpersonal situations, since we can become aware of and understand others only to the degree that we are aware of and understand ourselves.

We speak of an effective relationship as one in which the nurse and patient find a common ground and respond to one another. In establishing this type of relationship the nurse should examine both her motives and her attitudes. A sincere interest in the patient and a genuine desire to help him are prerequisite to establishing a harmonious relationship. The nurse, however, may find that she has negative motives and attitudes in caring for certain patients that will hinder the development of rapport.

The stages of nurse-patient relationship were considered in terms of an initial phase in which the nurse and patient get acquainted, a second phase characterized by a rather well-established feeling of trust, a third phase in which the patient does considerable acting out of his problems in his relationships, and the final phase wherein the relationship is terminated.

Both intrapersonal and interpersonal relationships were discussed as well as the spheres in which the nurse interacts—namely, with her patients, her co-workers, her family and friends, herself and the community.

Bibliography

Freud, Sigmund: *Group Psychology and Analysis of the Ego.* London, International Psychoanalytic Press, 1922.

Fromm-Reichmann, Frieda: *Principles of Intensive Psychotherapy.* Chicago, University of Chicago Press, 1950.

Fromm-Reichmann, Frieda: *Psychoanalysis and Psychotherapy.* Chicago, University of Chicago Press, 1959.

Hoffman, Gerhart: "Principles of Psychotherapy." Lecture given at Western Reserve University, 1948.

Meerloo, Joost A. M.: *Conversation and Communication.* New York, International Universities Press, Inc., 1952.

Mullahy, Patrick, ed.: *The Contributions of Harry Stack Sullivan.* New York, Hermitage House, Inc., 1952.

Reik, Theodor: *Listening with the Third Ear.* New York, Grove Press, Inc., 1956.

Rogers, Carl: *Client Centered Therapy.* Boston, Houghton Mifflin Co., 1951.

Rogers, Carl: *Counseling and Psychotherapy.* Boston, Houghton Mifflin Co., 1942.

Slavson, S. R.: "Types of Relationships and Their Application to Psychotherapy." *Am. J. Orthopsychiat., 15*:267-277, 1945.

Sullivan, Harry Stack: *Conceptions of Modern Psychiatry.* New York, W. W. Norton & Co., Inc., 1953.

Sullivan, Harry Stack: *The Interpersonal Theory of Psychiatry.* New York, W. W. Norton & Co., Inc., 1953.

Sullivan, Harry Stack: *The Psychiatric Interview.* New York, W. W. Norton & Co., Inc., 1954.

Suggestions for Further Reading

Alfano, Genrose: "What Rapport Means to Me." *Nursing Outlook, 3*:326-327, 1955.

Arnstein, Margaret: "Balance in Nursing." *Am. J. Nursing, 58*:1690-1693, 1958.

Badgeley, Elizabeth Wadleigh: "Making Friends with Children." *Am. J. Nursing, 57*:1558-1560, 1957.

Bojar, Samuel: "The Psychotherapeutic Function of the General Hospital Nurse." *Nursing Outlook, 6*:151-153, 1958.

Byron, Edna: "About Mary Murray." *Am. J. Nursing, 59*:527-528, 1959.

Copp, Laurel, and Copp, John Dixon: "Look to the Pattern of Relationships." *Am. J. Nursing, 60*:1285-1286, 1960.

Fagin, Claire M.: "Psychotherapeutic Nursing." *Am. J. Nursing, 67*:298-304, 1967.

Fernandez, Theresa M.: "How to Deal with Overt Aggression." *Am. J. Nursing, 59*:658-660, 1959.

Fries, Olive, H., and McLellan, Mary Lou: "Helping Patients Get Well." *Nursing Outlook, 7*:654-655, 1959.

Godboùt, Rose, and Patrick, Arlene: "The Child in the Nurse." *Nursing Outlook, 6*:460-461, 1958.

Gregg, Dorothy E.: "The Therapeutic Roles of the Nurse." *Perspectives in Psychiatric Care, 1*:18-24, 1963.

Hale, Shirley L., and Richardson, Julia: "Terminating the Nurse-Patient Relationship." *Am. J. Nursing, 63*:116-119, 1963.

Hart, Betty L., and Rohweder, Anne W.: "Support in Nursing." *Am. J. Nursing, 59*:1398-1401, 1959.

Highley, Betty Lee, and Norris, Catherine M.: "When a Student Dislikes a Patient." *Am. J. Nursing, 57*:1163-1166, 1957.

Hobart, John E.: "The Problem of Silences in Nurse-Patient Relationships." *Perspectives in Psychiatric Care, 2*:29-34, 1964.

Holmes, Marguerite J.: "What's Wrong with Getting Involved?" *Nursing Outlook, 8*:250-251, 1960.

Hyde, Robert W., and Coggan, Norma E.: "When Nurses Have Guilt Feelings." *Am. J. Nursing, 58*:233-236, 1958.

Ingles, Thelma: "Case Study—The Worst Patient on the Floor." *Nursing Outlook, 6*:99-100, 1958.

Jensen, Hellene N., and Tillotson, G.: "Dependency in Nurse-Patient Relationships." *Am. J. Nursing, 61*:81-84, 1961.

Jersild, Arthur T.: "Compassion." *Nursing Forum, 1*:61-72, 1962.

Johnson, Jean E., Dumas, Rhetaugh G., and Johnson, Barbara: "Interpersonal Relations: The Essence of Nursing Care." *Nursing Forum, 6*:324-334, 1967.

Jourard, Sidney M.: "How Well Do You Know Your Patients?" *Am. J. Nursing, 59*:1568-1571, 1959.

Levine, Myra E.: "The Four Conservation Principles of Nursing." *Nursing Forum,* 6:45-59, 1967.

Ludemann, Ruth S.: "Empathy — A Component of Therapeutic Nursing." *Nursing Forum,* 7:275-287, 1968.

Nichols, Claude R., and Bressler, Bernard: "Anaclitic Therapy." *Am. J. Nursing, 58*:989-992, 1958.

Post, Jerome, Swanson, JoAnne F., and Grinspoon, Lester: "Cyclic Staff Responses to Chronic Schizophrenic Patients." *Perspectives in Psychiatric Care, 2*:13-19, 1964.

Rohweder, Anne W., and Hart, Betty L.: "How Attitudes Are Taught and Caught." *Am. J. Nursing, 60*:806-809, 1960.

Rouslin, Shelia: "Coping with Chronic Helpfulness." *Ment. Hosp., 61*:10-12, 1961.

Schwartz, Doris: "Uncooperative Patients." *Am. J. Nursing, 58*:75-77, 1958.

Shea, Frank, and Hurley, Elizabeth: "Hopelessness and Helplessness." *Perspectives in Psychiatric Care, 2*:32-38, 1964.

Speroff, B. J.: "Empathy Is Important in Nursing." *Nursing Outlook, 4*:326-327, 1956.

Tudor, Gwen: "Sociopsychiatric Nursing." *Am. J. Nursing, 52*:1225, 1952.

Whiting, J. Frank: "Patients' Needs, Nurses' Needs, and the Healing Process." *Am. J. Nursing, 59*:661-665, 1959.

Wolfe, Nancy A.: "Setting Reasonable Limits on Behavior." *Am. J. Nursing, 62*:104-106, 1962.

Wolff, Ilse S.: "The Educated Heart." *Am. J. Nursing, 63*:58-60, 1963.

Chapter 9 Nurse-Patient Interaction Analysis

Data on nurse-patient interaction in psychiatric nursing are most commonly collected by a nonstructured method of observation known as *participant observation*. This chapter is concerned with the analysis of narrative data obtained by participant observation for the purpose of planning nursing care.

Once the "what," "where," "how," "when" and "why" have been determined tentatively and the flow of data in narrative form begins to accumulate, the student of nursing is faced with the question, "What do I do with it?" How should the data be classified so that they can be used in planning future nursing care? After reading over the observations for two or three periods of interaction with a given patient, the nurse may speculate about trends in patient behavior. If these trends can be identified and substantiated by observational facts, then they may be utilized for formulating goals for that patient's nursing care. Involved in arriving at trends in the patient's behavior which have application for nursing care is the process of interpreting.

THE BASIS FOR DEVELOPING SKILL IN INTERPRETING

Interpretation means to clarify, to explain, to tell the meaning of or to elaborate with reference to a point of view. Therefore, when we

123

interpret behavior we may elaborate by adding details in order to make the incident more clear and distinct or we may speculate about specific behavior by thinking it through and determining what particular meaning it has for us. On the other hand, we may analyze a certain action or feeling in terms of some related model that we accept and then develop the meaning from the discernible similarities and differences.

Everyone speculates about the behavior of others and has done so since the earliest days of his life. He has done so in order to determine his own reactions to those with whom he has interacted. The individual's basic philosophy about people and the world in general has evolved from these early experiences with the significant adults in his life. All these experiences more or less form a frame of reference by which the individual can measure his current experience and come to some conclusion as to what is going on. The results of these experiences or this frame of reference is sometimes called the "common-sense psychology" by which people operate. We should, therefore, expect everyone to have some degree of understanding of people and their behavior from these early experiences in interaction, although the degree of understanding will be quite varied. There are some people who have a much keener sensitivity to others and seem to make fairly valid interpretations intuitively. This intuition is also a result of early experience in interacting with others, so that everyone at least has the capacity for developing intuitive understanding. The fact that we so often function according to intuition, is illustrated in the "hunches" that we have about people or specific situations. The soundness of these "hunches" as they are substantiated or repudiated by the reality situation offers some clue as to the degree of understanding that an individual has. This understanding that we have been discussing thus far is most sound and helpful in situations with which we are already familiar. Lack of familiarity may be one of the reasons why the young nurse in psychiatry oftentimes finds that the patients' behavior "just doesn't make sense." The standards or criteria by which she has hitherto measured situations are not applicable to these patients. In order for the nurse to refine her interpretative skills and to apply them in gaining an understanding of the psychiatric patient, she must add some theoretical knowledge involving the principles and the dynamics of human behavior to the backlog of intuitive knowledge that she already possesses.

STEPS IN FORMULATING TRENDS OF BEHAVIOR

Before we can analyze we must first examine and classify our facts, impressions and hunches about a given situation according to some systematic form. Our next step is to analyze the information and to form generalizations about the data in each classification. We are then ready to check the reliability of our generalizations. We may do this in several ways. We may ask an expert to classify our data and then compare our outcomes to see wherein we agree or differ. We can reason through our data from the generalizations to our specific facts and then again reason from the specific facts to the generalizations and check to see if we reach the same conclusions in both instances. In addition, we can continually check our interpretations in terms of new data that are available, since our interpretations of human behavior can seldom lead to a final, definite conclusion and are always subject to change in the light of new evidence.

DATA AVAILABLE FOR FORMULATING TRENDS OF BEHAVIOR

The data with which the nurse will be primarily concerned in this instance will be information about the patient. This information is available from the following sources:

Patient's history — medical and social
Results of physical and psychologic examinations
Laboratory data
Nurses' notes
Progress notes by physician
Reports from other members of team, i.e., occupational therapist, psychologist
Personal observations of patient and the socioenvironmental context of behavior
Observation and contact with patient's relatives
Conferences in regard to patient's plan of care
Observations of social system if social scientist is a member of clinical team

In addition to these specific sources of information about the patient there will be information about the community from which he came, the community facilities that may be used in his care, textbooks, and the latest research on problems similar to that of the patient.

With such a wealth of material available to the nurse, she may find it helpful to classify it according to some system that makes it easier for her to utilize this information. Information as such is seldom helpful unless the nurse can organize it in a manner that is logical to her. It may be helpful to the nurse to group this information according to the present, past and future status of this individual.

PRESENT STATUS
Age
Nationality
Marital status
Children: age and sex

Physical handicaps
Intelligence
Predominant emotional tone
Special talents or abilities
Special interests and dislikes
Religion preference
Attitudes
Concept of self
Special problems
Plan of therapy and past and present response
Behavior from day to day

PAST STATUS
Childhood
Formal education
Occupational and work history
Economic and social status
Past interests and activities
Health pattern
Predominant emotional tone
Attitudes, values and general outlook
Religious preference
Community
Additional information (anything else about his usual life pattern)

FUTURE STATUS
Goals of other members of the health team
Plans for rehabilitation
Adjustments indicated (on part of patient and on part of his family)

The nurse then utilizes these data to gain an understanding of this individual's usual life pattern — that is, how he usually functioned. This understanding, in turn, helps to clarify his present behavior in the hospital situation.

FACTORS THAT HINDER SKILL IN INTERPRETING

When we interpret behavior, our data consist of facts, and we must be careful to examine them to be certain that they are facts. For example, we observe Joe, who is a very thin, undernourished boy trying out for the football team. Mary says, "Joe is stupid" and Jane says, "I think so, too." This agreement does not necessarily make it a fact that Joe is stupid. This is merely an agreement in judgment. It is true that both Mary and Jane stated that Joe is stupid and it is true that Joe, who is thin and undernourished, tried out for the football team; but it is not a fact that Joe is stupid.

Another important factor that may hinder our skill in interpretation is that we tend to ignore anything in our environment that is not unusual. For example, Mr. J. was a patient on a particular ward for a period of three weeks. He had very little to say, did everything that was asked of him and seldom made any special requests. Suddenly one day he refused to take his treatment. When the staff tried to understand his behavior, they were amazed to find out that no one really knew anything about this patient's reactions since his hospitalization; their interpretations were nothing more than vague generalities. In order to understand this patient's behavior and to make a fairly valid interpretation it would be necessary to consider all the details of his reactions, whether they were what was anticipated or what was unusual.

In spite of our intentions, we sometimes find that something besides the available objective data has influenced our conclusions. For example, Mary Jane had a friend whom she admired and whom she had discussed at length with Betty. This friend planned to spend her vacation with Mary Jane and everyone was pleased since Betty had not yet had the opportunity to meet her. A few days after the friend arrived, Betty was heard to say, "Gee, I had you pictured as a 'drip'— why, I don't know." Betty did not recall intentionally figuring out these expectations, but nonetheless she had a preconceived image of what she had anticipated Mary Jane's friend would be like. We have all had experiences similar to Betty's; being alert to these factors will aid us with the interpretations that we consciously and intentionally make.

Generalization in Nursing Situations

We all tend to form our conclusions too quickly before we have enough information to support them. It is true we may make a generalization on the basis of very little data, but it should remain tentative until we can verify it. The fact that some one does something once does not necessarily mean that we can generalize and say that the act is a part of his general pattern of behavior.

We may find that the reliability of our generalizations may also be affected because we lack sufficient knowledge about the data we are considering. For example, suppose we were observing two children playing and one of them suddenly slapped the other. We would not be able to determine just what went on or give any meaning to this occurrence unless we had additional information about each of the children and also some understanding of child psychology.

Unless we understand ourselves and how we feel in a given situation, we may find that we introduce our own thoughts and/or feelings into the situation. For example, the nurse may have had a difficult time with Mrs. J. that morning and may have become impatient with her because she couldn't decide what to wear. The nurse in recording the incident may note: "Mrs. J. was very irritable and impatient this morning and finally got dressed with much prodding." From the incident and facts available, it would seem that the note was a more accurate description of the way the nurse felt and she was apparently projecting her feelings onto the patient.

We may also forget to re-examine our generalizations in the light of new or recent facts that we have collected. For example, when a new patient first enters the hospital, we may know very little about him; nonetheless, we must care for him. After we gather more information about him, we can then re-examine our facts and see what changes need to be made in our tentative plan for nursing care.

Another factor which may hinder our skill in interpreting is that we may fail to reason logically. We may find ourselves doing syllogistic thinking. To illustrate, we may believe psychiatric patients are hopelessly ill; Mr. S. is a psychiatric patient; therefore, Mr. S. is hopelessly ill.

A lack of sensitivity may also hinder us. For example, if the nurse is acutely aware of what the patient is saying but is not aware of the feeling the patient is communicating, her interpretation will probably be inaccurate.

SPECULATION IN NURSING SITUATIONS

Although the nurse may not always be aware of it, she uses speculation constantly in her daily work with patients. Probably the least obvious and most important is in determining her own reaction to the patient, in reflecting the feelings of patients and in establishing effective nurse-patient relationships.

OBSERVATIONS	SPECULATIONS
4:00 P.M. Mrs. T. was standing near the window facing the street. There were many cars passing. Suddenly she walked rapidly over to the water fountain, took a drink, and returned at the same pace to the spot by the window. She repeated this pattern about five times in a period of one-half hour.	Mrs. T. had been fairly relaxed up until this time. It could be something that she saw from the window that initiated this restlessness. Her going back to the window may be an attempt to either disprove or validate the stimulus.
7:00 P.M. Nurse approached Mrs. T., "You enjoyed your supper tonight, Mrs. T.?" "Yes, very much. I ate the meat, too. I know that it wasn't right to (began to twist a lock of hair) but I did anyway. I don't always keep from eating the things I should anyway."	She appeared to be enjoying her food and ate with much relish. Now appears to be feeling guilty because of her religious taboos. May be a sign of rebellion against standards—could be masochism.

The nurse also determines the immediate nursing care in terms of how she interprets the situation. For example, assume that the nurse has been notified that a new patient is being admitted. The nurse can begin collecting information in regard to the patient the moment he enters the hospital. At first she may have only a minimum of information, but regardless of the amount of data she has she must care for the patient in the present situation. She can base the patient's immediate nursing care upon the few data that are available and formulate a tentative plan. As she gathers additional data her interpretations may change her nursing plan. To illustrate, the nurse through observing the patient collects the following data:

Mr. S. is accompanied by his wife who holds his hand until she has him safely seated in a chair in his room. He says very little but occasionally looks at his wife as she relates details about his illness, e.g., how much he has suffered from his abdominal pain, how tired he is, how they had put off going to the doctor, how he hadn't wanted to come to the hospital, etc. The wife then goes over to the bed, feels the mattress, examines the sheets, looks in the closet and the adjoining bathroom.

Mr. S. is thin and there is an obvious fine tremor of his hands. His skin and lips are dry and warm to touch.

From the admission sheet, the nurse learns that Mr. S. is 55 years of age, is a Catholic of Irish decent, and is a farmer from a nearby rural community.

On the basis of these data, the following speculations are a few which the nurse may make in regard to Mr. S.:

1. Mr. S. is very dependent upon his wife.
   Is this his usual pattern or is it a result of his present illness?
2. Mrs. S. is overprotective of her husband.
   Does she feel responsible for his illness?
   Is this a projection of her own feelings?
3. Mrs. S. has many fears in regard to her husband's hospitalization.
   Does Mr. S. have these fears, too?
   What has been their previous experience with hospitals?
   What does the hospital represent to them?
   −the door toward regaining health?
   −the door toward death?
4. Mr. S. is dehydrated and may have an elevated temperature which is probably related to his recent abdominal distress.
5. Mr. S., although weak and fatigued, is not experiencing acute pain at present.
6. Mr. S. is mildly depressed and has a feeling of worthlessness.

On the basis of these speculations, which represent her interpretation of the situation, the nurse would determine her actions. The first speculation will probably indicate to the nurse that she should be solicitous during the patient's initial adjustment to the hospital. She will be alert to any detail that may make him more comfortable and will see that he is not left alone for any length of time without someone stopping in. She will show interest in him so that he will feel that he is being adequately cared for. She will observe him carefully to try to determine how he responds to her solicitous attitude. Does he seem comforted by it or does he resent it?

On the basis of her second speculation the nurse may wish to encourage the wife to wait in the visiting room where she will join her later so that the patient will not be further influenced by what she says. Then, too, the wife may feel more free to express herself away from her husband. The nurse may also wish to discuss with the doctor Mrs. S.'s apparent overconcern.

On the basis of the third speculation the nurse will probably want to familiarize Mr. S. with his immediate environment and what to anticipate in the near future. In her contacts with him she may wish to encourage him to talk so that she can get some clues about how he feels about his illness and hospitalization. Also, if the nurse imparts this information to the physician, he may wish to talk with Mrs. S. before she leaves the hospital.

On the basis of the fourth speculation the nurse will check Mr. S.'s temperature, pulse and respiration and withhold anything by mouth until definite orders from the physician are obtained. She will also inquire about his fluid intake.

The fifth speculation will indicate that she will assist him in getting into bed and will arrange his environment so that a minimum of exertion will be necessary. She will probably ask him to remain in bed until seen by the physician and will also observe him for distention and any indication of recurring abdominal pain. She will carry out the remainder of the admission routine for that particular hospital.

The sixth speculation would indicate that she will be alert to further indications of depression and will prevent any self-injury which he might attempt.

In this situation we see that the nurse formed her speculations on a minimum of data because it was necessary to determine her immediate action. Then, as the nurse cares for Mr. S. and gains a better understanding of him as an individual and talks with his physician, she will change her plan for his care in relation to the long-term goals for his hospitalization as well as the immediate needs that he manifests.

Let us consider another illustration in which the nurse determines her action on the basis of speculation about the patient's behavior: She goes into the room of a patient who is on forced fluids and intake and output and observes that his intake for the day is quite low and that his pitcher is empty. Her interpretation of the situation would probably be that the patient needed more fluids; her action would be to provide him with additional fluids and to encourage him to consume them. On further analyzing the above situations, we find that what the nurse really did was to determine the patient's needs and then to plan her nursing care in an attempt to fulfill those needs.

As was implied in the example of Mr. S., the nurse communicates her information about the patient to the physician and other members of the staff. Whether or not certain information would be communicated would depend on whether the nurse regarded the data as being significant.

In interpreting a given situation, the first requirement is that we get an over-all picture of what happened. In other words, we try to reconstruct the occurrence, and we always think in terms of a particular person in a particular environment.

The immediate situation (observed data):

Mr. B. stands in the doorway of the dayroom. Several times he has started to take a step forward but has not followed through. He has just come from a conference with his doctor, with whom he has a very good relationship. The doctor was heard to suggest to him that he socialize with other people in the dayroom activities. Miss A., his favorite nurse, is in the dayroom playing bridge with two other patients and has been trying to find a fourth player. A variety show is on television at the time, and Mr. B. has been heard to make several derogatory remarks about such "idiotic" programs. Mr. B. has declined many offers to play bridge, saying that he could never win.

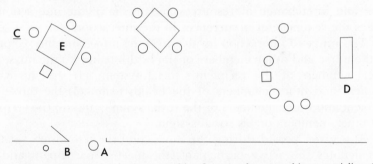

Key: *A*, The patient; *B*, the doctor (a positive factor), who wants him to socialize; *C*, the nurse (a positive factor that attracts him); *D*, television set (a negative factor that repels him); *E*, bridge game (a negative factor that repels him).

On the basis of the available data, the nurse may pose the following questions. What probably happened to Mr. B.? What does he want? How much does he want it? How does he perceive the situation? What are both the positive and negative factors operating in the situation? What additional data will be needed to clarify this situation?

After reconstructing the situation and weighing the influencing factors, both negative and positive, the nurse could better understand what Mr. B. perceived was happening to him and also have some basis for speculating about his response in the future.

In research, much more rigorous methods are utilized in classifying data. Sometimes well-defined codes in relation to the variables in nurse-patient interaction are used so that data can be quantified and hypotheses can be tested. Before such a task is undertaken in nursing research, nursing must be conceptualized in such a manner that it can be measured, and hypotheses related to a theory must be stated. In the following paragraphs, the authors present a conceptualization of nursing that may be helpful to researchers.

CONCEPTUALIZATION OF NURSING[1]

If nursing is to push against the frontiers of knowledge, a conceptual framework must be developed so that hypotheses can be deduced and tested. The following concept, although only a beginning, is suggested as a basis for further development.

Nursing is a process of verbal and nonverbal interaction directed toward the attachment of a recipient[2] to his social system within either an institution, a health agency or the community.

The significant dimensions of the social system are characterized by the range or number of persons involved, the temporary relationship of those involved, the duration of the relationship, the employment and interchange of resources and media of the interaction, as well as the sequence of occurrences in the interaction.

The range of interaction involves: (1) the nurse and the recipient; (2) the nurse and other members of the health team; (3) the nurse and other members of the recipient's social system; (4) the nurse, the recipient and other members of the health team; (5) the nurse, the recipient and other members of the social system; and (6) the recipient and other members of his social system.

At a given period during the interaction the temporary relationship denotes the active participant, the inactive participant and the initiator of either an activity, communication or feeling.

Involved in the resources of interaction are the employment and interchange of persons, objects, self, functions, abstractions and feelings brought into various combinations in a given unit of interaction, all of which are manifest through the media of either verbal interaction, nonverbal interaction or combinations of these components. Verbal components of the interaction may be either watched, transferred, requested or offered in the form of information, suggestion or direc-

---

[1]This conceptualization of nursing grew out of the research project, GN 5535, sponsored by the National Institutes of Health.

[2]The term recipient refers to either an individual or a group receiving the services of a nurse.

tion. Nonverbal components of interaction, on the other hand, may be either watched or employed.

Nursing functions, another resource of the social system, have three subclasses: bodily, psychologic and cultural. Functions that pertain to bodily care are those tasks that are necessary because of age, disease or condition. Psychologic functions take into consideration idiosyncratic preferences, self-identity, privacy, autonomy, emotional support, self-sufficiency and expression of feelings. Cultural functions are concerned with the norms and values of the social system as well as such cultural constants as material objects, speech, religion, economics, knowledge and other abstractions, government, family, kinship, food habits, art, transportation, war or degree of group dissension.

The duration of the temporary relationship of the actor and recipient refers to the amount of time of a given unit of interaction, whereas the sequence of interaction takes account of the recipient's responses to requests and offers, as well as the series of other occurrences in a continuous period of interaction.

The changes in the range, temporary relationship, duration, resources, media and sequence in a continuous interaction are the indicators of the degree of the recipient's attachment to his social system.

The *direction* (increase or decrease) of the desired change along any given dimension of the social system is a judgment of the health team; however, one might hypothesize that the *degree* of change in the desired direction is a function of the nurse's ability to modify the sequence and the foci of resources of nursing techniques, communications and feelings related to intimate life situations of daily living which involve: (1) biologic needs inherent in all people, as well as those requirements unique to individuals with *biologic* health problems concerned with either disease, disability or condition; (2) the psychologic requirements common to all persons, the idiosyncratic requirements of the individual, and the *psychologic* health problems manifested in disease, disability or condition; (3) the requirements related to an individual with a given socio-economic status and those requirements peculiar to the recipient's cultural group.

A MORE ADVANCED APPROACH

EXPLORING PREVIOUSLY LEARNED PRINCIPLES

In the initial phase of data collection the student reexamines all of the "what," "where," "how," "when" and "why." The last is of special importance in the analysis of data, because it is within the framework of the "why" that analysis of data takes place. For example, the student may be exploring Homans'[3] hypothesis (from a course in sociology) that "the more frequently persons interact with one another the stronger their sentiments (feelings) are apt to be." In such an instance, the student may confine her analysis to the range or number of persons with whom her patient interacts and the sequence of the interaction — that is, with whom did the patient interact first, with whom did he interact next and so forth. She also may be interested in the patient's interactional role, such as that of listener or active participator. Then, too, the duration and frequency of the interaction would be very important, as well as the feeling manifested by the patient and others with whom he interacted.

An analysis of data classified according to the aforementioned dimensions of social interaction may assist the student in exploring Homans' hypotheses about interaction. There are ways in which observations can be coded so that such data can be quantified; such systems are discussed in the pages that follow. The student may test the hypotheses set forth in other sciences to which she has been previously introduced.

PLANNING INTERVENTION

A very common reason for collecting data about patients is to plan the nursing intervention and to predict, to some degree, the effects of nursing intervention. If the effects of nursing intervention are to be ascertained, the nurse must know exactly what it is she does for the patient and under exactly what circumstances. With an experimental design, variables can be controlled so that it is possible to evaluate the effects of nursing care given in specified situations in a specified manner; however, the practitioner of psychiatric nursing need not treat every patient as though he were a statistic in a random sample of a target population. Some of the thought processes, on the other hand, that are appropriate for research might be useful in planning the nursing care for the psychiatric patient.

The nurse who collects data about her patient by the method of participant observation needs to find ways of classifying and analyzing such data. By observing trends in interaction over a period of time, some guesses can be made about the patient's response to stimuli and thus his response to nursing intervention. In most cases the nurse will want to know who initiated the interaction, who participated and how. The code in the Appendix has been helpful in reducing participant

---

[3]George C. Homans: *The Human Group.* New York, Harcourt, Brace and Co., 1950, p. 112.

observations to smaller units so that they can be analyzed with greater ease.

An example of the code is as follows: if the nurse said to the patient "How about wearing your pink dress today?" the unit is coded as NOfSuP (nurse offers suggestion to patient).

The nurse may wish to know how many requests a patient initiates and to whom such requests are directed. Needless to say, the patient's problem must be identified first and then the nurse may speculate about how he will react under certain circumstances. By using the above code or one which the nurse develops for herself, the number of times a patient responds in a given way can be ascertained. Then, if the nurse wishes to know the percentage of time the patient responds in a specified way, it can be calculated.

Along with each component of behavior about which the nurse wishes to make some generalization or prediction, the nurse must decide (usually with assistance from others) what change in behavior should be induced and in what direction. For example, it may be considered desirable for a patient to verbalize more than he does now, and so the goal might be to offer opportunity to the patient to verbalize more. In such an instance, the nurse's goal is to increase verbalization. When is the goal achieved? What if the patient talks too much or the effects of nursing intervention have induced too great an increase in the extent of patient verbalization? Usually, the nurse asks an expert to go over her observations with her and then independently checks her planned nursing intervention with another. If there is agreement that verbalization is increased, then the nurse can ascertain that the degree of change was in the *desired direction*. Frequent comparision of the results with others will help make sure that the patient's verbalization will be increased only to the desired level. If perchance the patient's verbalization is maximized to an extent that is beyond the desired level, then the nurse may have to provide less opportunity for the patient to verbalize; however, in her analysis of data, the nurse would measure how far away the patient is from the desired level of verbalization.

Prior to coding observation, the nurse may wish to classify her data into categories that were not predetermined. In such instances, she may wish to record her observations and leave a wide margin so that generalizations about the patient's behavior can be made. From these, she may then identify the patient's needs, which is the first step in any nursing intervention.

A classification of needs made by Ashley Montagu offers a good basis for nursing need identification. The classification and definitions are as follows:

(1) Vital Basic Need: Any biological urge or need of the organism which must be satisfied if the individual or the group is to survive. Examples are the

need for oxygen, food, liquid, activity, rest, sleep, bowel and bladder emptying, escape from danger, avoidance of pain, and conjugation.

(2) Emotional (Nonvital) Basic Need: Any biological urge or need which is not necessary for the physical survival of the organism, but which must be satisfied if the organism is to develop and maintain adequate mental health. Examples are the need to be loved, the need to love, the need to be with others, communication, and tactile and kinesthetic stimulation.

(3) Derived or Socially Emergent Need: Any need which arises out of the process of satisfying basic needs, which is not necessary for the physical survival of the organisms, and which is not biologically, though it may under certain conditions become socially, necessary for the maintenance of mental health. Examples are the need for proper clothes, grooming, shelter, the development of skills or the acquisition of knowledge, creative work, etiquette and religion.

(4) Acquired Need: Any need which does not arise directly out of the process of satisfying basic needs, which is not necessary for the physical survival of the organism, but which grows out of the person's relation to the derived or socially emergent needs, and is not usually necessary for the maintenance of mental health.

Acquired needs are individual, personal, idiosyncratic needs — idiosyncratic in that the acquired needs may differ from person to person within the same culture, whereas the derived needs are usually the same for all persons in all cultures, no matter how their form may differ. In the same culture some persons need tobacco, others do not; and so it is for all acquired needs.

Satisfaction of needs makes for health and cooperativeness; frustration of needs for disorder or disease and hostility, whether the needs be basic, derived, or acquired.[4]

There are, of course, numerous ways of analyzing data, and each one must be appropriate for the purpose of evaluating the effects of proposed nursing care. The nurse interested in research may consult the texts and articles on research methodology.

While the foregoing theory provides a framework for the development of other hypotheses which may be tested by experimental or other types of design, the practitioner of nursing may wish to evaluate the effects of her nursing care along any one of several dimensions. The burden of evaluation can become lighter if the units for analysis are much larger; thus the practitioner may wish to evaluate the patient's change in behavior by evaluating units based on time. The time period may be every thirty minutes or every hour or every twenty-four hours, but each time period should be the same for comparison. The following method for evaluating effects of nursing intervention has been found helpful.

---

[4]M. F. Ashley Montagu: *The Direction of Human Development.* New York, Harper & Brothers, 1955, pp. 150-151.

Schematic Presentation of Methodology for the Evaluation
of the Degree of Change Induced by the Nurse

NURSING DIAGNOSTIC PROCESS

Identification of that aspect of malfunction in the process of need-satisfaction
sequence appropriable to the nurse role.
Determination of direction in which change should take place in relation to dimensions of interaction (often in collaboration with appropriate
disciplines).

INTERVENING PROCESS

I. ORIGIN OF NURSING ACTIVITY

a. Nurse originated.
b. Physician originated.
c. Setting originated.
d. Patient originated.
e. Other.

II. UTILIZATION OF RESOURCES AVAILABLE TO SOCIAL SYSTEM

a. Bodily care (alterations necessary because of age, disease or
condition)
b. Psychologic functions or idiosyncratic preferences (identity,
privacy, autonomy, emotional support, self-sufficiency, expression of feelings)
c. Cultural constants (material objects, speech, religion,
economics, scientific knowledge and other abstractions, government, family, kinship, food habits, art, transportation, war or
degree of group dissention)

III. INVOLVEMENT OF RESOURCES IN SOCIAL SYSTEM

a. Perceives resources.
b Employs resources.
c. Imparts information about resources.
d. Makes suggestions and directions for use of resources.
e. Differentiates role in relation to use of resources.
f. Evaluates role in relation to use of resources.

IV. CONTROL OF RESOURCES IN SOCIAL SYSTEM

a. Quality (how good)
b. Quantity (how much)
c. Sequence (when)

Evaluation of Nursing Intervention and Its
Effects on Patients

BEGINNING OF INTERVENTION						DIMENSIONS OF INTERVENTION	END OF INTERVENTION					
Patient			Nurse				Patient			Nurse		
+	0	−	+	0	−		+	0	−	+	0	−
						1. (To be filled in by student) 1.						
						2. 2.						
						3. 3.						
						4. 4.						
						5. 5.						
						6. 6.						
						7. 7.						
						8. 8.						
						9. 9.						
						10. 10.						
						11. 11.						

Evaluation of Nursing Intervention (For Advanced Students)

If the focus of patient care is to be on nursing, then it follows that the content should stem from conceptualization of nursing. In the methodology for the evaluation of the degree of change induced by the nurse, there are at least three steps which can be identified: (1) nursing diagnosis; (2) nursing intervention; and (3) evaluation of the effects of the intervention.

If nursing is a process of verbal and nonverbal interaction[5] directed toward the attachment of a recipient to his social system within either an institution, a health agency or the community, it becomes

---

[5]Interaction refers to the influence of the behavior of one person in relation to another. Total behavior configuration deals with the internal functioning of a person as well as interpersonal relationships. For example, the administration of insulin by the nurse and the patient's physiologic response is considered an interaction.

necessary to conceptualize the dimensions of nurse-patient interaction so that the nurse's skill can be evaluated in terms of the degree of change induced in the appropriate direction.

The schematic presentation within this section is a modification of a more complex system developed in the study, *The Effects of Skilled Nursing Care Upon Personalization of Older Patients* (GN 5535).[6]

The nursing diagnosis in the aforementioned instrument is in itself a method of evaluation which, once made, forms the basis for the nursing intervention. The nursing diagnosis is concerned with a malfunction of the need-satisfaction sequence that is appropriable to the nurse role. The nurse attempts to reduce tension through nursing methods that are directed toward control of the resources in the social system.

The nursing diagnosis is limited to the aspect of the malfunction of the process in the need-satisfaction sequence of the intimate life situations of daily living for the recipient who has a disease, disability or health condition which affects the degree of attachment to the social system.

In the nursing intervention prescribed by the nurse, the practitioner is involved in noting the origin of the activity, in utilizing the resources available to the social system, in determining the extent of the involvement of resources and in establishing some capacity for the control of such resources. The theory pivots on the idea that as the individual becomes better acquainted with a resource the more apt he will be to exercise control over it. In the nursing methodology, the nurse is concerned with the control of sequential events in interaction. The variables listed in nursing intervention and the effects upon patients are not considered to be exhaustive. Thus, the graduate student may define and explore other variables of interest to her.

The diagram on evaluation of intervention is an attempt to ascertain the dimensions of nurse-patient interaction. With respect to the nurse practitioner, the significant dimensions of interaction are those which reflect stimulation (or restraint or reversal) of what the nurse does. With respect to patients, the significant characteristics are the effects upon patients in term of the manifestations of attachment to the social system.

In the initial phase of the interaction, the practitioner should determine the direction in which change should take place in any one of the several dimensions. It is recognized that it may be necessary for the nurse to collaborate with others in certain cases in order to determine the direction of change. Opposite each dimension the nurse

---

[6]Brown, Martha, *et. al.: The Effects of Skilled Nursing Care Upon Personalization of Older Patients* (GN 5535). Unpublished. 1961.

should indicate the direction of change by using a plus symbol if the activity along a given dimension is to be increased. A minus symbol is used if the behavior is to be decreased, and a zero is used if the behavior is to be maintained. In the same fashion, the nurse should determine the direction of change in relation to her own behavior. For example, it may be desirable that the extent of the patient's verbalization be increased, whereas the goal of the nurse's behavior is to decrease verbalization. The symbol Y is used when the dimension is not applicable to the situation and the symbol X is used in instances in which there is not enough information for making a decision. The three broad behavioral spectra in nursing methodology (diagnosis, intervention and evaluation of effects) are viewed not as independent but rather as mutually interacting and interdependent.

Summary

Interpretation has been described as a process through which clarification and meaning develop. It was implied that the interpretation of behavior is a highly individualized process since we tend to interpret situations according to our needs at the moment, our past experiences, and what we perceive is going on at the time. It was suggested that the nurse is apt to encounter many barriers as she attempts to refine her skills in generalizing; becoming alert to these factors is an essential step in the development of these skills. In conclusion, the various ways in which the nurse utilizes speculations in providing care for patients were discussed with an illustration of how a situation might be reconstructed in order to comprehend all the important factors operating. A conceptualization of nursing was presented for researchers who may wish to develop it more fully. A more advanced approach to the analysis of nurse-patient interaction was presented for graduate students.

Bibliography

Becker, H. S., and Geer, B.: "Participant Observation: The Analysis of Qualitative Data." In Adams, R. N. and Preiss, J. J. (eds.): *Human Organization Research.* Homewood, Ill., Dorsey Press, 1960. pp. 267–289.

Brown, Martha, *et al.:* "The Effects of Skilled Nursing Care Upon Personalization of Older Patients." (GN 5535). Unpublished, 1961.

Guest, R. H.: "Categories of Events in Field Observations." In Adams R. N. and Preiss, J. J. (eds.): *Human Organization Research.* Homewood, Ill., Dorsey Press, 1960. pp. 225–239.

Hayakawa, S. I.: *Language in Thought and Action.* New York, Harcourt, Brace and Co., 1949.

Homans, George C.: *The Human Group.* New York, Harcourt, Brace and Co., 1950.

Kreuter, Frances: "What Is Good Nursing Care?" *Nursing Outlook,* 5:302–304, 1957.

Lindzey, Gardner, ed.: *Handbook of Social Psychology,* Vol. I. Cambridge, Mass., Addison-Wesley Publishing Co., Inc., 1954.
Montagu, M. F. Ashley: *The Direction of Human Development.* New York, Harper & Brothers, 1955.
Peplau, Hildegarde E.: *Interpersonal Relations in Nursing.* New York, G. P. Putnam's Sons, 1952.
Reik, Theodor: *Listening with the Third Ear.* New York, Farrar, Straus and Co., 1948.
Sullivan, Harry Stack: *Conceptions of Modern Psychiatry.* Washington, D.C., William Alanson White Psychiatric Foundation, 1947.
Weiss, James, M. A. (ed.): *Nurses, Patients and Social Systems.* Columbia, Mo., University of Missouri Press, 1968.

Suggestions for Further Reading

Butler, Herbert J., and Flood, Frances R.: "Evaluating Nursing Care in a Mental Hospital." *Am. J. Nursing, 62*:84-85, August, 1962.
Dye, Mary C.: "Clarifying Patients' Communications." *Am. J. Nursing, 63*:56-59, August, 1963.
Gilbert, Doris C., and Wells, Fred L.: "A Ward Socialization Index." *Am. J. Nursing, 57*:59-61, January, 1957.
Godek, Isabelle: "Three Keys to Significant Behavior." *Am. J. Nursing, 59*:1564-1565, November, 1959.
Hale, Shirley L., and Richardson, Julia H.: "Terminating the Nurse-Patient Relationship." *Am. J. Nursing, 63*:116-121, September, 1963.
Hayes, Joyce Samhammer: "The Psychiatric Nurse as a Sociotherapist." *Am. J. Nursing 62*:64-67, June, 1962.
Herzog, Elizabeth: "Some Guide Lines for Evaluative Research." Washington, D.C., U.S. Department of Health, Education, and Welfare, Social Security Administration, Children's Bureau, 1959.
Hurteau, Phyllis: "The Psychiatric Nurse and the Mute Patient." *Am. J. Nursing, 62*:55-60, June, 1962.
Jensen, Hellene N., and Tillotson, Gene: "Dependency in Nurse-Patient Relationships." *Am. J. Nursing, 61*:81-84, February, 1961.
Lambertsen, Eleanor C.: *Education for Nursing Leadership.* Philadelphia, J. B. Lippincott Co., 1958, pp. 94-104, 133-180.
"Let Your Light So Shine." Roche Laboratories, Nutley, N.J., 1967.
Lewis, John A.: "Reflections on Self." *Am. J. Nursing, 60*:828-830, June, 1960.
Macgregor, Frances Cooke: *Social Science in Nursing.* New York, Russell Sage Foundation, 1960, pp. 285-309.
Peplau, Hildegarde E.: "Interpersonal Techniques: The Crux of Psychiatric Nursing." *Am. J. Nursing, 62*:5-54, June, 1962.
Sherlock, Basil J.: "Acquisition of the Nursing Role and the Transmission of Nontherapeutic Orientations." *Nursing Res., 12*:182-185, Summer, 1963. Abstract.
Wolfe, Nancy Anderson: "Setting Reasonable Limits on Behavior." *Am. J. Nursing, 62*:104-107, March, 1962.

Part Two   High-Visibility
Nursing Functions in the
Care of Psychiatric
Patients

Chapter 10 High-Visibility Nursing Functions in Patient Requirements

IMMEDIATE NEEDS

Like any other need, an immediate need evolves from a state of disequilibrium which gives rise to tension and can be relieved only by achieving some goal which re-establishes equilibrium, thereby creating a minimum tension state known as satisfaction. An immediate need, similar to other needs in our culture, is satisfied primarily through interaction with another person or a group of persons. Although an immediate need is more of an end in itself, it is also a means to an end in relation to the long-term goals of the person involved. The patient's day-to-day structure must provide for the satisfaction of immediate needs regardless of whether long-term goals have yet been formulated. In this respect, the nurse may often find that she is caring for a patient about whom she knows very little, and she may be unable to obtain any further information about him; nonetheless, she goes ahead in an attempt to provide for his immediate needs as she perceives them in the particular situation.

The area of immediate needs is one in which many problems are encountered, both with patients about whom little is known and with patients about whom adequate information is available and for whom an over-all plan of care has been formulated. It may help to elaborate on what constitutes a problem, since the ideas tend to be varied. We think of a problem as anything that is not solved most effectively by an instantaneous, almost automatic response. Therefore, anything that requires consideration, deliberation or forethought would be classified as a problem, as would anything that might be performed in a more economical, effective way. Only those areas in which the nurse is most likely to encounter problems with patients in general, as she attempts to assist them in meeting their needs, will be considered in the following material.

THE PROBLEM-SOLVING APPROACH. The nurse will find it most helpful if she utilizes a problem-solving approach in any attempt to plan for the patient's needs. This approach involves the following: observing the patient, both as a spectator and as a participant, then generalizing about the data in terms of what the patient was doing, and why, and what he was trying to accomplish. Then on the basis of these generalizations, the next step is deciding upon a plan of action that will help the patient meet his needs, then implementing the plan. If it is not beyond the capacity of the patient involved, it is desirable to bring him in on the planning and the implementing of the action. Then, after the plan has been carried out, the next step is evaluating the total approach, from the generalizing about the data to the outcome of the plan, including the patient's response.

PERSONAL HYGIENE

The problem of assisting the patient in matters of personal appearance is sometimes a challenge to the nurse. Someone must be responsible for determining what clothing and other articles the patient needs in order to become an acceptable member of the group. Relatives are usually glad to bring these articles to the patient if they are informed of his needs. In instances when it is not feasible for relatives to participate in this manner, there are usually some provisions made by the hospital to furnish clothing and other necessities for the patient. Too often, however, the patient is left to shift for himself in this respect.

A nurse with initiative can do much to help make these provisions for the patients. A ward manicure set consisting of various shades of nail polish and other necessary articles might be donated by some interested person. Deodorants and a kit for oral hygiene can usually be made up from articles obtained from the hospital supply room and the pharmacy. After determining what is needed for each patient and what is needed by the group, the next step is to find some way to make these articles accessible to the patients.

Clothing is sometimes kept in the patient's locker or in a special clothing room. It is important that the patient have some voice in the selection of his daily wearing apparel. There are, of course, some patients who are too ill to make such a decision; the nurse may find it necessary to decide for such a patient until such time as he is able to do so for himself. Patients who feel unworthy or who are destructive may take on renewed interest if their appearance is made attractive to them as well as to others.

Provisions must also be made to care for soiled clothing until it can be laundered. A paper bag labeled for each patient usually is sufficient. The soiled articles can then be taken home by relatives, taken to the patients' laundry, or sent to a commercial laundry. Care should be taken to list all articles of clothing that are sent out of the hospital.

On large wards in psychiatric hospitals, certain days may be set aside for manicuring, shampooing and bathing. In some instances, patients are given the opportunity to go to the hospital beauty shop. It is much nicer, however, and more interest is usually developed by the patient, if mass-production routines are not established. However, an alert and creative nurse can make almost any routine fun if she uses every opportunity to deviate from monotony.

Cosmetics can usually be made available by providing a box for each patient. Patients may enjoy designing their own boxes, which is less expensive. Some provision is necessary for the patient to have access to her cosmetics, and the nurse may sign the boxes "in" and "out" as the patients use them.

If patients have access to all the necessities for improving their appearance, the nurse must also provide the time for the patient to use them. Patients who require more than the usual amount of time may be encouraged to begin a little before the others. The nurse should also anticipate when the patient will probably want to use the articles. Usually he will want them upon arising and retiring, before meals, before his visitors arrive and before any other social occasion.

While some patients need to be encouraged to make their appearance more acceptable to others, there are some patients who may constitute a problem in the opposite direction. How these specific problems can be met by the nurse will be dealt with in other chapters.

Another problem in relation to personal hygiene that may require special attention on the part of the nurse is that of toileting certain patients. The aged or confused patient may not be able to care for his own needs in this respect and may require special attention. Sometimes just reminding the patient will be sufficient. In other instances it may be necessary for the nurse to record the patient's habits of urinating and defecating so that she can help the patient establish a pattern.

Once the pattern is established she can assist him to the bathroom or, if he is confined to bed, offer him the bedpan at a scheduled time.

PROMOTING AND MAINTAINING SAFETY FOR THE PATIENT

Attempts at self-injury may range from a slight abrasion to the destruction of life. The reasons for such attempts are numerous. In one instance, the patient's aim may be actual self-destruction; in another, he may be making a gesture in an attempt to further control his environment. On the other hand, he may mutilate himself because of some bizarre belief that a certain part of his body no longer belongs to him or he may think he hears someone telling him to commit such acts. Whether the patient's action is primarily to punish himself, to punish others or for other reasons, he usually gives many clues which will enable the nurse to anticipate his behavior.

Oftentimes the patient will comment about life not being worth living, or he may actually state his intention to commit suicide. These comments are apt to be disregarded and considered merely as the patient's attempt to gain attention rather than as a true statement of the way he feels. The latter seems to be the more accurate interpretation, because many times patients follow through on these threats. Frequent comments about the high cost of hospitalization or any kind of self-depreciating remarks should serve to warn us of the patient's self-destructive thoughts.

Usually the patient with these tendencies is placed under special observation, as are all newly admitted patients until sufficient knowledge is gained about their behavior. When a patient is ordered on special observations or precautions, it is essential to clarify the degree of precaution necessary. It may be that only the most obvious precautionary measures will be indicated; on the other hand, constant observation may be necessary, and this order means that someone must know what the patient is doing at all times. Most hospitals provide for some kind of routine check on all patients at specified times. The check may be at the change of shifts, it may be routinely every half hour, or it may be more frequent. Regardless of the frequency of the check, each room is usually inspected and the activity of each patient determined at the specified time.

If a patient is intent on injuring himself, there are certain articles that would obviously be kept away from him, such as sharp instruments, small items which might be swallowed and articles which might be used to strangle or choke, such as belts and strips of clothing. There are, however, many ways in which attempts at self-injury may be carried out. In addition to the usual injuries which may be inflicted by sharp instruments, the patient may try to drown himself in a very small amount of water or he may attempt suffocation by using the pillow or other bedclothing. If the patient is desperate, almost any article may be used as a weapon to achieve his goal. For specific care of patients in emergency situations, the student is referred to a textbook on first aid.

Similar problems may be encountered in caring for the patient with assaultive or homicidal tendencies. In addition to the articles mentioned previously, anything which might be thrown is also a hazard. It is usually wise to protect such a patient from group interaction when these tendencies are very active. Although there may be many reasons for a patient becoming assaultive, the most common one seems to be that of fear. The patient may misinterpret his environment and feel certain that someone is going to harm him unless he takes active steps to defend himself. Such a patient will oftentimes feel much safer if he is separated from the group until the intensity of these fears diminishes. As a rule, such behavior is not continuous but is rather spontaneous and erratic. Close observation may reveal that the patient's assaultive tendencies are evoked by certain routines, by certain patients or members of the personnel, or at specified times during the day or night.

Another closely related problem is that of caring for the patient who attempts on his own to terminate his hospitalization. These attempts may be motivated by several factors. First, the patient may lack any understanding of his true condition and feel that he is being held without cause. Second, he may wish to leave the structured situation in order to carry out suicidal or homicidal impulses. Third, he may just wander away because of an extreme state of confusion. These patients may attempt to go out the door with visitors or hospital personnel who are unfamiliar with them. They may also check the locked doors frequently to find one that has accidentally been left open, or they may attempt to secure the keys forcefully. While away from the hospital for activities with the group, these patients should be observed very carefully. It is most helpful if the nurse accompanying such a group remembers exactly how each patient is dressed, so that she can determine their location at all times. If, in spite of precautions, a patient is successful in leaving the group, the nurse's responsibility is to remain with the group of patients; another member of the personnel should be delegated to follow the departed patient. Each hospital usually has its own established policy to give direction to personnel in such instances.

In providing safety for patients with problems such as those we have just discussed, the care of keys is very important, as is the checking of all doors that are to be kept locked. Any loss of keys should be reported immediately, so that extra precautions may be instituted. Since these patients are very sensitive to the locked doors and keys in general, the way in which the nurse uses her keys may do much either to aggravate or to alleviate their problems in this area. Although restraints have not been mentioned as a measure in the care of these patients, they are sometimes used. The important thing to remember in the use of restraints is the manner in which they are applied and the attitude of the person using them. It has been the experience of the authors that, when fear is the primary motive underlying the patient's action, the application of restraints usually only intensifies the fear. The nurse may sometimes find it very difficult to remain calm and patient with someone who continually manifests assaultive or self-destructive behavior; however, she will be able to help the patient most if she can refrain from reprimanding him for his actions or showing any other indication of disapproval. There is usually provision made for the reporting of incidents of this nature, and from the legal standpoint these reports should be both accurate and detailed.

ENERGY RESTORATION

The primary problems in this area are centered around nutritional intake, rest and the overt expenditure of energy. In relation to nutritional intake, it is important that the nurse know what the patient eats, how much he eats, and when and how. Until the nurse is sufficiently familiar with the patient's pattern, she may want to keep a written record of these facts. She will be interested not only in the patient whose intake is inadequate but also in the patient who takes too much. The weight record of the patient will provide an index to the problem.

Regardless of the problem involved, the nurse will want to consider the culture from which the patient comes and the influence it has on his eating habits. She will be able to act constructively only when she knows the reasons for patients' particular eating patterns and understands the underlying dynamics of these patterns. It is sometimes helpful to make provision for the patient to eat alone if his behavior is such that it is repulsive to other patients or if it makes him appear ridiculous to them. Certainly, if it became necessary to spoon-feed or tube-feed a patient, the nurse would carry out these procedures in the patient's room where he would not be observed by other patients. Many patients are able to function much better on a schedule of interval feedings wherein small amounts of food are served more frequently. Obtaining an adequate fluid intake sometimes poses a problem, and it may be necessary occasionally to take the patient to the water fountain and remind him to drink some water, as well as to serve additional fluids. It will usually be found that there is a great variety in the degree of assistance needed by different patients in order for them to maintain an adequate nutritional intake.

Some patients may have difficulty securing an adequate amount of rest and sleep; in such instances it will be helpful for the nurse to become familiar with the usual sleep pattern of these patients. There are usually many factors which interfere with the patient's sleep, such as noises created by the personnel, other patients or the usual routines of the hospital. The routine or time of retiring may be quite different from the patient's former pattern. If any degree of discomfort is experienced by the patient shortly before bedtime, the nurse should anticipate that he may not be able to sleep. On the other hand, if he is hungry or is not tired or sleepy, he may also be restless. If he is afraid of certain patients or of the situation in general, he will not be likely to go to sleep.

Elderly patients or others who tire easily may require more rest than younger and more active individuals. It is often helpful to provide a short period after lunch when these patients may rest if they desire. There is also the patient who seeks withdrawal from group interaction by going to sleep; he, too, poses problems for the nurse.

ROUTINE AND DIAGNOSTIC MEASURES

In general, the patient comes to the hospital because he feels, or his relatives feel, that he may not or will not be able to carry on his usual way of life. The medical patient who comes to the hospital for diagnostic tests does so because he feels that he may have something wrong with him which, if left untreated, may interfere with his usual activities. The psychiatric patient, too, may come to the hospital because he feels that if his symptoms continue he may not be able to retain his rightful place in the community. Unfortunately, however, the psychiatric patient is often admitted not for diagnostic measures but because he already has a serious illness which makes it impossible for him to carry out his functions either at work or at home. Until general practitioners in medicine, nursing and the allied professions recognize early symptoms of psychiatric disorders, the psychiatric patient will probably be sent to the hospital in the later stages of his illness. Even though the psychiatric patient may recognize his problem early and ask for care, he is sometimes denied admission because of lack of facilities or lack of personal funds to pay for such care.

Before we can intelligently care for any patient, we must have some understanding of why and how he came to the hospital. In general, the nurse is usually familiar with why and how the medical or surgical patient is admitted to the hospital, but she has little knowledge about the special ways in which the psychiatric patient may be admitted. We shall digress for the moment, therefore, to discuss some of these possibilities so that we can have a better understanding of the patient's needs when he is placed under our care.

Special legislation has been passed in each state to deal with the admission of patients to psychiatric hospitals. Even though the specific legislation differs from state to state, psychiatric patients can usually be admitted by one of two ways—as voluntary or involuntary patients. The voluntary patient comes to the hospital because he has elected to do so and can leave when he desires. Most hospitals require that a patient entering in this manner give advance notice of his intention to leave. The voluntary patient is not deprived of his civil rights and does not go through any legal procedure in order to be admitted to the hospital. The involuntary patient, on the other hand, is committed to a specific institution through legal proceedings and loses all his civil rights. His legal status is somewhat similar to that of a child in that he cannot vote and cannot enter into contractual agreements such as in business or marriage.

Patients who are committed to psychiatric institutions are usually admitted from their homes, a psychiatric or nonpsychiatric ward of a general hospital or, because of lack of other facilities, from jails. In most instances the patient comes from places where his behavior has not been understood. If the nurse understands how the patient has perceived his previous treatment, it will enable her to orient him to his new hospital environment in a more effective manner.

It is important that the new patient be greeted by the nurse and be made as comfortable as possible. Every hospital has its own specific routines for admitting patients, but there are also general factors that need special consideration. Every patient has a need to belong. The nurse will introduce the new patient to members of the patient group as well as her own co-workers. She will also spend time in acquainting him with what is expected of him, what will happen to him, and other facts such as the location of the bathroom and dining room and the time certain ward activities occur. It may be that these steps will be taken over a period of days or in a few hours, depending, of course, upon the patient's condition.

The nurse can also do much to make the relatives feel better. Often the relative has considerable guilt feelings in regard to bringing the patient to the psychiatric hospital because of the stigma attached to such illness. If the nurse explains the ward routines and, in general, explains what will happen to the patient, the relative usually is somewhat comforted. The nurse will, of course, refer specific questions in regard to the patient's condition and treatment to the doctor.

In most hospitals the new patient's possessions are taken from him. His clothing is usually removed from his room so that it can be listed and marked. The clothing that is suitable for wearing in the hospital is returned to him. Articles that are unusually expensive or considered inappropriate may be returned to the relatives to be taken home. Valuables may be sent home or placed in the safe, while articles that are hazardous for the patient to keep in his immediate possession are stored and made available for his use under supervision.

If the patient is not given an admission bath and shampoo, his skin and scalp should be observed as soon as possible after admission. The nurse should record any marks, abrasions or bruises and note the condition of the scalp. Detailed notations may prevent serious misunderstandings at a later date in regard to the care given the patient and will also call the physician's attention to conditions that need immediate treatment.

Since little information is available about the average new patient, the nurse will want to observe him closely so that he will not have the opportunity to injure himself or others. It is important that the nurse remain with the new patient and not leave him alone with his possessions, since he may attempt to conceal something. She will carefully examine the clothing that he has removed before it is returned to him. She will also want to record as many other observations as possible in order to provide data to aid in diagnosing the patient's condition as well as in establishing an effective nurse-patient relationship.

Shortly after his arrival, the new patient will probably be examined by the physician. When the patient is undressed for the examination, the nurse will have a good opportunity to examine unobtrusively both his skin and his clothing. She will also want to explain the examination to the patient in such a manner as to instill confidence. The tray for the physician should not be brought to the room until it is to be used unless the nurse plans to remain with the patient. When the examination is completed, she should make sure that all articles are accounted for and the tray removed. If an empty syringe or needle is left in the room, it may be used as a weapon by the patient for self-injury.

It may be necessary to obtain the admission urine specimen under direct supervision or by catheterization if the patient is too confused to comprehend directions. We cannot overemphasize the necessity for collecting routine specimens and assisting the physician with routine examinations, since the patient's general state of health may be somewhat impaired. Then, too, the patient may not be able to describe all his symptoms to the physician, and the only clue may be through the routine data obtained during the admission procedure. Since the psychiatric patient is usually ambulatory, every effort should be made to rule out any infectious condition that could be transmitted to other members of the patient group.

Summary

The concept of the patient's immediate needs has been formulated as being similar to any need in that they evolve from a state of disequilibrium that gives rise to tension and can be relieved by achieving a goal that re-establishes equilibrium. Although the patient's immediate needs may appear to be an end in themselves, they do constitute a step in achieving a greater goal, that of recovery. Since a problem-solving approach has been taken, the concept of what constitutes a problem has been discussed.

Areas in which the nurse may encounter problems in meeting the patient's needs center around those that deal with personal hygiene, promoting safety, the restoration of energy, and routine diagnostic measures. The area of promoting safety was elaborated upon from the point of view of injury to the self and injury to others. Restoration of energy was discussed in regard to the problems of food and fluid intake, rest and sleep. Routine diagnostic measures such as those that take place during the admission procedure were described. Only a general discussion of these problems has been presented here, since the reader will find more specific applications in the chapters that follow.

Bibliography

Ingram, M. E.: *Principles of Psychiatric Nursing*, 5th Ed., Philadelphia, W. B. Saunders Co., 1960.

Kalkman, Marion: *Psychiatric Nursing*, 3rd ed., New York, McGraw-Hill Book Co., Inc., 1967.

Render, Helena Willis: *Nurse-Patient Relationships in Psychiatry*, 3rd ed., New York, McGraw-Hill Book Co., Inc., 1959.

Suggestions for Further Reading

Anderson, Barbara J.: "The Nurse's Role in Individualizing the Admission Process in a Psychiatric Hospital." *Am. J. Psychiat.*, *120*:890-893, March, 1964.

Ingram, M. E.: *Principles of Psychiatric Nursing*, 5th Ed., Philadelphia, W. B. Saunders Co., 1960, pp. 82-94, 95-104.

Kalkman, Marion: *Psychiatric Nursing*, 3rd ed., New York, McGraw-Hill Book Co., Inc., 1967.

Render, Helena Willis: *Nurse-Patient Relationships in Psychiatry*, 3rd ed., New York, McGraw-Hill Book Co., Inc., 1959.

Rykken, Marjorie B.: "The Nurse's Role in Preventing Suicide." *Nursing Outlook*, 6:377-378, 1958.

Shneidman, Edwin S.: "Preventing Suicide." *Am. J. Nursing*, 65:111-116, May, 1965.

Shneidman, Edwin S., and Farberow, Norman L., eds.: *Clues to Suicide.* New York, McGraw-Hill Book Co., Inc., 1957.

Shneidman, Edwin S., and Farberow, Norman L.: "A Socio-Psychological Investigation of Suicide." In Henry P. David and J. C. Brengelmann, eds.: *Perspectives in Personality Research.* New York, Springer Publishing Co., Inc., 1960, pp. 270-293.

Chapter 11 High-Visibility Nursing Functions in Physiochemical Therapies

In this chapter only those psychiatric treatments that are induced by either chemical or physical methods and used in rather typical situations will be considered. The nurse will better comprehend her role is she knows something of how the treatment developed and how it is used in the average situation. An understanding of the patient's reaction throughout the treatment is also essential if the nurse is to anticipate the changes in his behavior and to provide for his needs.

INSULIN THERAPY

Although insulin was first used by Steck and others in an attempt to increase the patient's weight and to influence excitement states, particularly in the treatment of morphine addiction, the method as practiced today is largely due to the work of Sakel, which was first reported in 1933. Sakel introduced the hypoglycemic coma in the treatment of schizophrenia after he had observed improvement in the condition of psychiatric patients who were receiving insulin for symptomatic treatment, but who had accidentally progressed into deep hypoglycemic states during this procedure.

The use of insulin therapy for individuals with nonchronic schizophrenia is still considered the best somatic treatment available,

155

although its therapeutic effects are not as dramatic as in the use of electroshock for individuals with depressions or involutional melancholia.

Many believe that it is still too early to toss out insulin therapy as an important method of treatment for conditions about which there are still so many unanswered questions. It is true that many patients seem to respond favorably to some of the antipsychotic drugs, but in many respects this form of treatment is as yet experimental. We still know too little about individual responses to and irreversible side effects of many of the compounds.

PREPARATION OF THE PATIENT AND HIS ENVIRONMENT

Preparing a patient for insulin therapy is similar to the preparation of any patient who is expected to become unconscious during the procedure. Food is withheld, but small sips of water may be permitted. If the patient has long hair, it is usually braided and all bobby pins are removed; dentures or bridges are removed; mouth care is given or supervised; temperature, pulse and respiration are checked, and deviations are reported. The patient should be toileted and dressed in pajamas, robe and slippers prior to the injection of the drug. If it is the patient's initial treatment, some explanation and reassurance may be indicated. The patient's weight is checked before the first treatment and each week thereafter.

The nurse is usually responsible for preparing the patient's environment during the treatment. The bed is equipped with a rubber sheet and a rubber-covered pillow and should be ready for the patient before he receives the initial injection of insulin. The room should be darkened, warm, adequately ventilated and free from drafts. An oral gavage tray should be readily accessible, equipped with litmus paper as well as the other necessary equipment. An intravenous tray should be prepared with $33\frac{1}{3}$ per cent glucose, ampules of emergency drugs, and both 50 cc. and 2 cc. syringes. A mouth gag, hand towels, mouth wipes and drinking water should be placed on the bedside table of each patient. Extra linen and blankets should be available as needed to keep the patient dry and warm, and it would also be helpful to have a screen available for each patient receiving treatment. If special forms are used for recording the treatment, they, too, will be in the treatment unit. The room should be equipped with a rectal thermometer tray, sphygmomanometer and such other equipment as will be needed, depending upon the procedure of the specific hospital. Throughout the treatment an atmosphere conducive to relaxation should be maintained. This will involve keeping external stimuli at a minimum and possibly restricting the people in the room to those who are immediately involved in administering the treatment.

The care of patients receiving insulin coma therapy requires considerable skill and experience; therefore, it is suggested that a qualified graduate nurse be in attendance in the insulin unit and that student nurses not be given the total responsibility of the care of these patients. Because of the possibility of rapid change in the patient's condition, he should remain in bed throughout the treatment, and a nurse should be in the room at all times. It is also preferable that a physician be accessible in the insulin unit, especially during the second phase of the treatment. It is also customary to have some sort of emergency signal in the room, so that the nurse may obtain additional supplies or assistance without leaving the patient. When such signals are utilized, it is imperative that other nurses or other personnel be alert for them and follow through immediately.

RELATIONSHIP TO OTHER THERAPIES

Insulin therapy is usually used in combination with other therapies, since many authorities consider it only of symptomatic value in and of itself.

In any treatment in which the patient remains in bed, he becomes more dependent upon others to assist him in meeting his needs. During insulin therapy the patient not only becomes dependent but also regresses to a more primitive level of behavior. Some psychiatrists utilize this regressive state psychotherapeutically and request that the nurse play a prescribed therapeutic role. A plan for this type of therapy requires considerable skill and also a close working relationship between the nurse, physician and other co-workers concerned with the care of the patient. A commonly accepted role ascribed to the nurse is that of a solicitous mother figure who manifests an active interest in the patient; however, this role will not be effective with all patients and its use could precipitate a panic state because of differences in the dynamic factors of the patient's psychiatric disorder.

Insulin therapy is also used in combination with electrotherapy, which may be given either to terminate the insulin coma or on alternate days; or a series of convulsive treatments may be given either prior to or following a course of insulin therapy. Many variations of insulin therapy itself are commonly used, such as ambulatory insulin, in which the patient receives small doses of insulin and is permitted to be up and about; precoma insulin, wherein the treatment is terminated before the coma phase is reached; and coma insulin (insulin shock therapy), in which the patient is allowed to reach varying degrees of a comatose state.

In many instances insulin therapy is considered only a part of the total plan of treatment, since it is believed to increase the patient's accessibility for other therapies. In addition to the use of psychotherapy, a planned program of occupational and recreational therapy is considered vital in facilitating the patient's progress toward a quicker and more effective rehabilitation.

HYDROTHERAPY

Hydrotherapy was one of the earliest methods used for the symptomatic treatment of psychiatric patients, and many psychiatrists and psychiatric nurses believe that it should be available to those patients who, for some reason or other, cannot be treated with medication. Although hydrotherapy departments may no longer be considered an essential part of many psychiatric units, the use of water in various forms to facilitate relaxation and to help reduce the individual's level of tension is still as effective today as it was many years ago. The physiologic effects of heat and cold and the principles underlying the care of the patient are the same even though the standard equipment is not utilized. The use of swimming pools and various water games for patients is a fairly new innovation in hydrotherapy and can have either a relaxing or a stimulating effect as desired.

ELECTROTHERAPY

Pharmacologic convulsive therapy was first introduced by Von Meduna in 1935 with the use of camphor and later the use of Metrazol. With the introduction of electrotherapy in 1938 by Cerletti and Bini, a simpler method was discovered which was less feared by most patients. However, many variations in both electrical and pharmacologic methods of treatment have been developed in recent years.

In preparing the patient for electrotherapy, the usual plan is either to restrict food intake prior to treatment or to limit it to a light breakfast, to allow intake of fluid and the usual morning hygiene, to remove hairpins and other metal objects and to braid the patient's hair if long, to remove any dentures and/or gum from the mouth. If the patient is hospitalized he is dressed in pajamas; otherwise, any tight clothing which he may be wearing is removed. The patient should be toileted and also have his temperature, pulse and respiration checked before the treatment. In addition, the nurse should check the chart for the preliminary laboratory data and the treatment permit and give any preshock medication that has been ordered, such as sedatives or atropine or Dramamine to prevent nausea and excessive salivation.

Depending upon the physical structure of the hospital, the treatment may be administered either in the patient's room or in a special unit. It is believed that patients who are receiving treatment should not observe one another immediately before, during or following the treatment.

There are many modifications of machine and electrodes as well as methods for using them. In most situations, however, the temporal region of the patient's head is swabbed with alcohol and/or saline, and electrode jelly is applied. The nurse should take precautions to avoid irritating the patient's eyes with these solutions. The residue of electrode paste should be removed from the patient's head immediately after the treatment, not only because it is much easier to remove at this time but also because, if left on, it will stimulate much added concern about the treatment.

Usually the nurse checks the machine to see that it is in working order. She then places the patient in the desired position (there is much experimenting being done with regard to position), which will differ depending upon the physician and the situation. Either the physician or an experienced nurse should insert the mouth gag so that the patient will not bite or swallow his tongue. If the patient has loose or missing teeth, a special mouth gag may be necessary. The person who holds the mouth gag then exerts pressure on the patient's chin so that fracture or dislocation of the jaw will be averted. During the convulsion, the patient's shoulders and extremities are held gently in order to prevent fractures.

If the treatment is not given in the patient's own bed, precaution should be taken in placing him in his bed after the treatment. The patient's respiration should be checked carefully until normal breathing and color are re-established, and artificial respiration should be administered if indicated. An ashen gray color indicates serious complications and should be reported immediately. Some patients may manifest a period of excitement and may become combative if the nurse tries to control them. For these patients, additional assistance or restraints may be necessary. Since the patients are often confused following treatment and tend to misinterpret environmental stimuli, they should be kept in bed until fully reacted. The nurse may clarify the degree of orientation by the way in which the patient answers simple questions. It may be necessary for her to assist the patient in dressing, walking and eating his breakfast. Since the patient may experience a blurring of vision, it will probably be best if activities that require close, distinct visual perception or concentration are avoided. The patient is also apt to experience nausea, dizziness and headache following the treatment; if these symptoms are reported promptly, the physician may order palliative drugs. The nurse should also be alert to any symptoms of fracture, although all muscular and joint pain of which the patient may complain is not indicative of such a complication. A common reaction which is of concern to both the patient and his relatives is his loss of memory: the nurse should reassure them that this memory difficulty is only temporary. She may also assist the patient in recalling recent events and other facts of general interest to him.

Electrotherapy is commonly used in conjunction with various pharmacologic preparations such as curare and barbiturates. Although it is used for the treatment of persons with varied problems, it is most effective for those with depressions or strong suicidal tendencies. The nursing care for patients receiving modified forms of electrotherapy may require some adaptation of the points discussed.

PSYCHOPHARMACOLOGY

Although much has been learned in the field of psychopharmacology in the past few years, a constant state of change is still characteristic of both theory and practice. As many classifications and subclassifications have been coined as there are drugs available. The recent tendency to use the terms antipsychotic agents, antidepressant agents and antianxiety agents seems the simplest as well as the most logical organization in terms of chemical structure and clinical reactions to the drugs. It will be helpful to become familiar with both the generic name and the trade name of each of the drugs, because references discussing the drugs often combine usage of these terms.

ANTIPSYCHOTIC AGENTS

Chemically, there are four major classes of drugs thought to be of value as antipsychotic agents: phenothiazine derivatives; *Rauwolfia* alkaloids; thioxanthenes; and butyrophenones (not available commercially in U.S.).

The phenothiazines are further divided into three subgroups:

GENERIC NAME	TRADE NAME
1. Aliphatics	
Chlorpromazine	Thorazine
Promazine	Sparine
Triflupromazine	Vesprin

GENERIC NAME	TRADE NAME
2. Piperidines	
Thioridazine	Mellaril
Mepazine	Pacatal
Piperacetazine	Quide
3. Piperazines	
Trifluoperazine	Stelazine
Perphenazine	Trilafon
Prochlorperazine	Compazine
Thiopropazate	Dartal
Fluphenazine	Prolixin
Carphenazine	Proketazine
Acetophenazine	Tindal
Butaperazine	Repoise

The *Rauwolfia* alkaloids are represented by five commonly used drugs:

GENERIC NAME	TRADE NAME
1. Reserpine	Serpasil
Rescinnamine	Moderil
Deserpidine	Harmonyl
Syrosingopine	Singoserp
Alseroxylon	Rauwiloid

The thioxanthene derivatives are represented by three drugs:

GENERIC NAME	TRADE NAME
1. Chlorprothixene	Taractin
Thiothixene	Navane
Clopenthixol	Sordinal

The butyrophenones are a class of drugs which have a completely different chemical structure than others of the antipsychotic agents. There is one significant representative:

GENERIC NAME	TRADE NAME
1. Haloperidol	Haldol

Phenothiazine Derivatives

The first subgroup of the phenothiazines is the aliphatics. Chlorpromazine hydrochloride, more commonly known by its trade name, Thorazine, was introduced in the United States in 1954 and is still the most widely used of these. This synthetic compound was developed in a research laboratory in France and was first reported in 1952 by Delay, Deniker and Harl. While the compound was originally used in anesthesia to potentiate preoperative medication or to alleviate postoperative shock, it was soon noticed that patients who were given the drug seemed to become strangely detached from their surroundings. Observation of this detachment led to the evaluation of the drug for treatment of the psychiatric patient.

Thorazine is a white, crystalline powder and is readily soluble in water. It may be given orally or by deep intramuscular injection and is available in 10, 25, 50, 100 and 200 mg. tablets; 25 and 50 mg. ampules; syrup, 10 mg./5 cc.; suppositories, 25 and 100 mg.; and a concentrate, 150 mg./5 cc. This drug has proved to be of value in varying degrees in the treatment of patients with schizophrenia, manic-depressive reactions, manic phase, organic brain syndromes, acute alcoholism, delirium, senility, psychoneuroses and psychosomatic disorders. Throughout the literature it is emphasized that the clinical picture presented by the patient is more significant than his diagnosis in determining whether or not he may be helped by a particular drug. Thorazine has proved most helpful for patients for whom rapid sedation is required, as in states of extreme excitement, terror, agitation, destruction, open hostility or assaultiveness. Many chronic psychotic patients who had apparently failed to respond to other forms of treatment have become quiet and orderly and are making a better hospital adjustment with the administration of Thorazine.

For acutely disturbed patients for whom quick sedation is required, Thorazine 25 mg. is usually administered by deep intramuscular injection into the upper outer quadrant of the buttock. The solution is injected very slowly and the site of injection massaged for several minutes. Sometimes physiologic salt solution and/or 2 per cent procaine solution is given simultaneously with the Thorazine to minimize the local irritation and pain of the injection experienced by some individuals. If at all feasible, the patient should remain in bed for one-half hour following the injection because of the possibility of a rapid lowering of blood pressure, which may produce a feeling of faintness and dizziness. Occasionally, a marked hypotensive effect occurs, producing a shocklike condition, in which case the patient's head should be lowered, his feet elevated and other nursing measures carried out as would be indicated in any state of shock. As a rule, one may expect the patient to become drowsy within twenty minutes after the initial injection. The drug reaches maximal action about one hour after administration, but the effects continue for approximately six hours. If the first injection is not effective, an additional injection of 25 mg. is sometimes given within an hour.

When treatment is instituted by parenteral injections of Thorazine, oral therapy is usually started within a few days and is gradually regulated to the maintenance dose that is necessary to bring about the desired change in the patient's symptoms. Although there is no standard dose of Thorazine, maintenance doses for patients who have been acutely disturbed usually vary from 500 to 800 mg. daily. It will be important for the nurse to observe the patient carefully and to report any sign of his symptoms recurring, because the physician may want to increase the medication.

For patients who are less acutely excited, treatment is usually initiated with oral administration of 25 to 50 mg. of Thorazine three times a day with a gradual increase until maximal effect is achieved. Some patients have been able to stabilize on a maintenance dose of 50 mg. per day, whereas others have required up to 500 mg. daily.

Although there is still controversy in regard to just how the effects of chlorpromazine are produced, it is agreed that the drug induces a state of tranquility and calmness, which makes the patient more amenable to other forms of therapy. What can the nurse anticipate from the patient receiving Thorazine?

First of all, the more erratic and bizarre the behavior, the more pronounced will be the influence of the drug and the more marked the changes that will occur. During the first few days of treatment, the patient will probably be quite drowsy and may sleep much of the time. It will be easy to arouse him, and he will usually respond readily to questions. If all goes well, this somnolence should disappear by the end of the second week of treatment. Because of a lowering of body temperature and also the basal metabolic rate, the patient may complain of feeling weak and cold. On the other hand, during the early phase of treatment some patients develop a slight elevation of temperature, which usually subsides spontaneously.

Another frequent occurrence is a dryness of the mucous membranes, an unpleasant taste in the mouth, nasal congestion and, occasionally, either a marked contraction of the pupils or a marked dilatation. The foregoing manifestations are thought to be the effect of the drug on the autonomic nervous system.

What influence does Thorazine have on delusions and hallucinations? We are apt to find the previously loud, aggressive, hostile individual sitting quietly staring off into space. As we said previously, he usually responds readily when we speak to him but he seldom offers conversation spontaneously. It may seem that both his delusions and hallucinations have disappeared, but studies indicate that the only change is that they no longer perturb the patient, so he neither reacts to his hallucinations nor assertively expresses his false beliefs. This indifference which the patient shows toward his symptoms carries over to his surroundings, and he will need a great deal of encouragement to participate even passively in activities.

To what other factors does the nurse need to be alert with patients receiving Thorazine? Some patients experience tachycardia, palpitation, headaches and pains in the legs and abdomen. Many suffer from constipation, and fecal impactions may be quite common unless special attention is given. Many physicians order daily laxatives for patients receiving Thorazine. Symptoms of parkinsonism that should be watched for are unsteady gait, a slowing of movements, fine tremor of hands, and often excessive salivation and drooling.

Usually between the second and sixth weeks of treatment, there is a possibility of patients' developing jaundice, and any elevation of temperature or change in color of urine or stool would be significant. Between the third and tenth weeks, the nurse should be alert to indications of developing agranulocytosis, such as an elevation of temperature, sore throat, lesions in the mouth or any sign of infection. A further complication that may occur at any time is an allergic skin reaction with redness, itching, edema, vesicles, macules or papules.

The nurse or others giving Thorazine injections or concentrate may also develop a dermatitis, so precautions should be taken to prevent getting the solution on either skin or clothing. This contact dermatitis usually clears up when there is no further exposure to the solution.

Two of the other aliphatics commonly used are promazine (Sparine) and triflupromazine (Vesprin). Promazine is usually given in fairly large doses of 25 to 1000 mg. daily, while triflupromazine is given in doses of 20 to 150 mg. They both tend to produce drowsiness, feelings of apathy and lethargy and retarded psychomotor activity.

The piperidines, the second subgroup of the phenothiazines, includes only one compound that is now available in the United States: Thioridazine (Mellaril) given in doses of 30 to 800 mg. daily is thought to have marked sedating and tension-reducing effects. This drug is also believed to have a low incidence of extrapyramidal and autonomic side effects and is safer than the stronger agents in outpatients in borderline states and in patients in follow-up and aftercare regimes. Patients do frequently gain considerable weight and have headaches while on Thioridazine. Mepazine (Pacatal), once widely used, has been withdrawn from the market because of the high incidence of blood dyscrasias associated with its use.

The third subgroup of phenothiazine derivatives is the piperazines, and the most commonly used drug in this group is prochlorperazine (Compazine), which has been used in the treatment of psychiatric patients since 1956. Compazine is much more potent than Thorazine, and reports indicate fewer side effects from the drug unless large doses are required. Usually patients are started on Compazine with 5 to 10 mg. orally three or four times daily. Some are able to achieve optimum results on 50 to 75 mg. daily, while others require 100 to 150 mg. daily. Compazine does not have a sedative effect like Thorazine and is, therefore, not so effective with the acutely excited patient; otherwise, the range of patients who have been treated with this drug is about the same. Patients receiving Compazine are usually alert and more actively interested in their surroundings. The development of symptoms of parkinsonism is more common with this drug, and the patient's tremors may be so marked that he will be unable to perform detailed activities that require the use of fine movements. Some patients may also become restless and have difficulty in sleeping. If the extrapyramidal symptoms become severe enough, the patient may manifest symptoms of the dystonic type, such as opisthotonos, in which the patient's back is arched and only his heels and head are touching the bed; his eyes may roll back in his head; he may have spasms of his neck or shoulder muscles which twist his neck and head similar to torticollis; he may have difficulty in swallowing and opening his mouth if the muscles of his face and mouth are affected. Patients on Compazine therapy have also developed allergic skin reactions and occasionally blurred vision. At the first indication of any of these symptoms, they should be reported so that proper treatment may be instituted.

Trifluoperazine (Stelazine) has been used since 1958 and has proved helpful in the treatment of patients who are withdrawn and apathetic. One advantage of this drug is supposedly its long action, which allows for effective results with only two doses a day. Patients are usually started on Stelazine therapy with 2 mg. orally three times a day or 5 mg. twice a day. After receiving the medication for three weeks, most patients do well with a maintenance dose. Most of the side effects of Stelazine occur within the first weeks of therapy. During the early period, patients may become restless and have difficulty sleeping, and the dose of the drug is not increased until these symptoms subside. Other patients have experienced drowsiness, dizziness, weakness of muscles, skin rash and loss of appetite, but these symptoms are usually transient. Extrapyramidal symptoms are more common than with Thorazine, and any indication of these should be noted early and reported.

A common occurrence in premenopausal women being treated with any of the antipsychotic agents is nonpuerperal galactorrhea frequently accompanied by some degree of breast enlargement. The incidence reported has been quite variable — from zero to 80 per cent. The size of the dose does not seem to be significant, and the condition may occur as early as eight days after the beginning of treatment. This condition, although not serious or irreversible, may certainly increase the stress for the individual concerned and may be the basis for new delusional ideas or reinforce old ones.

Any of the phenothiazines may produce a hyperglycemic effect in some patients and thereby trigger diabetes in patients who have been known as latent or prediabetic. They can also produce such a relaxation of peripheral resistance that a drastic fall in both systolic and diastolic blood pressure may occur and a state of shock may ensue. This condition naturally calls for immediate action to prevent further complications. If patients are also taking antihypertensive medications, they must be observed carefully, because the phenothiazines potentiate the effect of these drugs. Thorazine has been reported to produce hyperthermic coma in patients with myxedema, and intensified tachycardia in patients with hyperthyroidism.

The piperazines, the newer phenothiazines, produce a very high incidence of extrapyramidal effects much greater than those seen when either Thorazine or Mellaril is used.

Since most of the psychotropic drugs potentiate the sedative action of the barbiturates, the opiates and alcohol, the nurse should be especially alert for indications of exaggerated depressant action if the patient has consumed any of the above. Since all of the phenothiazine derivatives have an antiemetic action, any condition that is usually accompanied by nausea and vomiting, such as a toxic or neurologic condition, could be easily masked.

Rauwolfia Alkaloids

This group of drugs is composed of derivatives of the plant *Rauwolfia serpentina* Bentham. The *Rauwolfia* plant grows in India, and the natives have used the root of this plant for many years as a medicinal herb thought to have many healing properties. The experimental use of reserpine, a crystalline alkaloid of *Rauwolfia*, began in the United States in 1953, and it proved to be a successful drug in the treatment of patients with psychiatric disorders.

Reserpine, marketed under the trade name of Serpasil, is thought to be effective in the treatment of adult patients with both acute and chronic schizophrenia, senility accompanied by increased tension, irritability and hostility, chronic asthma with fear and restlessness, and children with brain injuries who are overactive. The treatment is usually initiated by the administration of 5 mg. intramuscularly once a day for ten days and 1 mg. orally twice a day. The oral dose may be increased gradually to 10 mg. daily and continued indefinitely, although more than 15 mg. should not be given within any twenty-four-hour period.

The action of reserpine is much slower than chlorpromazine, although it has a similar relaxing and quieting influence. Most patients become drowsy and lethargic, and there is danger of their blood pressure dropping low quite rapidly. The occurrence of a serious drop in blood pressure is more frequent than with chlorpromazine. Some patients experience a transitory rise in body temperature and many become edematous. Others develop gastrointestinal symptoms owing to increase in both the amount and the acidity of the gastric juice.

During the period between the second and the eighth week of treatment, the development of extrapyramidal symptoms may occur.

The parkinsonism associated with reserpine is much more exaggerated than that produced by chlorpromazine.

As with the phenothiazine derivatives, the patient receiving one of the *Rauwolfia* derivatives may develop any of the side effects discussed previously, and the nurse should be alert for the first indication of such an occurrence so that corrective measures may be instituted.

Rauwolfia alkaloids are not used as extensively as formerly, although they are still utilized for patients who have not responded to or for some reason cannot take other drugs. They are especially appropriate in the treatment of hostile, very agitated or hypertensive patients who are unmanageable.

Thioxanthene Derivatives

The thioxanthene derivatives were discovered during a search for more effective antipsychotic agents with fewer side effects. The first and primary drug of this group is chlorprothixene (Taractin), which produces a clinical effect similar to that of chlorpromazine (Thorazine). It is given in doses of 10 to 600 mg. daily and so far has proved to be less toxic and to produce fewer and milder side effects in relation to the eyes, the liver and the blood. It does, however, produce extrapyramidal side effects. Taractin seems to have both relaxing and stimulant qualities.

Butyrophenone Derivatives

The butyrophenone derivatives are represented by haloperidol (Haldol) in the United States. This drug has a completely different chemical structure than the other antipsychotic agents. It is given in doses of 3 to 50 mg. daily and has a calming, quieting effect on agitated patients without inducing a hypnotic effect. It does, however, have the highest potential for inducing extrapyramidal side effects of all the antipsychotic agents.

ANTIDEPRESSANT AGENTS

In 1957, two new classes of drugs were introduced that had originally been tried in the treatment of patients with schizophrenia but were found more effective in treating patients with apathy and depression. Representing these two classes were imipramine (Tofranil) and iproniazid (Marsilid). Since then Marsilid has been removed from the market because the gravity of its side effects outweighed its effectiveness. Many new compounds have been added in the last few years which are thought to be effective in the treatment of individuals with depression, and many of them are still being studied. There is still substantial disagreement in the results of the studies and there are many areas which need to be clarified through further research.

There are at present four broad classes of antidepressant agents: tricyclics, monoamine oxidase inhibitors, amphetamine-like stimulants and a miscellaneous group.

The tricyclics are divided into three groups:

GENERIC NAME	TRADE NAME
1. Iminodibenzyl derivatives	
Imipramine	Tofranil
Desipramine	Pertofrane
	Norpramine
Trimeprimine	Surmontil
2. Dibenzocycloheptane derivatives	
Amitriptyline	Elavil
Nortriptyline	Aventyl
Protriptyline	Vivactil
3. Dibenzoxepin derivatives	
Doxepin	Sinequan

The monoamine oxidase inhibiting group can be subdivided into two classifications: the hydrazines and the nonhydrazines.

GENERIC NAME	TRADE NAME
1. Hydrazines	
Isocarboxazid	Marplan
Nialamide	Niamid
Phenelzine	Nardil
2. Nonhydrazines	
Pargyline	Eutonyl
Tranylcypromine	Parnate

The group of amphetamine-like or psychomotor stimulants is divided into the amphetamines and the amphetamine-like compounds.

GENERIC NAME	TRADE NAME
1. Amphetamines	
Amphetamine	Benzedrine
Dextroamphetamine	Dexedrine
Methamphetamine	Methedrine, Desoxyn, Syndrox, etc.
2. Amphetamine-like compounds	
Methylphenidate	Ritalin
Pipradrol	Meratran

The fourth subclass of antidepressant agents includes several miscellaneous drugs:

GENERIC NAME	TRADE NAME
1. Lithium carbonate	Lithium
Meprobamate with benactyzine	Deprol
d-Amphetamine with amobarbitol	Dexamyl

Tricyclic Compounds

Imipramine hydrochloride (Tofranil), one of the first antidepressants to be available commercially in the United States, is one of the most thoroughly studied of the antidepressant drugs. A review of most of the studies of Tofranil's effectiveness, both inpatient and outpatient, shows that negative results equal positive results. Many of the studies on hospitalized patients with psychotic depressions indicate that placebos are just as effective as Tofranil. The results of studies of the overall antidepressant group are just as contradictory and may reflect problems in methodology.

The dosage of Tofranil may range from 75 to 200 mg. daily, and, in general, effects may not be evident for five to ten days. A daily dose of 150 mg. is thought to be optimal. Many prefer to divide the dose and administer it three times daily, with the last dose no later than 6:00 p.m. to avoid too much evening stimulation. Others prefer a single daily dose; the evidence related to an increase in side effects with this method is contradictory.

Although Tofranil is recommended for the treatment of both exogenous and endogenous depressions, most studies indicate that it is superior for patients with periodic endogenous depression. The drug has been used for patients in all age groups, with all types of depression or depressive symptoms. It has been used alone and in combination with other drugs.

In general, how do patients with depression respond to Tofranil? If effective, the drug produces a gradual but definitive elevation of mood. This gradual change is thought to be more "normal" than the sudden artificial swing which might be produced by the action of amphetamines. There is a lessening of somatic and vegetative disturbances and a gradual increase of self-confidence and interest in self and environment.

Possible side effects of Tofranil are multiple but are generally reversible if detected early and if the dosage is adjusted. Symptoms similar to atropine reactions are common, e.g., blurring of vision, dry mouth, constipation and tachycardia. Dizziness and agitation have also been reported. There may be coarse tremors or sudden jerks of muscles while lying in bed before going to sleep. Any of these experiences would be disconcerting to the patient, to say the least. If he is allowed to talk about how he feels and to understand that these experiences are a reaction to his medication he will usually feel relieved.

There are also more serious complications which may develop, depending upon the patient's total state of health. Any cardiovascular, thyroid or liver problem would indicate close observation. Any indication of urinary retention should be reported immediately because it can be reversed by lowering the dosage or discontinuing the drug if necessary.

As the patient improves he may experience a state of hypomanic excitement which would require immediate action. He may become confused and some may experience excessive sunburn if exposed to direct sunlight.

Although Tofranil is the most studied of all the antidepressants, there are still too few controlled studies to permit statistical accuracy in stating the number of patients who improve with the drug. In general, improvement in controlled studies varies between 50 and 70 per cent, while in uncontrolled studies the rate varies between 60 and 85 per cent. Clinically it is believed that this drug is safe and can be used for a large variety of depressed patients with positive results.

Amitriptyline (Elavil), another of the tricyclics, was first used in the United States in 1960. Although widely used there are relatively few reports as yet published on its usage. Elavil is thought to be more effective in endogenous than in reactive depressions. It is also thought to be as effective as an antidepressant as Tofranil and somewhat less sedating. It may even have some stimulating action and produce side effects less frequently.

The dosage of Elavil is 75 to 150 mg. daily, with maintenance levels between 40 and 150 mg. daily. The initial response to the drug takes place between six and 21 days. Although it was earlier believed that Elavil would prove superior to Tofranil, patients' responses and the possible complications seem very similar.

Desipramine (Pertofrane) was introduced in 1967 with the claim that it was more rapid-acting than Tofranil. Two controlled studies, however, showed no difference in terms of effectiveness or speed of effect. Pertofrane and Norpramine as well as nortriptyline (Aventyl) have been found very effective in the treatment of patients with acute panic reactions associated with phobias.

Monoamine Oxidase Inhibitors

A number of monoamine oxidase (MAO) inhibitors have been developed since 1957. Many psychiatrists view this group of drugs as interesting but relatively unsafe compared to the other drugs available. This group contains the first antidepressants to become available for psychiatric use. Phenelzine (Nardil) is considered the most toxic of the group, followed by isocarboxazid (Marplan) and nialamide (Niamid). Any of the MAO inhibiting agents may cause a hepatitis similar to viral hepatitis but with a much higher mortality. Another complication is hypertensive crises followed by cerebral hemorrhage. Milder side effects are excruciating headaches, confusion and hyperactivity.

Isocarboxazid (Marplan) is given in doses of 10 to 30 mg. daily. In general it is considered safe but it does produce side effects similar to those mentioned earlier. Phenelzine (Nardil) is given in divided doses of 30 to 60 mg. daily. In addition to the more serious complications, it commonly produces dizziness, drowsiness, dry mouth, postural hypotension and weakness. Nardil is contraindicated in patients with liver damage and epilepsy. Nialamide (Niamid) is given in doses of 75 to 300 mg. daily. It produces fewer and milder side effects than other drugs in this group but its effect on depression is minimal. In many studies its effects are no different from those of placebos.

Tranylcypromine (Parnate) is given in doses of 10 to 30 mg. daily. In addition to its action as an MAO inhibitor, it has an amphetamine-like action. Although quite potent it produces blood and liver disorders less frequently than other MAO inhibitors, but its potentiation effect is much greater. It is thought to act more rapidly than other antidepressants and some patients respond to it who have not responded to other antidepressants. Pargyline (Eutonyl) is given in doses of 25 to 75 mg. This drug is thought to have definite antidepressant properties, but sufficient studies are not yet available to indicate whether its benefits outweigh its disadvantages.

Certain foods should not be eaten by patients taking any of the drugs in the monoamine oxidase inhibiting group. For reasons not yet clear, severe hypertensive crises followed by death may be precipitated by the ingestion of aged cheeses, especially Cheddar, Limburger, Gouda and Stilton, or Chianti wines, chicken livers or broad beans.

Amphetamine-like Stimulants

This group is the oldest of the effective drugs used for the treatment of patients with depression.

Racemic amphetamine (Benzedrine) is given in doses of 5 to 30 mg. daily. It is used very little today because of the distressing side effects and other disadvantages. The side effects of this stimulant are insomnia, severe anorexia and jitteriness.

Dextroamphetamine (Dexedrine) and methamphetamine (Desoxyn and Methedrine) have similar but less intense side effects. The daily dose of the former is 5 to 15 mg., the latter, 2.5 to 20 mg. Deanol (Deaner) is given in doses of 25 to 75 mg., but its usefulness has proved to be meager.

The disadvantages of this group of drugs are many: their effects wear off in three to four hours and a worse slump is experienced; a tolerance is built up fairly rapidly and larger doses are required; habituation may occur and a psychotic-like reaction similar to paranoid schizophrenia may result. The drugs in this group are favorites of many drug abusers, who take them for "kicks."

In spite of the disadvantages, it is believed by many that amphetamine-like stimulants still have a place in the treatment of persons with mild depressions or who are waiting for the delayed action of a drug in the tricyclic group.

Methylphenidate (Ritalin) is given in doses of 10 to 20 mg. three or four times daily. At first it was believed that this drug would do away with the problems created by the amphetamines but, in the meantime, studies reveal that all of the complications are similar. The same conclusions are reached in the case of pipradol (Meratran), which is given in doses of 2 to 7.5 mg. daily. This drug is believed to have definite stimulant properties with little or no euphorizing action.

Among the miscellaneous drugs of the fourth classification, lithium carbonate (Lithium) is given in doses of 750 to 2500 mg. daily and has just been made available in the United States as an investigational drug. Lithium has been used in Australia and in various European countries for several years in the treatment of manic states, and one of the first studies of its effectiveness was published in 1949. There must be a certain level of Lithium in the tissues before it is effective. The full effect of the drug is not reached for five to ten days after treatment is initiated. Blood serum levels must be checked three times a week, and when a maintenance dose is reached monthly blood checks are thought to be sufficient. Lithium intoxication is one complication which can be avoided if the blood serum levels are always checked. During the first few weeks of treatment side effects may occur, such as muscle weakness, thirst, polyuria, sluggishness and varied gastrointestinal symptoms which usually disappear as the patient adapts to the treatment. Many studies report a 70 to 90 per cent remission in patients with manic states. There are indications that this drug not only produces remission but also prevents a recurrence of the manic state. Further studies are required before anything more definite will be known.

Meprobamate with benactyzine, in a ratio of 400 mg. of the former to 1 mg. of the latter (Deprol), was thought to be outstanding when first introduced. It is now believed to be of little value in the treatment of patients with depression although it is helpful when some degree of sedation is indicated. Deprol is considered quite safe, with the main side effect being drowsiness.

Amphetamine with amobarbitol (Dexamyl) comes in tablet, Spansule and liquid forms. The Spansules are most commonly used now because of the sustained effect over a 10 to 12 hour period. Spansule No. 1 contains 10 mg. amphetamine and 65 mg. amobarbitol, while Spansule No. 2 contains 15 mg. amphetamine and 97 mg. amobarbitol. The time until the effect is felt is the same for both, but the intensity of the effect is greater with No. 2. Dexamyl is rapid in action, usually producing effects in 30 to 60 minutes. It has proved effective in persons with mild depressions, discouragement, pessimism, loss of interest, sensations of exhaustion and undue preoccupation with somatic "problems." Many physicians prefer this drug because it is safe and it produces neither a dulling nor an exciting effect. The only side effects, which are infrequent, are insomnia and increased motor activity.

ANTIANXIETY AGENTS

GENERIC NAME	TRADE NAME
1. Benzodiazepines	
Chlordiazepoxide	Librium
Diazepam	Valium
Oxazepam	Serax
2. Glycol or Glycerol derivatives	
Meprobamate	Equanil, Miltown
Tybamate	Solacen
Phenaglycodol	Ultran
Oxanamide	Quiactin
3. Diphenylmethane derivatives	
Hydroxyzine	Atarax, Vistaril
Benactyzine	Suavitil, Phobex
Captodiamine	Suvren
Azacylonol	Frenquel
Buclizine	Softran

There are three main drugs in the subgroup of benzodiazepines: Chlordiazepoxide (Librium) was first introduced in 1957, and by 1969 it was prescribed more frequently in the United States than any other drug. It is usually given in doses of 5 to 10 mg. three times daily but can be increased to 75 to 125 mg. daily for patients in severe anxiety states. Librium is the most sedating and motor inhibiting of this group, and it also has anticonvulsant properties. It has proved effective for individuals with symptoms of increased tension, agitation, hyperactivity and anxiety. It has only a slight effect in reducing hostility but reduces hyperactivity in almost 50 per cent of the subjects. The most common side effects of this whole group are drowsiness and ataxia.

Diazepam (Valium) has a higher potency per milligram than Librium and is usually effective in doses of 2 to 5 mg. three times a day. It also has the most stimulant-like qualities and has been helpful in hypoactivity. Valium is increasingly being used in intravenous form for status epilepticus. The newest drug of the benzodiazepine group is oxazepam (Serax), which has a lower milligram potency than Librium or Valium. The usual dose for mild anxiety is 10 to 15 mg. daily. Serax is also very effective in reducing hostility and is fairly effective in reducing hyperactivity.

The glycol or glycerol derivatives include four main drugs: Meprobamate (Equanil or Miltown) was the first antianxiety drug, introduced about 1954. It is given in a dose ranging from 1600 to 2400 mg. daily. Equanil may produce drowsiness and ataxia but has no autonomic side effects. It has proven helpful in patients whose anxiety is accompanied by insomnia. There have been many reports of dependence and withdrawal symptoms with Equanil.

Tybamate (Solacen) is relatively new and is given in doses of 750 to 1200 mg. daily. There have not been too many studies done on this drug, but some do indicate its effectiveness in reducing anxiety. One group of researchers was unable to produce any withdrawal symptoms, so in this respect it may be safer than the other glycol or glycerol derivatives.

Phenaglycodol (Ultran) is usually given in doses of 200 to 400 mg. three times daily. It is believed to have definite tranquilizing properties, to be fairly rapid in action and, thus far, to be safe enough that no absolute contraindications have been established. It has been found helpful for individuals with chronic apprehension, hyperexcitability and marked tension. Oxanamide (Quiactin), another of this group, is usually given in doses of 250 to 400 mg. three times a day and usually produces results similar to those of Ultran.

The diphenylmethane derivatives are many, but only one will be discussed here because it seems characteristic of the group. Hydroxyzine (Atarax) was one of the earlier tranquilizers and is still frequently prescribed. The usual dose is 30 to 50 mg. three times a day. It does have some potentiating qualities, especially in relation to meperidine (Demerol) and phenobarbital, and caution is indicated. It has been helpful in the treatment of patients with extreme anxiety, tension and psychomotor agitation. It is also used frequently for patients who have definite organic pathology and whose degree of apprehension is so high that it interferes with the healing process and the rest required. There have been few side effects, and studies carried over a period of four years indicate the absence of toxicity.

As is well known, it is impossible to even estimate the number of the populace who are taking one or more of the antianxiety agents and who are functioning as if they were drug free. Even the so-called "minor tranquilizers" produce periods of drowsiness, and studies definitely indicate an impairment of driving ability and judgment, concentration and visual acuity. Many believe that these drugs are both prescribed and used indiscriminately. The use of such drugs is sometimes really a "cop out" that frees the physician from having to listen to people who are having difficulty coping with the realities. There is no easier way to "turn a patient off" than to prescribe a drug that is going to make him "feel better." Often nothing is really solved, and the patient is apt to reach the point where he believes that any elevation of tension or experience of anxiety is "bad"; he may even begin to increase his dose or to add alcohol to maintain what he thinks is a comfortable level of tension.

These drugs are thought to be helpful as an adjunct to psychotherapy, but many psychiatrists are beginning to doubt their value unless the patient is in an almost constant state of acute anxiety or has a phobia which is becoming paralyzing in relation to his life activities. Other than the facts that most of the antianxiety agents can lead to dependence and habituation and that they potentiate the effects of alcohol, very little is known about them. With the pharmaceutical companies turning out new drugs so rapidly in their competition for the lucrative consumers market, it is difficult to keep abreast of the new discoveries and to really have time to evaluate them.

As soon as there is a remission of symptoms and maintenance dosage is established, the patient is usually allowed to return home with instructions about his continued medication. If the physician or nurse has a continuing relationship with the patient, it is essential that home visits be arranged and that his family be oriented so that he will continue his medications as ordered. Some type of monitoring or supervision is essential if the patient is to remain symptom-free. It has been estimated that 20 per cent of hospitalized patients do not take their medication consistently even though they are supervised.

In general, drug therapy has changed the picture in both psychiatry and psychiatric nursing considerably, although it is not considered to be the final answer to the many problems which still persist. The antipsychotic agents have been perhaps the most dramatic in bringing about the remission of symptoms for many chronically ill patients. The antidepressant agents are considered helpful in the treatment of many depressed patients, but electrotherapy is still the treatment of choice in patients with profound depression or marked suicidal tendencies. The antianxiety agents are of benefit if used discriminately.

Summary

The physiochemical therapies have been defined as specialized psychiatric treatments that are induced by either physical or chemical means and wherein emphasis is placed primarily upon the techniques selected. Although some of the older treatments may not be used to the same extent today, they should remain part of the overall means of treatment available because some patients do not respond to drug therapy or for some reason they cannot be given drugs.

A few introductory comments in regard to the history and use of insulin therapy were made. The nurse will find that the preparation of the patient for this treatment is somewhat similar to that of preparing a patient for general anesthesia. The importance of meeting the patient's needs by creating an effective static and dynamic environment has been discussed. In administering the insulin the nurse should review problems in dosage and become familiar with symptoms of hypersensitivity to the drug. It was also emphasized that during the treatment period the nurse should be able to anticipate the reaction of the patient so that she can adequately provide for his needs. The nurse's role in observing the patient has also been elaborated.

The continuous tub bath and the wet sheet pack were considered as the two most widely used hydrotherapy procedures. The preparation of the patient for these treatments is similar. The nurse will find that these procedures can be modified considerably to meet the needs of the individual patient, provided she observes the usual safety precautions and measures for promoting the patient's comfort and relaxation.

Psychopharmacology has been discussed in detail, with a suggested classification of three major groups: the antipsychotic agents, the antidepressant agents and the antianxiety agents. If one is to be involved in the use of these drugs over a period of time, it is helpful to remember the generic names of the subgroups because they do not change as often as the trade names. As the pharmaceutical companies continue their research, there will be new drugs available, each with a different name, although the basic chemical formulas are similar. There is a continual search for new antipsychotic and antidepressant agents with fewer and less dangerous side effects and for antianxiety agents that will not lead to habituation. The various drugs were considered in relation to their background, effects, dosage and side effects in order to provide some tangible basis for knowing what to anticipate when an individual is on a drug regimen.

Considerable experimentation is still taking place in most hospital situations in regard to both electrotherapy and psychosurgical methods. Electrotherapy is still the treatment of choice for many patients with depression, and newer methods of psychosurgery are being developed and used that are not as drastic as the prefrontal lobotomy. The writers have attempted to point out the more prominent needs for nursing care as they exist in the typical situation. The nurse who understands her patient and the treatment he is receiving will be able to make minor adaptations and variations in procedures as the need arises.

Bibliography

Aivazian, G. H.: "Chlorpromazine in the Withdrawal of Habit-forming Drugs in Addicts." *Dis. Nerv. System,* 16:57–60, 1955.
Arieti, Silvano: *American Handbook of Psychiatry.* Vol. II. New York, Basic Books, Inc., 1959.

Arieti, Silvano: *American Handbook of Psychiatry*. Vol. III. New York, Basic Books, Inc., 1966.

Barsa, J. A.: "The Dual Action of the Tranquilizers." *Am. J. Psychiat., 114*:74-75, 1957.

Barsa, J. A., and Kline, N. S.: "Use of Meprobamate in the Treatment of Psychotic Patients." *Am. J. Psychiat., 112*:1023-1025, 1956.

Beck, Aaron: *Depression*. New York, Harper & Row, 1967.

Beckman, Harry: *Pharmacology*, 2nd Ed., Philadelphia, W. B. Saunders Co., 1961.

Borrus, J. S.: "Study of Effects of Miltown on Psychiatric States." *J.A.M.A., 157*:1596-1598, 1955.

Bowes, H. A.: "The Ataractic Drugs: The Present Position of Chlorpromazine, Frenquel, Pacatal and Reserpine in the Psychiatric Hospital." *Am. J. Psychiat., 113*:530-539, 1956.

Brooks, W., Deutsch, L., and Dickes, R.: "The Use of Chlorpromazine Hydrochloride in the Treatment of Barbiturate Addiction with Acute Withdrawal Syndrome." *Am. J. Psychiat., 111*:696-698, 1955.

DiMascio, Alberto, and Shader, Richard (eds.): *Clinical Handbook of Psychopharmacology*. New York, Science House, 1970.

Diethelm, Oskar: *Treatment in Psychiatry*, 3rd Ed., Springfield, Ill., Charles C Thomas, Publisher, 1955.

DiPalma, J. R.: *Drill's Pharmacology in Medicine*, 3rd Ed., New York, McGraw-Hill Book Co., Inc., 1965.

Feldman, Paul E.: "A Comparative Study of Various Ataractic Drugs." *Am. J. Psychiat., 113*:589-594, 1957.

Ford, H., and Jameson, G. K.: "Chlorpromazine in Conjunction with Other Psychiatric Therapies: A Clinical Appraisal." *Dis. Nerv. System, 16*:179-185, 1955.

Gearren, J. B.: "Trifluoperazine in Emotionally Disturbed Office Patients." *Dis. Nerv. System, 20*:66-68, 1959.

Goldman, D.: "Treatment of Psychotic States with Chlorpromazine." *J.A.M.A., 157*:1274-1278, 1955.

Goodman, Louis S., and Gilman, Alfred: *The Pharmacological Basis of Therapeutics*. 3rd Ed., New York, Macmillan Co., 1965.

Havens, Leston L.: "Some Difficulties in Giving Schizophrenic and Borderline Patients Medication." *Psychiatry, 31*:44-50, 1968.

Hayes, R. H., and Warbner, I.: "Chlorpromazine in the Treatment of Symptomatically Refractory Conditions in General Paretics." *Dis. Nerv. System, 17*:48-52, 1956.

Himwich, Harold: *Brain Metabolism and Cerebral Disorders*. Baltimore, Williams & Wilkins Co., 1951.

Hollister, L. E., Stannard, A. N., and Drake, C. F.: "Treatment of Anxious Patients with Drugs." *Dis. Nerv. System, 17*:289-293, 1956.

Hollister, L. E.: "Clinical Use of Psychotherapeutic Drugs: Current Status." *Clin. Pharmacol. Therap., 10*:170-198, 1969.

Kalinowsky, Lothar B., and Hoch, Paul H.: *Somatic Treatments in Psychiatry*, New York, Grune & Stratton, Inc., 1961.

Kinross-Wright, Vernon: "Chlorpromazine—A Major Advance in Psychiatric Treatment." *Postgrad. Med., 16*:297-299, 1954.

Kinross-Wright, Vernon: "Chlorpromazine Treatment of Mental Disorders." *Am. J. Psychiat., 111*:907-912, 1955.

Korn, R. J., Rock, W., and Zimmerman, H. J.: "Studies of Hepatic Function in Patients Receiving Promazine." *Am. J. M. Sc., 235*:431-436, 1958.

Kurland, A. A.: "Chlorpromazine in the Management of the Institutionalized Aged Psychiatric Patient with Chronic Brain Syndrome." *Dis Nerv. System, 16*:366-369, 1955.

Lehmann, H. E., and Hanrahan, G. E.: "Chlorpromazine: New Inhibiting Agent for Psychomotor Excitement andManic States." *Arch. Neurol. & Psychiat., 71*:227-231, 1954.

Lemere, F.: "Combined Chlorpromazine-Reserpine Therapy of Psychiatric Disorders." *Arch. Neurol. & Psychiat., 74*:1-2, 1955.

Lesse, Stanley: "An Evaluation of Promazine Hydrochloride in Psychiatric Practice." *Am. J. Psychiat., 113*:984-987, 1957.

McAfoos, L. G. Jr.: "Prochlorperazine in Emotional Disturbances." *Dis. Nerv. System, 18*:430-433, 1957.

Myers, J. B., and Rosen, H. B.: "Psychiatrists' Current Attitudes about Psychiatric Treatment." *Compr. Psychiat.*, 7:232-239, 1966.

Noce, R. H., Williams, D. B., and Rapaport, W.: "Reserpine in the Management of the Mentally Ill." *J.A.M.A.*, *158*:11-15, 1955.

Perlstein, M. A.: "Use of Meprobamate in Convulsive and Related Disorders." *J.A.M.A.*, *161*:1040-1044, 1956.

Pollack, B.: "The Effect of Chlorpromazine on the Return Rate of 250 Patients Released from the Rochester State Hospital." *Am. J. Psychiat.*, *112*:937-938, 1956.

Redlich, Frederick, and Freedman, Daniel: *The Theory and Practice of Psychiatry.* New York, Basic Books, Inc., 1966.

Rickles, K. E.: *Non-Specific Factors in Drug Therapy.* Springfield, Ill., Charles C Thomas, 1968.

Rosner, B. S., Fierman, L. B., and Kramer, J. F.: "Clinical Evaluation of Meratran and Frenquel on a Chronic Psychotic Population." *Am. J. Psychiat.* *113*:993-996, 1957.

Rudy, L. H., Himwich, H. E., and Tasher, D. C.: "Clinical Evaluation of Two Phenothiazine Compounds, Promazine and Mepazine." *Am. J. Psychiat.* *113*:979-983, 1957.

Scharmer, Bernice: "Insulin Shock Therapy." *Am. J. Nursing*, *41*:1154-1156, 1941.

Smith, J. A., Warner, R., Wolford, J. A., and Rutherford, A.: "Tranquilizing Medication in the Aged Mentally Ill." *Geriatrics*, *12*:549-552, 1957.

Thal, Nathan: "Clinical Evaluation of Chlorpromazine Therapy for Psychiatric Disorders." *Northwest Med.*, *55*:653-656, 1956.

Tourney, Garfield, Isberg, E. M., and Gottlieb, J. S.: "The Use of Reserpine in an Acute Psychiatric Treatment Setting." *Arch. Neurol. & Psychiat.*, *74*:325-328, 1955.

Wilson, W. P., and Glotfelty, J. S.: "Effect of Intravenous Promazine on Arousal Responses in Man." *Dis. Nerv. System*, *19*:307-309, 1958.

Wright, Rebekah: *Hydrotherapy in Psychiatric Hospitals.* Boston, Tudor Press, Inc., 1940.

Suggestions for Further Reading

Ayd, Frank J.: "The Chemical Assault on Mental Illness." *Am. J. Nursing*, 1965: "The Major Tranquilizers," *65*:70-78; "The Minor Tranquilizers," *65*:89-94: "The Antidepressants," *65*:78-84.

Behnken, Priscilla, and Merrill, Elizabeth Good: "Nursing Care Following Prefrontal Lobotomy." *Am. J. Nursing*, *49*:431-434, 1949.

Berblinger, Klaus, W.: "The Influence of Personalities on Drug Therapy." *Am. J. Nursing*, *59*:1130-1132, 1959.

Bross, Robert B.: "The Modern Mood-changing Drugs." *Am. J. Nursing*, *57*:1142-1143, 1957.

Caffey, Eugene C., Jr., Hollister, Leo, Kaim, Samuel, and Pokorny, Alex D.: "Drug Treatment in Psychiatry." *Inter. J. Psychiat.*, *9*:428-473, 1970-71.

Halliday, A. M., Davison, K., Brown, M. W., and Kreeger, L. C.: "A Comparison of the Effects on Depression and Memory of Bilateral E.C.T. and Unilateral E.C.T. to the Dominant and Non-dominant Hemispheres." *Brit. J. Psychiat.*, *114*:997-1012, 1968.

Harmer, Bertha, and Henderson, Virginia: *Textbook of the Principles and Practice of Nursing*, 5th Ed., rev., New York, Macmillan Co., 1955, pp. 608-653.

Hollister, Leo E.: "Choice of Antipsychotic Drugs." *Am. J. Psychiat.*, *127*:186-190, 1970.

Inglis, James: "Shock, Surgery and Cerebral Asymmetry." *Brit. J. Psychiat.*, *117*:143-148, 1970.

Ingram, Madelene Elliott: *Principles of Psychiatric Nursing*, 5th Ed., Philadelphia, W. B. Saunders Co., 1960, pp. 275-317.

Lynn, Frances H., and Friedhoff, Arnold J.: "The Patient on a Tranquilizing Regimen." *Am. J. Nursing*, *60*:234-240, 1960.

Maloney, Elizabeth M., and Johannesen, Lucile: "How the Tranquilizers Affect Nursing Practice." *Am. J. Nursing*, *57*:1144-1147, 1957.

Post, Felix, Rees, W. Linford, and Schurr, Peter: "An Evaluation of Bimedial Leucotomy." *Brit. J. Psychiat.*, *114*:1223-1246, 1968.

Sherman, Clinton C., and Charbonneau, Leon O.: "Electric Shock Therapy." *Am. J. Nursing, 48*:294-296, 1948.

Steele, Katharine McLean, and Manfreda, Marguerite Lucy: *Psychiatric Nursing,* 6th Ed., Philadelphia, F. A. Davis Co., 1959, pp. 459-489.

Valentine, Max, Keddie, K. M. G., and Dunne, David: "A Comparison of Techniques in Electro-Convulsive Therapy." *Brit. J. Psychiat., 114*:989-996, 1968.

Wharton, Ralph N.: "Electroshock Treatment: Two Novel Problems." *Am. J. Psychiat., 125*:397-398, 1968.

Whittington, H. G., Zahourek, Rorry, and Grey, Leslie: "Pharmaco-Therapy and Community Psychiatric Practice." *Am. J. Psychiat., 126*:551-554, 1969.

Chapter 12   Combined High- and Low-Visibility Nursing Functions in Various Therapies

In this chapter, a few of the more accepted and more widely used innovations, with which the nurse might have experience in her initial psychiatric nursing practice, are described. The degree to which her function is high or low visibility depends upon her level of understanding and the structure of the specific situation.

THE DAY OR NIGHT HOSPITAL

These facilities have been in existence for quite a while in certain areas but still exist merely on paper in too many instances. As the names imply, day and night hospitals are transitional facilities and provide care for the patient during the interim when he no longer needs complete hospitalization but is not yet ready to assume his full role at home or in the community. Some patients spend the day at home with their families or at work and then return to the hospital for the night. Other patients spend the night at home and return to the hospital for the day, usually an eight hour period.

In the day hospital there is usually a schedule of activities in which all patients participate. There is an opportunity for group meetings in which common problems can be discussed and an approach to solving these problems can be evolved. Sometimes members of the families are encouraged to come in for the day or one evening a week to become better oriented to the patient's problems and to be better prepared to help him in his readjustment at home when he is discharged.

Some day hospitals admit acutely ill patients and have a separate unit adjoining the convalescent unit for them. These units usually have a psychiatrist in attendance at all times, and treatment is started immediately. The activities on such a unit depend upon the degree of illness manifested by the patient population. Psychopharmacology, electrotherapy and other physiochemical measures may be used and then, as they are able, the patients join the groups in the regular day hospital for occupational and recreational therapy and discussions.

What is actually done and how it is done in a day hospital depend upon the basic philosophy and the underlying beliefs of those responsible for the unit. As a rule, uniforms are not worn by nursing personnel, who are encouraged to interact with patients on a friendly, supportive level.

BEHAVIOR THERAPY OR BEHAVIOR MODIFICATION

Underlying the development of this type of treatment are Pavlov's classical experiments on conditioning plus the learning theory constructs. To do justice to its evolution, a review of the development of experimental psychology would be necessary. One factor which served as an impetus to its development was the dissatisfaction of the clinical psychologist with his traditional role in the care and treatment of psychiatric patients. Many people describe behavior modification as a protest movement and many loaded comments have been exchanged by the various therapists.

One of the definitions of behavior therapy states that it is an attempt to change human behavior in a positive direction using the laws of modern learning theory. This raises the question of whether or not we have actually established "laws" in relation to the different levels of learning. Is complex human behavior just labeled according to the principles of conditioning? Or can it really be explained?

Behavior modification (the preferred term in the United States) is an approach to the treatment of behavior disorders with the intent of alleviating specific behavioral problems as quickly as possible by controlling the learning behavior of the individual. The focus of the treatment is upon overt behavior. Initially most of the procedures could be classified as operant, aversion or desensitization techniques; today there are many combinations of these as well as new techniques being used, i.e., modeling, coverant procedures, implosive devices, flooding and covert sensitization.

The actual practice in the field of behavior modification now draws more heavily from experimental psychology since there is some disagreement among therapists about the actual mechanisms (processes) of learning. Many suggest that the therapy not be identified by its techniques because its main attribute is an assessment strategy which reflects an empirical orientation that attempts to alter the behavior deficit observed in the individual case.

In general, the behavioral therapist says that he does not deal with value judgments, since behavior cannot be good or bad. Behavior invariably has consequences, however, which are labeled desirable (good) or undesirable (bad). This statement is neither new nor different from what has been believed and stated in many ways over the years.

One of the basic techniques of behavior therapy is to arrange contingencies between the patient's behavior and the consequences of that behavior. A good consequence is typically referred to as a reward (positive reinforcer), whereas a bad consequence is viewed as something that is undesirable (negative reinforcer). The environment is purposely structured so that behavior becomes the vehicle by which rewards are acquired or undesirable occurrences prevented.

The behavioral therapist insists that complete consistency be maintained in manipulating and structuring the patients' environment, making all necessities as well as luxuries of daily life contingent upon some behavior. All of this is provided for by a treatment plan which indicates the initial and terminal behavior involved in therapy—stated in specific terms of what and how the patient will act if he is progressing toward the goal; the reinforcers to be used for the specific patient—a list of the stimuli which function as reinforcers for that patient and can be used to strengthen behavior; a description of situations which are to serve as control stimuli—these can operate in two ways, to increase control or to relax control.

The nursing personnel have to be oriented to this form of treatment and the goals involved. Whether or not they help develop the plan for treatment depends upon the specific situation. They do, however, usually implement the plan, keep the records and help evaluate the results. In many ways, carrying out these techniques is similar to the step by step procedures that used to make up the bulk of traditional nursing care.

This type of therapy is still new, as practiced today, and is constantly changing; however, it will take several years to find out if it really "cures," if it facilitates remissions or if it has a place in prevention of behavior with undesirable effects. It has been used for patients with psychoses, neuroses, character disorders, mental retardation and organic brain syndromes within a wide range of ages. Some degree of success has been reported. It is now being used with "problem" children in kindergarten and first grade, who are rewarded for desirable behaviors.

THE WALK-IN CLINIC

The first walk-in psychiatric clinic was opened in New York City in 1956, and since then many more have been established throughout the United States. They are more apt to be found in the metropolitan areas, although there is a great need for them in all areas. As the name implies, the emphasis is on immediate treatment, which may be initiated from five minutes to two hours after application, and on short-term therapy, usually a fixed number of visits during a certain period that is arbitrarily determined. The organization of the clinic differs with the institution of which it is a part, but in general the services which they provide are similar.

An effective walk-in clinic requires an adequate staff, not only in terms of number but in terms of preparation. Here, if anywhere, is needed a smooth-functioning psychiatric team composed of individuals who are experts in their particular disciplines: psychiatrist, psychiatric nurse, social worker and psychologist. In addition to their expertise, they need some orientation to and understanding of the problems of the financially, educationally or socially deprived person. Knowledge about economic and housing problems, community pressures, jobs available or job training programs is invaluable.

The team, by pooling observations, interview data, test results and so forth must make an almost instant assessment of the presenting patient's situation and must develop a plan of action which will not only be "helpful" to the patient but will be perceived by him as being helpful. The initial visit is crucial in terms of reducing the patient's immediate stress, of determining whether he will return again and of stimulating hopeful expectations.

Walk-in clinics have been remarkably successful in providing services to a large segment of the population never before reached who have many immediate problems with which they must learn to cope. The degree of the clinics' success is not yet available in statistical form but can be reflected in the increase in the number of patients who "walk in." They apparently have received the word that help is available.

THE THERAPEUTIC COMMUNITY

The term "therapeutic community" was originated by Dr. Maxwell Jones, who has had over three decades of experience with therapeutic communities in hospitals. This concept is based on the premise that the social or interpersonal milieu can be an instrument in treatment.

The suggested basic characteristics of a positive environment for the hospitalized psychiatric patient have been reiterated over and over since chains and torture chambers were supposedly removed as methods of treatment. These characteristics, although not all-inclusive, suggest that the patient's environment be humanitarian (vs. oppressive), flexible (vs. rigid), democratic (vs. authoritarian) and treatment-oriented (vs. custodial). All of these ideas, plus the conceptualization of psychiatric illness as a social and interpersonal phenomenon, are incorporated into a therapeutic community. Anyone familiar with the writings of Dr. Harry Stack Sullivan will recognize this as one of his basic tenets.

In addition, the therapeutic community utilizes the total social structure of the hospital unit as the helping process. As Maxwell Jones has said, we can learn a great deal from observing the patient in his day-to-day social environment and from seeing how he relates to other people, how he reacts to stress and so forth. Dr. Jones believes that if at the same time the patient can be made aware of how he affects other people and can learn to understand some of the motivations underlying his behavior, the situation is potentially therapeutic. Furthermore, he believes that this can be considered the distinctive quality of a therapeutic community.

Within this community, there is an organization of groups and subgroups which meet daily or at various times each week to solve certain tasks. The "community meeting" consists of all of the staff and the patients involved in the unit, who get together to discuss whatever is relevant to the functioning of the group. The focus is upon two-way communication, group interaction, decision-making and shared responsibility. In a community that is functioning well, the atmosphere is characteristically warm, accepting, optimistic and friendly. In other words, all members of the group are encouraged to relate to each other as "real" people, to get involved in whatever is the center of the group's attention at the time and to work through, clarify and validate what has occurred or what is going on. In order to achieve this, however, it is essential to have well-qualified leaders who have an understanding of the dynamics of groups and interpersonal interaction and are able to interact with the members in a non-threatening way. Such group leaders must have considerable self-understanding and must be sensitive to people and their needs. After a community meeting, it is essential that the staff have an opportunity to get together with a skilled leader to reflect on and clarify what they, as members of the group, were doing and to validate their motivations. In this way the total community grows.

This system of groups, through which patients interact in a variety of situations with other patients and staff, provides great possibilities for an adequate feedback so that all involved may become more aware of their actions. The basic assumption of the whole concept of the therapeutic community is that the "leader," more than any other member of that society, knows what he is doing and why.

In addition to the various meetings, there is usually a schedule of activities in occupational therapy, recreational therapy, industrial therapy and vocational rehabilitation to occupy the rest of the patients' day.

The basic principles underlying the development and maintenance of a "truly" therapeutic community must be accepted by the professional staff and other personnel on more than a verbal level. It involves a belief in the dignity of the patient as a person, in his common humanness and in his potentials for growth and more productive living. It requires an absence of ridicule, disparagement, disgust, hopelessness and indifference.

It is doubtful if Dr. Maxwell Jones would agree with the label of "therapeutic community" for many of the situations which have adopted this name merely because they have group meetings between the personnel and the patients. The activities which go on within some of these situations are not even therapeutic for the non-patient members and only serve as sanctions to reinforce the acting out of their own "hang-ups." In these situations we often hear the following cliches: "Let's get things on the table!" "We must be truthful!" Who is "we?" The patient and personnel or just the patient? We must be truthful with whom? With others, with ourselves or with both?

A therapeutic community is not a medium for true confession! It is not a license for the acting out of staff problems! It is not a means to elevate the egoistic esteem of the self-designated "therapist" or manipulator! It is not a method for evoking or increasing the anxiety and the fears of patients by backing them into a corner or by coercing them to do what is thought to be best for them. A high quality of custodial care provided by nursing personnel who were really concerned about the patients would be far superior to this "therapeutic community."

A real therapeutic community can be called a school for living; as Sullivan stated, all psychiatric hospitals should be places where both patients and personnel grow in the skills and understandings necessary for more effective living. An effective therapeutic community requires the skills of collaboration of the total staff involved. These are skills acquired only on the highest level of interpersonal interaction. In a setting characterized by collaboration, the energy and potential of all members are directed toward a common goal. A feeling of "we" and a sensitivity to the feelings of others permeates the group. We all know how difficult it is to get a group of people to even cooperate, a social skill that should be developed in the juvenile or latency period of development. We are in dire need of more methods of helping people to grow up, to mature and to develop their inherent potentials.

Bibliography

Ackerman, Nathan: *The Psychodynamics of Family Life.* New York, Basic Books, Inc., 1958.
Anthony, E. James, and Benedek, Therese (eds.): *Parenthood: Its Psychology and Psychopathology.* Boston, Little, Brown & Co., 1970.
Arieti, Silvano (ed.): *American Handbook of Psychiatry.* Vol. III. New York, Basic Books, Inc., 1966.
Bandura, A.: *Principles of Behavior Modification.* New York, Holt, Rinehart & Winston, 1969.
Cumming, John, and Cumming, Elaine: *Ego and Milieu.* New York, Prentice Hall, 1962.
Edelson, Marshall: *The Practice of Sociotherapy.* New Haven, Yale University Press, 1970.
Franks, C. M.: *Behavior Therapy: Appraisal and Status.* New York, McGraw-Hill, 1969.
Jones, Maxwell: *The Therapeutic Community: A New Treatment Method in Psychiatry.* New York, Basic Books, Inc., 1953.
Jones, Maxwell: *Beyond the Therapeutic Community: Social Learning and Social Psychiatry.* New Haven, Yale University Press, 1968.
Mowrer, O. Hobart: *Learning Theory and Behavior.* New York, John Wiley & Sons, Inc., 1960.
Rapoport, Robert: *Community as Doctor.* Springfield, Illinois, Charles C Thomas, 1960.
Sullivan, Harry S.: *The International Theory of Psychiatry.* New York, W. W. Norton and Co., Inc., 1953.
Yates, Aubrey J.: *Behavior Therapy.* New York, John Wiley & Sons, Inc., 1970.

Suggestions for Further Reading

Ackerman, Nathan, and Behrens, Marjorie: "The Family Approach and Levels of Intervention." *Amer. J. Psychotherapy, 22:*5-14, 1968.
Agras, W. S.: "Behavior Therapy in the Management of Chronic Schizophrenia." *Amer. J. Psychiat., 124:*240-243, 1967.
Barnard, R. I., Robins, L. L., and Tetzlaff, F. M.: "The Day Hospital as an Extension of Psychiatric Treatment." *Bull. Menninger Clin., 16:*50-56, 1952.
Brady, J. P.: "Psychotherapy, Learning Theory, and Insight." *Arch. Gen. Psychiat., 16:*304-311, 1967.
Brody, Warren: "On Family Therapy." *Family Process, 2:*280-287, 1963.
Carmichael, Donald M.: "A Psychiatric Day Hospital for Convalescent Patients." *Mental Hospitals, 11:*7, 1960.
DeYoung, Carol: "The Nurse's Contribution in Family Crisis Treatment." *Nurs. Outlook, 16:*60-62, 1968.
Glaser, Frederick B.: "Our Place: Design for a Day Program." *Amer. J. Orthopsychiat., 39:*827-841, 1969.
Greenblatt, Milton, Levinson, David, and Williams: *The Patient and The Mental Hospital.* Glencoe, Illinois, The Free Press, 1957.
Haley, Jay: "Whither Family Therapy?" *Family Process, 1:*69-100, 1962.

Hogarty, Gerard E., Dennis, Helen, Guy, William, and Gross, Gertrude M.: "Who Goes There?—A Critical Evaluation of Admissions to a Psychiatric Day Hospital." *Amer. J. Orthopsychiat., 124*:934–944, 1968.

Lazarus, A. A.: "Behavior Therapy, Incomplete Treatment, and Symptom Substitution." *J. Nerv. Ment. Dis., 140*:80–86, 1965.

Libermann, Robert: "Behavioral Approaches to Family and Couple Therapy." *Amer. J. Orthopsychiat., 40*:106–118, 1920.

Lindemann, Erich: "Preventive Intervention in Situational Crises." *J. Cl. Psychol., 4*:69, 1962.

Normand, William, Fensterheim, Herbert, Tannebaum, Gerald, and Sager, Clifford: "Acceptance of a Psychiatric Walk-In Clinic in a Deprived Community." *Amer. J. Psychiat., 120*:533, 1963.

Papanek, Helen: "Therapeutic and Antitherapeutic Factors in Group Relations." *Amer. J. Psychotherapy, 23*:396–404, 1969.

Sadock, Benjamin, Newman, Lenore, and Normand, William C.: "Short-Term Group Psychotherapy in a Psychiatric Walk-In Clinic." *Amer. J. Orthopsychiat., 38*:724–732, 1968.

Sager, Clifford, J., Masters, Yvonne J., Rondall, Ruth E., and Normand, William C.: "Selection and Engagement of Patients in Family Therapy." *Amer. J. Orthopsychiat., 38*:715–723, 1968.

Satir, Virginia: *Conjoint Family Therapy.* Palo Alto, Science and Behavior Books, 2nd ed., 1967.

Visher, John S., and O'Sullivan, Maureen: "Nurse and Patient Responses to a Study of Milieu Therapy." *Amer. J. Orthopsychiat., 127*:451–456.

Warner, James: "Conjoint Family Therapy." *The Royal Society of Health J. 90*:262–263, 1970.

Wilder, Jack, and Coleman, Marshall: "The Walk-In Psychiatric Clinic, Some Observations and Follow-Up." *Inter. J. Social Psychiat., 9*:192, 1963.

Williams, Jack, Dudley, Harold K. and Guinn, Terry J.: "Use of Day Treatment Center Concepts with State Hospital Inpatients." *Amer. J. Orthopsychiat., 39*:748–752, 1969.

Zeilberger, J., Sampen, S. E., and Sloan, H. W.: "Modification of a Child's Problem Behaviors in the Home With the Mother as Therapist." *J. Appl. Behav. Anal., 1*:47–53, 1968.

Zeitlyn, B. B.: "The Therapeutic Community—Fact or Fantasy?" *Inter. J. Psychiat., 7*:195–200, 1969.

Zwerling, Israel, and Mendelsohn, Marilyn: "Initial Family Reaction to Day Hospitalization." *Family Process, 4*:50–63, 1965.

Part Three   The Psychiatric Patient and His Socio-Environmental Milieu

Chapter 13 Patients with Feelings of Anxiety and Stereotypic Responses

The greater the depth of understanding and the broader the frame of reference one has in relation to human motivation, needs, defenses, patterns of interaction and communication, and the greater the understanding of the processes of normal growth and development and the crises of each period which may lead to ineffective patterns of living, the better one will be able to understand oneself, the psychiatric patient and the people who have problems for which they must seek help. The patient has the same basic hierarchy of needs as each of us although his wants, desires and wishes may be different, depending upon the degree of his illness. As was implied in Chapters 4, 7, and 8, one does not have to be a psychiatric patient to distort reality and to live according to that distortion.

In order to plan and provide nursing care for patients with feelings of anxiety and stereotypic responses, the nurse must learn first to observe their behavior and then to interpret it in terms of their needs. This interpretation will, of course, involve an understanding of the basic dynamics underlying the behavior of these patients. Since it would not be feasible to discuss every possible neurotic manifestation, two patterns which pose many problems for the nurse have been selected, the anxious and the stereotypic.

UNDERSTANDING THE ANXIOUS PATIENT

The anxious patient, as a rule, is very restless. He may show this increase of tension by movement of his extremities, by pacing the halls, or by general fidgeting. The nurse will anticipate that his overt behavior pattern will become disorganized. Very often the patient expresses this feeling as being afraid something terrible is going to happen or as just not feeling well. He is unable to concentrate or to focus his attention on anything for any period of time.

By observing him closely, the nurse will be able to recognize cues to the many physiologic changes that occur during this period. His heart rate may increase and he may have tachycardia, which will tend to further increase his fears as his respirations also become more rapid. He will usually begin to perspire more, and if the nurse checks his blood pressure during this time it will undoubtedly be elevated. He may also experience a lump in his throat and complain about being thirsty. At any time during this acute phase, the patient may develop diarrhea and/or frequency of urination. His appetite, too, may be influenced—that is, he may suddenly lose his appetite or he may become extremely hungry. In general, the patient tends to behave as though his very existence were threatened, and he is completely helpless in coping with the situation.

What does this behavior of the anxious patient mean? What is he trying to communicate to us? What are his needs for nursing care? As his overt behavior informs us, this patient is frightened, and he acts as though the threat comes from the external environment. The various physiologic changes that he experiences are due to the action of the autonomic nervous system and are obviously preparations for activity, as though he could deal with this threat by attacking it or fleeing from it. All this preparation, however, is ineffective because the conflict is within the individual; he is unable to escape it although he has already tried through repression.

Throughout this period, the ego is more or less overwhelmed by all of this excitation. Since the ego has no immediately available means of coping with the situation as it is perceived, regression occurs. During the anxiety attack the patient is making an appeal for help so that he will not be injured, abandoned, ridiculed or condemned. Since there is regression, some of the individual's ego functions are disturbed, which further hinders his ability to cope with his environment.

NURSE-PATIENT INTERACTION

The role of the nurse during the patient's acute periods of anxiety is primarily supportive. Since the patient feels so lonely and threatened he will usually seek the company of the nurse, and the nurse should be very alert to what he is trying to communicate to her. As a rule this patient does not ask in so many words for the nurse to remain with him, but he is apt to make many picayunish requests and may become demanding if the nurse does not understand what he really wants. Because of his fears and increased tension, this individual usually wants to talk. The nurse can help him by listening and perhaps by offering comments that will encourage him to express his feelings. He wants to be taken care of, and the nurse's interest at this time will make him feel a little less threatened. It may help, too, for the nurse to offer him a cigarette, something to drink or a snack to eat, since his oral needs are very intense.

This patient has very little tolerance for stress or delay at any time, and, with his increased irritability, he tends to build up tension readily. The nurse, therefore, will try to fulfill his needs with as little delay as possible unless his physician has ordered otherwise. Other than during his acute periods of distress, the nurse will try to interest him in participating in activities. She will select something that can be accomplished fairly quickly, which is not beyond his current capacity for concentration. Since he is extremely sensitive to noise, it is helpful for the nurse to minimize environmental stimuli at specified times to enable this patient to get adequate rest.

UNDERSTANDING THE PATIENT WITH STEREOTYPIC RESPONSES

The patient with stereotypic behavior is usually a rigid, meticulous person who is overtly considerate of others. He may be slow and precise about everything that he does. He may also show great concern about doing what is "right" and question the nurse about many minor details in an attempt to reassure himself that what he does is all right. We also anticipate that this individual will have some kind of ritual that he will have to carry out periodically regardless of the activities in the over-all situation. In this way he may appear very possessive and controlling of the objects in his environment; this behavior, in turn, may often arouse the resentment of other persons in his environment. At the same time he may become very upset if there is any change in the routine or usual schedule of activities.

This individual's interpersonal relationships may show many other distortions. His general attitude is one of doubt and indecision, with considerable vacillation toward those to whom he relates. In addition, he appears rather cold and abstract and seems to lack genuineness and warmth in his relationships.

What does this behavior of the ritualistic patient mean? Why does he act this way? Just as in all other neurotic manifestations, the ritualistic behavior of this patient evolves from conflicts that he has not been able to resolve. Some of the major alternatives that are usually involved are aggressiveness and submissiveness, disorder and order, dirtiness and cleanliness. This individual is so torn between what to do and what not to do that the constant increase of tension threatens to disintegrate him entirely. He consequently attempts to arrange his world so that nothing unexpected can happen that will require a spontaneous decision. Only when he feels that everything is under control can he gain any feeling of being safe. One of his constant fears seems to be that of losing control; therefore, many of his rigid patterns are the result of reaction formations that are to reinforce his control over his real impulses and feelings.

At the same time he fears being controlled by others and tries to maintain his relationships on a superficial level. Another pattern that he uses extensively is that of isolation; this pattern gives him that cold, detached manner in his interaction with others. His general attitude toward himself is one of helplessness and worthlessness, which further increases his tendency toward passivity. His ritualistic behavior may sometimes be for the purpose of atonement, it may be to prevent certain of his unconscious wishes from being fulfilled, it may be a form of punishment or it may be to postpone punishment. Regardless of the purpose involved, the patient has the feeling that he must perform the act or he will be overwhelmed by intense anxiety. Even though he knows and may say that the action is foolish, his tension continues to build up until he follows through with the ritual.

This individual is basically an extremely hostile person who anticipates that others are, in turn, going to be hostile toward him. His intrapersonal relationships are dominated by his superego, which functions in a cruel, relentless, punishing manner. He seems overly ready to experience guilt at the slightest opportunity. In addition to the conflicts already mentioned, his regression revives further conflicts that he experienced during his years of development, and he now experiences increased guilt, anxiety and ambivalence as a result of them.

NURSE-PATIENT INTERACTION

In providing care for the patient with stereotypic responses, the nurse should anticipate that he may be slow and precise in everything that he does; therefore, she will make allowances for the time factor so that he will not feel unnecessarily pushed. It is helpful for the nurse to begin preparing this patient a little while before he is to be ready for specific activities, since his progress may be slowed down by his rituals or his meticulousness. The nurse should not try to interfere with or prevent this patient from carrying out his rituals unless specifically ordered by his physician. The nurse will remember that this patient may require others to fit into his rituals, and this behavior is a reflection of his need to control his environment. She will also be alert to the hostility that this control may evoke in others so that she can minimize these instances, since they will make the patient feel more guilty, which, in turn, will increase his need to control. Because he is extremely sensitive to rebuke or criticism and is overly ready to experience guilt, the nurse may also have to protect him in this area.

The nurse should be permissive and accepting of this patient and sincere in her contacts with him, even if he does become hostile. She will recall that he has a great deal of repressed hostility and that he anticipates that others will be hostile in return. Furthermore, this patient needs the opportunity to express his feelings; but since he is afraid of his hostility, he may be overwhelmed if too much is provoked before he can handle it. The nurse will anticipate that he may lack warmth in their interaction but she will continue to communicate her interest in him. She may tend to become discouraged by his apparent lack of responsiveness, but when she understands that this lack of genuineness is due to isolation of his feelings she will be more tolerant.

Since he also feels worthless and has a strong need for approval, the nurse will tell him when he does things well. She will select activities for him that have some value so he can gain a feeling of accomplishment.

Summary

Patients with two of the neurotic patterns, anxiety and stereotypic responses, were selected as representative of those with neurotic manifestations. Each of these patients was discussed in relation to usual behavior patterns, the meaning of this behavior and some of the main points in nursing care.

Bibliography

Alexander, Franz, and Ross, Helen, eds.: *Dynamic Psychiatry*. Chicago, University of Chicago Press, 1962.
Bergler, Edmund: *The Super Ego*. New York, Grune & Stratton, Inc., 1952.
Cameron, Norman: *The Psychology of Behavior Disorders*. Boston, Houghton Mifflin Co., 1947.
Deutsch, Helene: *Psychoanalysis of the Neuroses*. London, Hogarth Press, 1951.
Fenichel, Otto: *The Psychoanalytic Theory of Neurosis*. New York, W. W. Norton & Co., Inc., 1945.

Freud, Sigmund: *The Problem of Anxiety.* New York, W. W. Norton & Co., Inc., 1936.

Fromm-Reichmann, Frieda: *Principles of Intensive Psychotherapy.* Chicago, University of Chicago Press, 1950.

Fromm-Reichmann, Frieda: *Psychoanalysis and Psychotherapy.* Chicago, University of Chicago Press, 1959.

Horney, Karen: *Our Inner Conflicts.* New York, W. W. Norton & Co., Inc., 1945.

May, Rollo: *The Meaning of Anxiety.* New York, Ronald Press Co., 1950.

Odier, Charles: *Anxiety and Magic Thinking.* New York, International Universities Press, Inc., 1956.

Redlich, Frederick C., and Freedman, Daniel X.: *The Theory and Practice of Psychiatry.* New York, Basic Books, Inc., 1966.

Sullivan, Harry Stack: *Conceptions of Modern Psychiatry.* New York, W. W. Norton & Co., Inc., 1953.

Sullivan, Harry Stack: *The Interpersonal Theory of Psychiatry.* New York, W. W. Norton & Co., Inc., 1953.

Sullivan, Harry Stack: *Clinical Studies in Psychiatry.* New York, W. W. Norton & Co., Inc., 1956.

Suggestions for Further Reading

Arieti, Silvano (ed.): *American Handbook of Psychiatry.* Vol. I. New York, Basic Books, Inc., 1959, pp. 237-416.

Falstein, Eugene, and Sutton, Helen A.: "Childhood Schizophrenia." *Am. J. Nursing, 58:*666, 1958.

Friedman, David B.: "Obsessive Hyperamnesia and Free Association As a Transference Resistance." *Am. J. Psycotherapy, 21:*105-111, 1967.

Marks, I. M., Crowe, M., Drewe, E., Young, J., and Dewhurst, W. G.: "Obsessive Compulsive Neurosis in Identical Twins." *Brit. J. Psychiat., 115:*991-998, 1969.

Maslow, A. H., and Mittelmann, Bela: *Principles of Abnormal Psychology.* New York, Harper & Brothers, 1951, pp. 417-425, 426-430, 431-438, 439-453, 454-469.

Norris, Catherine M.: "The Nurse and the Crying Patient." *Am. J. Nursing, 57:*323-327, 1957.

Noyes, Arthur P., and Kolb, Lawrence C.: *Modern Clinical Psychiatry.* 6th Ed., Philadelphia, W. B. Saunders Co., 1963, pp. 425-430, 443-448.

Ruesch, Jurgen: *Disturbed Communication.* New York, W. W. Norton & Co., Inc., 1957, pp. 127-130, 134-137.

Thorner, Melvin: *Psychiatry in General Practice.* Philadelphia, W. B. Saunders Co., 1948, pp. 291-335.

Warters, Jane: *Achieving Maturity.* New York, McGraw-Hill Book Co., Inc., 1949, pp. 213-244.

Chapter 14 The Patient With Autistic Behavior

In order to plan and provide nursing care for the autistic individual, the nurse must first learn to observe his behavior and to interpret it in terms of his needs. This latter activity will involve an understanding of the patient's psychopathology and the dynamic factors that underlie his behavior.

This individual is called autistic because he appears absorbed in his fantasy to the exclusion of any interest in reality. Seclusive is another term that is sometimes used to describe this person—that is, he has withdrawn and isolated himself from his external environment. These patterns of autism and seclusiveness are apt to be manifested in many of the clinical syndromes. They are a prominent aspect of all schizophrenic reactions. They may also be evident in organic and toxic disorders, as in the older patient who encases himself in a shell and becomes indifferent to his surroundings. The individual with neurotic conflicts may also repeatedly attempt to solve his problems by temporarily secluding himself. In addition, these patterns may be the characteristic way in which some people habitually try to cope with any frustrating situation in everyday life.

While it would be impossible to portray accurately every individual who may manifest autistic behavior, an attempt will be made to describe the usual behavior of a patient who is autistic. At the same time, we will be inquiring: What is the meaning of this behavior? What is the patient trying to communicate to us? What does he anticipate from us? What are the implications for nursing care?

UNDERSTANDING THE AUTISTIC PATIENT

The overt behavior of the patient may be somewhat varied, depending upon whether he is on an antipsychotic drug regime. It would be wise to check the specific drug (many are elaborated on in Chapter 11) in order to know what to expect in the way of reactions to the drug. The drug may make the patient more amenable to forming a relationship; on the other hand, he may be so drowsy and lethargic that he has little response to anything.

This patient has secluded himself from his environment. He seems to have built a wall around himself to ensure that he will not be required to interact with his surroundings. He gives the appearance of indifference to everyone and everything and seems absorbed in his own thoughts or his own autistic community. He has difficulty relating to others; his object relations, if any, are on a very superficial level. Another closely allied factor is his difficulty in communication. Most obvious is his lack of feeling tone and warmth in his contacts with others, and he may seem entirely unresponsive. On the other hand, if he does express feeling, it may be entirely inappropriate to what he is saying or to the total situation. He may, at times, show a disunity of affect by both laughing and crying at the same time. His gestures, which are usually a valid clue to the feelings, may be entirely personal so that they have meaning for him alone, or they may be so repetitious that they are offered as a response to everything. In addition, his language, one of the major tools of communication, may show various disturbances. First of all, he may be mute. If he does respond, his responses may be irrelevant. He may join syllables together, producing new words. His speech may show a lack of coherence or unity in the trend of thought. Another thinking disturbance that may be revealed by his verbal communication is his inability to generalize or to classify objects according to principle. His thinking may also be literal or concrete—that is, he may react to only one property of the object or situation involved. Finally, he may form his conclusions on the basis of only a casual association between objects. For a more extensive elaboration on this subject, refer to J. S. Kasanin's book, *Language and Thought in Schizophrenia*.[1]

---

[1] J. S. Kasanin, ed.: *Language and Thought in Schizophrenia.* New York, W. W. Norton Co., Inc., 1964.

This patient may also reveal many symptoms by his muscular apparatus, such as a generalized muscular immobility, an increase or decrease of muscular tension, various postures and gestures. He may assume one position and remain that way for an indefinite period of time or may maintain any posture in which he is placed. His overt activity may range from periods of immobility to periods of extreme restlessness and hyperactivity, wherein he may become assaultive and destructive. He may, at times, seem very suggestible and perform almost automatically in response to requests and demands. At other times, he may do the opposite of what is requested or he may be completely passive as if unable to perform anything alone.

He may have many delusions, false ideas and beliefs concerning himself, things that he has done or is capable of doing, and/or the activities of others. (Refer to page 200 for an elaboration of the term delusion.) His ideas about himself may be very bizarre, such as that changes have occurred in his body organs, that he possesses great powers, that he has performed great feats or has yet to carry them out. On the other hand, he may speak of feelings of estrangement which may be in terms of the whole world being different or strange or of himself being changed. He may also have varied hallucinations in the form of peculiar odors or poisonous gases. Then, auditory and visual hallucinations are quite common as the process continues.

During this time, he may be quite indifferent to his personal needs such as food, fluids, rest, elimination and protection from heat and cold. Although he functions as if he were entirely uninhibited, at times he is unable to tolerate any restriction or interference in his activities.

What does the behavior of the autistic patient mean? Why does he act this way? First of all, let us consider his basic personality structure, since this individual is said to have a weak ego. It may be helpful at this time to review the material in Chapter 3 on the basic functions and characteristics of the personality structure and Chapter 4 on the early period of development.

This individual's withdrawal from reality is a reflection of his weak ego. It seems almost as though he had attempted to adjust to the reality situation but found it too difficult, too frustrating or too frightening; therefore, he gave up, withdrew from the situation and regressed to his earlier patterns of behavior. Nonetheless, his ego still tries to maintain some kind of connection with the world of reality, although it is often rather impulsive and aggressive.

With the regression to early ego patterns, both the ego and the superego are further weakened, so that sublimation and repression are often so reduced that his primitive drives are expressed without the former inhibitions. As he withdraws his interest and energy from objects in the environment, the world is apt to appear different or strange. Sometimes he expresses ideas that the world is coming to an end and, if he has regressed to the narcissistic stage, he may express the belief that he has destroyed everything and, in turn, is being destroyed. You will recall that, during the narcissistic stage of development, the infant's ego is not yet differentiated from the world of objects. In the same way, this individual's ego may show a marked permeability of boundaries wherein parts of the ego overflow into the outside world and parts of the external environment are experienced as belonging to the ego. This patient very often is afraid of close contacts for fear that he will merge with others and lose his identity completely. As the ego withdraws its energy, the libido, from its boundaries, the individual may also experience feelings of body changes, such as some of his organs no longer belonging to him; or the change may be extensive enough so that he says that he feels dead. These experiences lead to behavioral manifestations that we call *delusions*. A delusion is usually defined as a false belief that cannot be changed by appeal to reason.

Let us examine what usually happens in an individual who does not manifest delusions. His ego boundaries are invested with an adequate amount of energy, and this feeling enables him to sharply differentiate between that which is a part of him and that which is a part of the external world. When an idea or a thought representation of a "real" object impinges on this ego boundary, the individual can readily distinguish between his thoughts and that which is "real"—the object that exists outside this ego boundary. It is through the functioning of his ego that the individual is able to become aware of his thought processes and feelings and keep himself and the outside world separate. Refer to Chapter 3 for a further discussion of ego functions.

When the individual's ego boundaries have become weakened by a reduction of the energy invested in them, the ideas or thought representations of "real" objects that impinge on the boundary are experienced as having a different quality than his usual thoughts and ideas. Because his thoughts lack this former quality, the individual attributes to them the same quality of "real" objects that exist in the external world. Since this individual can no longer distinguish between the object and the thought representation of the object, his perception of reality is confusing. With this loss of energy he has also lost his awareness of his own thought processes and feelings.

The delusion, or false belief, is the individual's attempt to cope with the confused reality that he is experiencing. Through the delusion, he further distorts reality in an attempt to prevent his remaining ego functions from being overwhelmed. It sometimes appears that he is further distorting this "false reality" to make his other patterns of behavior appear more logical and acceptable.

As these experiences continue and loss of contact with reality becomes greater, the patient often feels more and more isolated and is haunted by his feelings of loneliness. At the same time, he is very frightened by these experiences, and his attempts to master his environment are overtly expressed as hostility and aggression. These feelings are usually intense and may threaten to overwhelm the already weakened ego. Added to this fear of his feelings is his fear of being disappointed and hurt; consequently, he represses all his emotions and gives the appearance of being cold and lacking any feeling. He also usually isolates all of the feeling from his ideas and experiences and represses it; therefore, he is able to relate his most traumatic experience without any display of feeling. These repressed feelings, however, may be displaced onto any accessible object if the pressures become too great. This displacement seems to explain some of the explosive, unpredictable behavior of these individuals over what appear to be trivial incidents.

In spite of the fears, loneliness and general insecurity of the autistic individual, he is apt to give the nurse the impression that he is self-sufficient and needs nothing from anybody. This may be a reflection of his regression to the narcissistic phase of development where he was all-omnipotent. If you will recall, during this period the infantile ego believes in omnipotence of thought, and a wish for something is equated with fulfillment. Although someone in his external environment is responsible for fulfilling the infant's needs, the infant seems to attribute the fulfillment to his own omnipotence, since he is as yet unable to comprehend any causal relations. Ferenczi describes this feeling of omnipotence as "the feeling that one has everything one wishes for and that nothing more is left for which to wish." This feeling may well be one that is familiar to the autistic individual and may account in part for his passive indifference to the everyday incidents of his life.

NURSE-PATIENT INTERACTION

The establishment of a positive relationship with the autistic patient is the basis for any further plan of therapeutic nursing care that may be attempted. Although this relationship is the most essential part of the nursing care, it is also the most difficult and is possible only if it is based on an understanding of this patient. However, in addition to understanding, the nurse must also have a sincere interest in and a desire to help this patient if she is to be successful. In other words, the nurse has to become aware of her true feelings about the patient so that she will be better able to recognize them as they change in her interaction with him. If she feels hostile and resistive toward him, he will immediately sense it and block her further attempts to get close to him. This autistic patient is extremely sensitive to the feeling tones of others even when they are unverbalized; he is often able to pick them up, even though the other person is not yet completely aware of them. This sensitivity may be partly due to his regression wherein, like the infant, he readily empathizes the underlying feeling tones of those about him. See Chapter 8 for a discussion of empathy.

After the nurse has been able to clarify her own feelings about the patient, she will find it helpful in approaching him if she recalls frequently that he has withdrawn because he is frightened and that his desire for contact with people is often as great as his fear. Recognizing that his past experiences with people have not been too satisfying, the nurse will not anticipate an immediate response to her overtures. However, she will continue to impart personal warmth and interest in her contacts with him and give him plenty of time to respond. She will avoid making hurried contacts with him if at all possible, since it may make him feel pushed. If the nurse is accepting and in no way criticizes or reprimands the patient, he will eventually accept her overtures and respond to her. It is essential that the nurse approach the patient on the level at which he is currently functioning. This level will be determined by his overt behavior, and the nurse may clarify and validate her interpretation by discussing it with the patient's physician. For example, if the patient is mute and to all appearances seems to have regressed to an infantile narcissistic level, the nurse's contacts with him may consist of merely sitting by him for long periods and doing little things for him like combing his hair or getting him a drink of water. Merely being in proximity and showing an interest in him may be all that it is possible for the nurse to do at the time to help lessen the gap between him and reality.

Once the nurse has penetrated the barrier of the autistic patient and has established contact with him, she can influence his behavior to a marked degree. Refer to Chapter 8 to review the phases of the nurse-patient relationship. As a sound relationship is established with this patient, it is inevitable that he will become dependent on the nurse, because he yearns for a protective mother who will give the needed security in spite of the fact that he resents the helplessness that the dependency implies. Therefore, the nurse can anticipate that considerable vacillation and ambivalence will be expressed by the patient in the relationship. Ambivalence refers to the simultaneous experiencing of contradictory feelings toward the same object or situation. The patient will have both positive and negative feelings about the nurse and will move toward her and then withdraw.

As the patient begins to feel secure in his relationship with the nurse, the nurse should gradually broaden the contact to include another patient or another member of the personnel. It is helpful for the nurse to evaluate her relationship with the patient periodically, but especially at this time. As the patient begins to trust the nurse, he tends to look upon her as the superior person. He is inclined to flatter her and try in every way to please her in hopes that he, too, will be lifted up to her level of superiority. The first tendency of the nurse is to accept this role of the superior being that is bestowed upon her by the patient. However, if the nurse does accept this role and finds herself feeling very inflated, she will find herself caught in a trap. She would be able to continue helping the patient for a while as he became increasingly dependent upon her, but simultaneously he would become increasingly controlling of her. He would soon be competing with other patients for all of the nurse's time and attention. Since the nurse's needs are involved as much as the patient's, the relationship would soon end in disaster. The nurse would have difficulty encouraging this patient to be independent or to broaden his contacts because, although unaware of it, she would want to keep him dependent upon her to satisfy her own egocentric needs.

If the nurse's relationship with the autistic patient is established and maintained on a therapeutic level, the nurse will function as an auxiliary ego for the patient by giving support and structure to his everyday pattern of living. Since his superego has also been weakened and he seems to be completely uninhibited at times, the nurse will also function as an external authority figure to help him re-establish some controls.

IMMEDIATE NEEDS.   In caring for the autistic patient, the nurse will usually find that he manifests problems in many areas because of his indifference and passivity. As a rule, he tends to neglect his personal appearance and may be entirely uninterested in whether or not he is even dressed. The nurse will usually have to provide some assistance, although the degree may vary. In working with a patient who shows marked muscular immobility and who is very regressed, the nurse may have to plan and also to carry out each step in regard to his personal care until he can get himself mobilized and do these things for himself. On the other hand, the patient may not be able to get dressed or carry out other hygienic activities because he cannot make a decision. In this instance, the nurse will merely offer her suggestions in a positive way whenever the patient is unable to progress further. Very often the nurse will find that patients like this cannot comprehend a complex request like "get ready for a walk" or "get dressed." The nurse will have to analyze these activities into the steps involved and assist the patient with each one. As the nurse consistently shows an interest in the patient's personal appearance he will usually show some response which, if nurtured, will ignite a spark of interest that is basic to self-motivation.

This patient may manifest problems in elimination by retaining both feces and urine; therefore, his habits in this respect should be closely observed by the nurse. Depending upon the degree of his regression, he may also be untidy and then smear his feces and urine. In this instance, the nurse will want to establish a habit-training schedule and toilet the patient at regular intervals. Since the autistic patient tends to be rather inactive and this lack of exercise may influence his eliminative functions, the nurse may plan for him to have exercise periods. This exercise will also be helpful indirectly in providing adequate rest periods, because many times patients have difficulty in sleeping when they have been inactive all day.

It may be quite a problem for the nurse to provide an adequate food and fluid intake for the autistic patient. Here it is essential for the nurse to discover the reasons for the patient's not eating or drinking fluids. He may just be indifferent to such trivial activities because he is busy with much more important things. He may be unable to make a decision about what to eat first and just sit there with his food in front of him. He will usually be able to eat if the nurse offers a suggestion about where to begin. The nurse may have to place the spoon in his hand and then guide him in taking the first few bites of food. On the other hand, if all other suggestions fail, it may be necessary for the nurse to spoon-feed the patient. In so doing, the nurse will take him to his room or some other place where he would not be observed by everyone. She will be most successful if her attitude is positive—that is, if she really feels that he is going to eat and then follows through, being firm and sure in her movements. An additional problem in this area is the swallowing of inedible substances, and the nurse will observe the patient closely to counteract this tendency.

If the patient is negativistic he is often unable to do as requested; he may do the opposite or he may not respond at all. In coping with the former instance, the nurse might request that he do the opposite. Although she would accomplish her immediate goal, it would be detrimental to the patient since it would strengthen this negative pattern. It is much better if the nurse can remove the pressure by letting the patient know that she is willing to wait. Very often this understanding is enough to enable the patient to go on and perform as requested.

The nurse may also encounter problems in providing optimum safety for the autistic patient. He will require protection from injuring both himself and others. Because of his bizarre delusions about his body, he may mutilate himself by attempting to remove an organ which he feels no longer belongs to him. Because of his vivid hallucinations, which change so rapidly during periods of excitement, the autistic patient may assault and injure other persons.

ACTIVITIES.   In planning and providing activities for the autistic patient, the nurse will utilize all the general information on the subject as presented in Chapter 25. In addition, the activities for the autistic patient should be simple but should provide enough variety to avoid monotony. Any activity that provides a creative experience for the patient will be helpful.

With this patient, it would be essential for the nurse to begin the activities on a level where the patient could function and then grade them upward from there. Since his shell of indifference is so strong, the nurse may find that an activity that utilizes his sense of touch is most successful. For example, finger paint or modeling clay gives the patient something concrete that he can manipulate and experience through his sense of touch. Experiences that require active participation are preferable, since they will help him re-establish and maintain contact with his environment.

Summary

It was emphasized that the nurse first has to learn to observe and interpret the behavior of the autistic patient in order to plan and provide nursing care that will meet his needs. The pattern of withdrawal as an attempt at coping with stress was seen to be quite common in both psychiatric disorders and in everyday life.

The usual behavior of an autistic patient was discussed, with an elaboration of the various possible meanings of this behavior. What does this patient want? What is he trying to communicate to us? We saw that, basically, this patient is one whose needs were deprived in early childhood; that he has neither the ego strength nor the interpersonal skills to live in a reality situation. His retreat from reality is somewhat like a fight for survival until a level of eqilibrium can be attained.

Various aspects of nurse-patient interaction have been elaborated upon, with emphasis on the early interaction and how it influences the establishment of a sound relationship. Developments that can be anticipated in this relationship were clarified, with suggestions for maintaining the relationship on a therapeutic level. Problems which the autistic individual may manifest were enumerated in relation to personal hygiene, elimination, food and fluid intake and safety, with alternative actions by the nurse illustrated. The passivity and apparent indifference of this individual offer a constant challenge to the nurse to break through this wall and establish contact with the person who lives behind it.

Bibliography

Arieti, Silvano: *Interpretation of Schizophrenia*. New York, Robert Brunner, 1955.
Arieti, Silvano (ed.): *The World Biennial of Psychiatry and Psychotherapies*. Vol. I. New York, Basic Books, Inc., 1971.
Bellak, Leopold: *Dementia Praecox*. New York, Grune & Stratton, Inc., 1947.
Bleuler, Eugen: *Dementia Praecox or the Group of Schizophrenias*. New York, International Universities Press, Inc., 1950.
Brody, Eugene, and Redlich, Fredrick, eds.: *Psychotherapy with Schizophrenics*. New York, International Universities Press, Inc., 1952.
Bychowski, Gustav: *Psychotherapy of Psychosis*. New York, Grune & Stratton, Inc., 1952.
Cameron, Norman: *The Psychology of Behavior Disorders*. Boston, Houghton Mifflin Co., 1947.
Canero, Robert: *The Schizophrenic Reactions*. New York, Brunner/Mazel, Inc., 1970.
Erickson, Erik H.: *Identity and the Life Cycle*. New York, International Universities Press, Inc., 1959.
Federn, Paul: *Ego Psychology and the Psychoses*. New York, Basic Books, Inc., 1952.
Fenichel, Otto: *The Psychoanalytic Theory of Neurosis*. New York, W. W. Norton & Co., Inc., 1945.
Ferenczi, Sandor: *Further Contributions to the Theory and Technique of Psychoanalysis*. New York, Basic Books, Inc., 1952.
Freeman, Thomas, Cameron, John L., McGhie, Andrew: *Chronic Schizophrenia*. New York, International Universities Press, Inc., 1958.
Freud, Sigmund: "On Narcissism: An Introduction." In: *Collected Papers, IV*. London, Hogarth Press, 1950, p. 30.
Freud, Sigmund: "On the Transformation of Instincts with Special Reference to Anal Erotism." In: *Collected Papers, II*. London, Hogarth Press, 1950, p. 164.
Fromm-Reichmann, Frieda: *Principles of Intensive Psychotherapy*. Chicago, University of Chicago Press, 1950.
Fromm-Reichmann, Frieda: *Psychoanalysis and Psychotherapy*. Chicago, University of Chicago Press, 1959.
Guntrip, Harry: *Schizoid Phenomena, Object Relations and The Self*. New York, International Universities Press, Inc., 1969.
Hoskins, R.: *The Biology of Schizophrenia*. New York, W. W. Norton & Co., Inc., 1946.
Jackson, Don D., ed.: *The Etiology of Schizophrenia*. New York, Basic Books, Inc., 1960.
Kasanin, J. S., ed.: *Language and Thought in Schizophrenia*. New York, W. W. Norton & Co., Inc., 1964.
Odier, Charles: *Anxiety and Magic Thinking*. New York, International Universities Press, Inc., 1956.
Piaget, Jean: *The Origins of Intelligence in Children*. New York, International Universities Press, Inc., 1952.
Piaget, Jean: *The Construction of Reality in the Child*. New York, Basic Books, Inc., 1954.
Rosen, John: *Direct Analysis*. New York, Grune & Stratton, Inc., 1953.
Ruesch, Jurgen: *Disturbed Communication*. New York, W. W. Norton & Co., Inc., 1957.
Schilder, Paul: *Introduction to a Psychoanalytic Psychiatry*. New York, International Universities Press, Inc., 1951.
Sechehaye, Marguerite: *Symbolic Realization*. New York, International Universities Press, Inc., 1951.
Sechehaye, Marguerite: *A New Psychotherapy in Schizophrenia*. New York, Grune & Stratton, Inc., 1956.
Sullivan, Harry Stack: *Conceptions of Modern Psychiatry*. New York, W. W. Norton & Co., Inc., 1953.
Sullivan, Harry Stack: *Clinical Studies in Psychiatry*. New York, W. W. Norton & Co., Inc., 1956.
Sullivan, Harry Stack: *The International Theory of Psychiatry*. New York, W. W. Norton & Co., Inc., 1953.

Suggestions for Further Reading

Arieti, Silvano (ed.): *American Handbook of Psychiatry.* Vol. I. New York, Basic Books, Inc., 1959, pp. 455–507.

Falstein, Eugene I., and Sutton, Helen A.: "Childhood Schizophrenia." *Am. J. Nursing, 58*:666-670, 1958.

Fernandez, Theresa M.: "How to Deal with Overt Aggression." *Am. J. Nursing, 59*:658–660, 1959.

Fodor, Nandor, and Gaynor, Frank, eds.: *Freud: Dictionary of Psychoanalysis.* New York, Philosophical Library, Inc., 1950.

Fries, Olive H., and McLellan, Mary Lou: "Helping Patients Get Well." *Nursing Outlook, 7*:654-655, 1959.

Gravenkemper, Katherine Hepp: "Hallucinations." *Nursing World, 132*:6, 16-17, 1958.

Gregory, Elizabeth M.: "How to Help a Patient During an Emotional Crisis." *Nursing World, 132*:8-11, 1958.

Hart, Betty L., and Rohweder, Anne W.: "Support in Nursing." *Am. J. Nursing, 59*:1398-1401, 1959.

Hayter, Jean: "Reassure the Patient." *Nursing World, 134*:21-32, 1960.

Katz, Philip: "The Therapy of Adolescent Schizophrenia." *Am. J. Psycchiat., 127*:132-137, 1970.

Knowles, Lois N.: "How Can We Reassure Patients?" *Am. J. Nursing, 59*:834-835, 1959.

Lidz, Theodore: "The Influence of Family Studies on the Treatment of Schizophrenia." *Psychiatry, 32*:237-251, 1969.

Marshall, Margaret A.: "Hopelessness." *Nursing World, 133*:30-31, 1959.

Maslow, A. H., and Mittelmann, Bela: *Principles of Abnormal Psychology.* New York, Harper & Brothers, 1951, pp. 515-535.

May, Philip R. A.: "The Hospital Treatment of the Schizophrenic Patient." *Internat. J. Psychiat., 8*:699-722, 1969.

Nichols, Claude R., and Bressler, Bernard: "Anaclitic Therapy." *Am. J. Nursing, 58*:989-992, 1958.

Noyes, Arthur P., and Kolb, Lawrence C.: *Modern Clinical Psychiatry.* Philadelphia, 6th Ed., W. B. Saunders Co., 1963, pp. 325-364.

Pullinger, Walter F., Jr.: "Remotivation." *Am. J. Nursing, 60*:683-685, 1960.

Rodnick, Eliot H.: "The Psychopathology of Development: Investigating the Etiology of Schizophrenia." *Am. J. Orthopsychiat., 38*:784-798, 1968.

Rohweder, Anne W., and Hart, Betty L.: "How Attitudes Are Taught and Caught." *Am. J. Nursing, 60*:806-809, 1960.

Ruesch, Jurgen: *Disturbed Communication.* New York, W. W. Norton & Co., Inc., 1957, pp. 130-134.

Schwartz, Doris: "Uncooperative Patients." *Am. J. Nursing, 58*:75-77, 1958.

Sechehaye, Marguerite: *Autobiography of a Schizophrenic Girl.* New York, Grune & Stratton, Inc., 1951.

Speroff, B. J.: "Empathy Is Important in Nursing." *Nursing Outlook, 4*:326-327, 1956.

Thorner, Melvin: *Psychiatry in General Practice.* Philadelphia, W. B. Saunders Co., 1948, pp. 250-290.

Wexler, Milton: "Schizophrenia: Conflict and Deficiency." *Psa. Quart., 40*:83-99, 1971.

Chapter 15   The Patient With Feelings of Distrust

The nurse will find the care of the patient with feelings of distrust quite challenging as she learns to analyze her patterns of interaction with him. When she begins to understand what he is doing and why he is doing it, she will then be able to translate this data in terms of his needs for nursing care.

The patient with feelings of distrust is one who is characterized by marked skepticism, a tendency to mistrust others and doubts about everything in general. This pattern of distrust or suspicion is common and can be readily recognized in many of the clinical syndromes, although it is more prominent in some than in others. In all the paranoid conditions, suspicion is one of the predominant characteristics. It is also commonly manifested by patients with organic reactions such as general paresis and senility. Suspicion may also be evident in patients with toxic conditions, such as reactions to infectious disease, drugs or alcohol. The person who develops defective hearing after reaching middle age often gets the idea that other people are talking about him when he can no longer clearly hear what they are saying. In addition, there is the individual who habitually becomes suspicious whenever the pressures become too great; he projects his doubts and fears on others as a means of relieving his anxiety.

Since here, too, it would not be feasible to portray an accurate picture of every individual who may show evidence of suspicion, an attempt will again be made to describe the usual behavior of a patient with feelings of distrust.

UNDERSTANDING THE DISTRUSTFUL PATIENT

The suspicious individual perceives his environment as hostile; therefore, his reaction, overt or otherwise, is usually one of anger and resentment. There are two main ways in which these feelings are expressed overtly. First, the suspicious individual who is passive and overtly submissive is unable to express any of his hostility directly but keeps it all within him. His primary means of discharging tension is through his hallucinations and the autistic world that he inevitably creates. However, if situations become threatening enough, this patient is apt to become very explosive. Then there is the suspicious individual who is aggressive and who overtly expresses his hostile, resentful attitude toward the social community. This individual believes himself to be persecuted and spends all his time trying to get even with his persecutors or trying to counteract the attacks that he believes they make against him. This patient will very often become grandiose and will make all sorts of claims to distinction. In addition, the suspicious patient is asocial and has always been more or less what people call a lone wolf. He gives others the impression that he is solitary, cold and reserved. This patient also tends to be very demanding and to make his requests with a dogmatic, arrogant attitude. Another characteristic of his behavior is his impulsiveness. He seems to act very quickly, as though his thought and action occurred almost simultaneously.

From the characteristics presented thus far, we readily see that the suspicious patient will manifest disturbances in his interpersonal relations. He not only tends to dominate a situation but is also usually very competitive in a destructive sort of way. His contact with reality will vary, depending upon the stability of his autistic community and the degree and kind of false ideas or delusions that he has about himself and others.

He may be able to take care of his own personal hygiene and health needs with little assistance. On the other hand, he may be so preoccupied with his inventions, his persecutors or his special missions that he has no time for such commonplace matters as eating, sleeping or caring for his personal appearance.

What does this behavior of the suspicious patient mean? Why does he act this way? The suspicious individual also has a weak ego and his level of functioning indicates regression to an earlier phase of development. He is threatened by both his own impulses and outside stimuli;

consequently, his ego feels weak and helpless. Unable to tolerate the tensions arising from these two sources, the ego resorts to projection, and by separating these painful perceptions from itself the ego is successful in repudiating them. Projection as the primary defense of the suspicious individual's ego indicates considerable regression to the level where his reality testing is defective and the boundaries between what is ego and what is nonego are rather permeable.

This throwing out of whatever the ego no longer wants to claim as its own further weakens its ability to carry out its functions, and the tendency to project is increased until the greater part of reality is dealt with by denial. The level of regression, the narcissistic stage, contributes to this patient's feeling of being all-powerful and omnipotent in his interaction with others. At the same time, anything that threatens him brings out his aggression, which is a reflection of his early ambivalence toward a world of objects that he could not control or, in other words, which did not satisfy his needs. Refer to Chapter 4, under "One to Three Years," for an elaboration of the term ambivalence.

NURSE-PATIENT INTERACTION

In establishing a relationship with a suspicious patient, the nurse's attitude is of primary importance. It is essential that she be nonpunitive in all her dealings with the patient. This attitude may be difficult to maintain because the nurse's security and self-esteem are more apt to be shaken while caring for the suspicious patient than with any other. This patient is extremely sensitive to the unconscious feelings of others, and he readily utilizes what he empathizes as an object for projecting his own impulses and feelings. It is helpful if the nurse frequently recalls that basically this patient is a very insecure person and that his domination and sarcasm are merely his attempts to compensate for the inferiority that he feels. Refer to Chapter 8 for a discussion of empathy.

The nurse will be most successful in her approach to the suspicious patient if she is calm and self-assured. She should speak clearly and concisely in an attempt to minimize any opportunity for the patient to misinterpret her comments. She should also avoid touching the patient, since he may misinterpret her action. In spite of his grandiose manner, the nurse should make a special effort to be accepting and to treat him with respect to which every patient is entitled. Because of his inflated concept of himself, the nurse will protect him from assuming responsibility which is beyond his current capacity.

It is wise for the nurse to avoid making promises to the suspicious patient; but should such an incident occur, she should make a definite attempt to follow through. The nurse will be consistent in her contacts with the patient and, if it becomes necessary to exercise authority, she will do so in a quiet, unassuming, but firm manner.

Because of the patient's psychopathology, he will undoubtedly manifest an attitude of superiority in his relationship with the nurse. He will tend to look down upon her as if she were his servant and will utilize every opportunity to depreciate her. At this time, as well as periodically, the nurse will evaluate the relationship and attempt to identify just how the patient makes her feel. The first response of the nurse may be that she feels challenged by this patient's arrogance and she is tempted to struggle for her authority. She naturally dislikes the position which the patient ascribes to her but, if she begins to assert herself, she will be caught in a trap. Then, at every contact thereafter, she and the patient will be striving to get the best of each other and to prove who is in control of the situation. The relationship from then on will be a struggle for superiority. On the other hand, if the nurse feels fairly adequate and understands what the patient is trying to do, she will be able to remain calm and self-assured. As the patient sees that his attempts at sarcasm cannot hurt the nurse, her feeling tone will be communicated to him and he will gradually feel more secure too. Then his need for constantly proving his superiority will decrease accordingly as he gains more confidence and feels more secure.

IMMEDIATE NEEDS. The problems that the nurse encounters in providing for the immediate needs of the suspicious patient will vary, depending upon the specific details of his behavior. This patient may care for his personal hygiene fairly well, and, if he does, he will resent any intrusion by the nurse. If oral hygiene poses a problem, the nurse may set up a schedule and provide a routine time for the activity. The patient will then usually be willing to brush his teeth if his toothbrush has his name on it and he is allowed to take the tooth paste from the container himself.

If he is either afraid of or antagonistic toward other patients, he may not be able to secure adequate rest if he is expected to sleep near them or in the same room. A problem may arise, too, in regard to maintaining an adequate food and fluid intake if the patient's delusions are involved. The nurse will, first of all, have to find out the particular idea that is interfering with the patient's intake. For example, if he believes that someone is trying to poison him, the nurse might arrange for him to either observe or assist with serving the food. It has also been suggested that such a patient be served food in the original condition or container if at all possible. It may also be helpful for the nurse to taste the food or, if necessary, to secure an identical serving and eat with the patient. On the other hand, the patient may be indifferent to his needs or be too preoccupied with other important matters. In this instance, the nurse should serve the food in a matter-of-fact way and inform the patient that his meal is ready.

The suspicious patient will manifest problems in the area of safety, since he is always potentially dangerous both to himself and to others. Because this patient is so impulsive, the nurse should always minimize the hazardous articles to which he has access. The nurse will also supervise this patient closely, but as unobtrusively as possible.

ACTIVITIES.   In providing experiences for the suspicious patient, the nurse should first of all consider the general factors involved in planning any activities. In addition, she should select activities which require fairly close concentration in an attempt to reduce the time available for the patient to dwell on his delusions. She will minimize the articles which the patient might use as weapons and always provide adequate supervision. She will select activities with a minimum of competition, since the suspicious patient always strives to prove his superiority and cannot tolerate losing.

At first it will be better for the nurse to provide activities that the patient can do alone or with one other member of the personnel until he is ready to become a member of a group. The nurse will avoid activities that require close physical contact and/or an overt display of aggression. The suspicious patient needs an opportunity to gain satisfaction from activities without other patients having to be placed under his domination.

Summary

It was emphasized that the nurse first has to learn to observe and interpret the behavior of the suspicious patient in order to plan and provide nursing care to meet his needs. The material presented on the behavior of the patient with feelings of distrust is to help provide more understanding of his psychopathology.

It was brought out that the pattern of distrust is commonly manifested by patients with psychoses as well as by others. The nurse-patient relationship was elaborated on, and it was pointed out that it should be evaluated periodically to determine the level of effectiveness of the interaction.

In addition, the immediate needs that are most apt to pose problems for the nurse were enumerated and examples given to illustrate how provision might be made for each. The types of activities suitable for the patient were discussed, with emphasis on the need to maintain a safe environment.

Bibliography

Bellak, Leopold: *Dementia Praecox.* New York, Grune & Stratton, Inc., 1947.
Bleuler, Eugen: *Dementia Praecox or the Group of Schizophrenias.* New York, International Universities Press, Inc., 1950.
Brody, Eugene, and Redlich, Fredrick, eds.: *Psychotherapy with Schizophrenics.* New York, International Universities Press, Inc., 1952.
Bychowski, Gustav: *Psychotherapy of Psychosis.* New York, Grune & Stratton, Inc., 1952.
Cameron, Norman: *The Psychology of Behavior Disorders.* Boston, Houghton Mifflin Co., 1947.
Erikson, Erik H.: *Identity and the Life Cycle.* New York, International Universities Press, Inc., 1959.
Federn, Paul: *Ego Psychology and the Psychoses.* New York, Basic Books, Inc., 1952.
Fenichel, Otto: *The Psychoanalytic Theory of Neurosis.* New York, W. W. Norton & Co., Inc., 1945.
Ferenczi, Sandor: *Further Contributions to the Theory and Technique of Psychoanalysis.* New York, Basic Books, Inc., 1952.
Freeman, Thomas, Cameron, John L., McGhie, Andrew: *Chronic Schizophrenia.* New York, International Universities Press, Inc., 1958.
Freud, Sigmund: "On Narcissism: An Introduction." In *Collected Papers, IV.* London, Hogarth Press, 1950, p. 30.
Freud, Sigmund: "On the Transformation of Instincts with Special Reference to Anal Erotism." In *Collected Papers, II.* London, Hogarth Press, 1950, p. 164.
Fromm-Reichmann, Frieda: *Principles of Intensive Psychotherapy.* Chicago, University of Chicago Press, 1950.
Fromm-Reichmann, Frieda: *Psychoanalysis and Psychotherapy.* Chicago, University of Chicago Press, 1959.
Hoskins, R.: *The Biology of Schizophrenia.* New York, W. W. Norton & Co., Inc., 1946.
Jackson, Don D., ed.: *The Etiology of Schizophrenia.* New York, Basic Books, Inc., 1960.
Kasanin, J. S., ed.: *Language and Thought in Schizophrenia.* New York, W. W. Norton & Co., Inc., 1964.
Odier, Charles: *Anxiety and Magic Thinking.* New York, International Universities Press, Inc., 1956.
Piaget, Jean: *The Origins of Intelligence in Children.* New York, International Universities Press, Inc., 1952.
Piaget, Jean: *The Construction of Reality in the Child.* New York, Basic Books, Inc., 1954.
Rosen, John: *Direct Analysis.* New York, Grune & Stratton, Inc., 1953.
Ruesch, Jurgen: *Disturbed Communication.* New York, W. W. Norton & Co., Inc., 1957.
Schilder, Paul: *Introduction to a Psychoanalytic Psychiatry.* New York, International Universities Press, Inc., 1951.
Sechehaye, Marguerite: *Symbolic Realization.* New York, International Universities Press, Inc., 1951.
Sechehaye, Marguerite: *A New Psychotherapy in Schizophrenia.* New York, Grune & Stratton, Inc., 1956.
Sullivan, Harry Stack: *Conceptions of Modern Psychiatry.* New York, W. W. Norton & Co., Inc., 1953.
Sullivan, Harry Stack: *Clinical Studies in Psychiatry.* New York, W. W. Norton & Co., Inc., 1956.
Sullivan, Harry Stack: *The Interpersonal Theory of Psychiatry.* New York, W. W. Norton & Co., Inc., 1953.

Suggestions for Further Reading

Arieti, Sylvano (ed.): *American Handbook of Psychiatry.* Vol. I. New York, Basic Books, Inc., 1959, pp. 508-539.
Chrzanowski, Gerald: "Cultural and Pathological Manifestations of Paranoia." *Perspectives in Psychiatric Care, 1:*34-42, 1963.

Fernandez, Theresa M.: "How to Deal with Overt Aggression." *Am. J. Nursing,* *59*:658-660, 1959.

Figelman, Matthew: "A Comparison of Affective and Paranoid Disorders in Negroes and Jews." *Internat. J. Social Psychiat., 14*:277-282, 1968.

Gravenkemper, Katherine Hepp: "Hallucinations." *Nursing World, 132*:6, 16–17, 1958.

Gregory, Elizabeth M.: "How to Help a Patient During an Emotional Crisis." *Nursing World, 132*:8-11, 1958.

Hart, Betty L., and Rohweder, Anne W.: "Support in Nursing." *Am. J. Nursing,* *59*:1398-1401, 1959.

Hayter, Jean: "Reassure the Patient." *Nursing World, 134*:21-32, 1960.

Knowles, Lois N.: "How Can We Reassure Patients?" *Am. J. Nursing, 59*:834–835, 1959.

Maslow, A. H., and Mittelmann, Bela: *Principles of Abnormal Psychology.* New York, Harper & Brothers, 1951, pp. 535-541.

Noyes, Arthur P., and Kolb, Lawrence C.: *Modern Clinical Psychiatry.* Philadelphia, W. B. Saunders Co., 1958, pp. 350-352, 409-412, 434-447.

Peplau, Hildegarde E.: "Themes in Nursing Situations." *Am. J. Nursing, 53*:1221, 1343, 1953.

Peplau, Hildegarde E.: "Utilizing Themes in Nursing Situations." *Am. J. Nursing, 54*:325, 1954.

Pullinger, Walter F., Jr.: "Remotivation." *Am. J. Nursing, 60*:683-685, 1960.

Rohweder, Anne W., and Hart, Betty L.: "How Attitudes Are Taught and Caught." *Am. J. Nursing, 60*:806-809, 1960.

Schwartz, Doris: "Uncooperative Patients." *Am. J. Nursing, 58*:75-77, 1959.

Schwartz, Morris S., and Shockley, Emmy Lanning: *The Nurse and the Mental Patient.* New York, Russell Sage Foundation, 1956, pp. 113-138.

Speroff, B. J.: "Empathy Is Important in Nursing." *Nursing Outlook, 4*:326-327, 1956.

Thorner, Melvin: *Psychiatry in General Practice.* Philadelphia, W. B. Saunders Co., 1948, pp. 337-363.

Wolowitz, Howard, and Shorkey, Clayton: "Power Motivation in Male Paranoid Children." *Psychiat., 32*:459-466, 1969.

Chapter 16　The Patient With Feelings of Worthlessness

Unless the nurse understands the behavior of the patient, there is little that she can do to help him progress toward the goal of recovery. The nurse collects data from the social history and other sources, from the physician and others working with the patient, and she will also have some acquaintance of the literature in the field. The following material will serve to provide such a background. The student, however, must be cautioned that all patients who are depressed will not necessarily follow this portrayal. The authors have attempted to select information which seems pertinent to understanding the behavior of the *typical* patient with feelings of worthlessness.

UNDERSTANDING THE PATIENT WITH FEELINGS OF WORTHLESSNESS

The overt symptom of depression is found to some degree in almost all psychiatric disorders, as well as in the average individual. In an individual with a psychiatric disorder the symptom is seen more commonly in such illnesses as the depressed phase of manic-depressive psychosis, involutional melancholia, and certain neurotic manifestations such as the reactive depression.

The depressed person is a very ambivalent individual in that he has both love and hate for many objects in his environment, including members of his family and his close friends. The attitude of ambivalence is founded upon frustrating basic nursing experiences in early infancy. Since it is the mother who gives love, food, and attention to the infant, it is apparently she who is involved in his frustrating experiences; therefore, his first feeling of ambivalence is toward her, his first love object.

During this early period the infant "takes" much but "gives" little. He incorporates or "takes in" much of his environment with little discrimination. However, he tends to give up what he does not want, and expels it from his body. He likes the feeling of being engulfed at the mother's breasts, and feels safe as though he were in hiding. When the individual is frustrated later in life he has a tendency to regress to the earlier patterns of behavior that gave him the most satisfaction. Similarly, the patient with feelings of worthlessness is said to regress to his former patterns of ambivalence, incorporation, desire to be engulfed and wish to expel unwanted objects.

The patient with feelings of worthlessness is suffering from the loss of a love object, either real or imagined, that he previously incorporated. He, therefore, behaves somewhat like the average individual who mourns his loss because of the death of a loved one. Because this patient incorporated his lost love object, the loss is felt within, and thus the patient often complains of a hollowness or emptiness inside. He usually expects others to share his grief over his loss, and is further disappointed with their apparent indifference. At times hostility is expressed in such statements as, "How could he leave me?"[1] Then he concludes that he is responsible for the loss and begins to feel guilty. His hostility is directed inward, and he begins to hate himself. Finally, he arrives at the conclusion that he is unworthy. Because of these delusions of self-depreciation, he tries to convince others that they should have nothing to do with him or they, too, will become tainted.

The ego of the patient is described as being weak. It appears as if the ego were almost fused with an engulfing and sadistic superego that is overwhelming in its criticisms. Thus the possibility of suicide is very great. At times we may hear him say that he wishes that he had never been born. Such a desire may go back to his wish to be engulfed by the mother's breast where he was safe. Frequently we find that this type of patient begs for punishment and expresses the desire to be dead.

Because of ambivalent feelings toward people and other objects in the environment, the patient has difficulty in establishing mature rela-

---

[1]Gustav Bychowski: *Psychotherapy of Psychosis.* New York, Grune & Stratton, Inc., 1952, p. 218.

tionships. He is unable to give love without getting something in return, and is also very dependent when it comes to receiving love and attention from others. His needs, like the infant's, are somewhat narcissistic, and his depression is just another "cry for love."[2] The slightest criticism or rebuff is intolerable, and he is apt to respond by becoming even more depressed. Since his first feelings of hostility are founded upon being frustrated at the breast, it is not surprising to find that the patient does not eat well. This response becomes his punishment for feeling hostile toward his mother.

Difficulty in sleeping is also an overt symptom of the patient with feelings of worthlessness. Bychowski explains this phenomenon on the basis of the individual being afraid to sleep because of the possibility of encountering his lost loved one in his dreams.

At times in the early phases of the illness, the patient is very ritualistic, in a way similar to the patient with obsessive-compulsive neurosis. The ritual is his way of trying to relieve his anxiety. By performing tasks, such as arranging his possessions in a very neat order, cleaning things about him and washing his body, he tends to wash away some of the guilt, which in the early stages of his illness may not be so convincing to him. His feelings of ambivalence seem more pronounced during the beginning of his depression, perhaps because he is more aware of them. Also in the early phases of his illness he is more apt to express his irritability by being hostile to others. Decisions are difficult because of his many ambivalent feelings, and he is very likely to become irritable when they are required. In the deeper phases of the illness, when all hostility is turned inward, and the patient is thoroughly convinced of his guilt, he is not so apt to express his hostile feelings openly. Here, too, decisions are difficult to make, but only because his thoughts are retarded. If he were able to express himself, he probably would deny that a decision was involved by making such a comment as, "Just let me die, and that will solve everything. It's the only solution."

During a period of depression, which is so characteristic of the patient with feelings of worthlessness, the patient's body processes become slower; he has difficulty with digestion, and often refuses food. He is inclined toward constipation, and is slow in speech and movement. His face is sad, and his muscles sag. His whole body droops as though he had the weight of the world upon him. He has little interest in his personal appearance or in doing things for himself. This tendency seems to stem from the fact that he feels unworthy of spending time upon himself, that he has used most of his energy in directing his

[2]Gustav Bychowski: *Psychotherapy of Psychosis.* New York, Grune & Stratton, Inc., 1952, p. 262.

hostile feelings inward. He may also complain that he feels tired, and that the sleep he gets does not rest him.

We have previously mentioned that the patient is unusually sensitive to everything around him. During periods in which he is not depressed he seems to be easily influenced by his environment, and engulfs much of it without discrimination; however, once he has incorporated, he seems equally capable of throwing off or losing the objects that he does not wish to keep. During his depression, however, he seems to be more selective in his incorporation; through a defect in his perception of reality he seems to magnify the "bad" objects in the environment and incorporate them into the self. As his feeling of worthlessness becomes more intense, almost everything in his environment appears buried in gloominess and despair. The more he incorporates these aspects of environment, the more hopeless he feels. The feeling of emptiness may then become a feeling of heaviness that causes him to bend with the weight.

We have implied that there are various degrees of the illness. Patients who are depressed may experience only a lack of interest in things about them. In this instance hospitalization may not be required. On the other hand, some patients become so depressed that they become stuporous, and hospitalization is essential.

The feeling of worthlessness may have an insidious onset, and may envelop the patient so slowly that he is unaware of what is happening to him; at other times the patient may become abruptly and acutely depressed almost overnight. While the average feeling of worthlessness lasts only a few months, there are a few patients who become chronically depressed, and their symptoms last for several years. After some patients experience a feeling of worthlessness they may have a feeling of elation, and this too may manifest itself in varying degrees.

SUMMARY OF CHARACTERISTICS

Before turning to the content relevant to the development of the nurse-patient relationship, a summary of the major characteristics of patients with feelings of worthlessness may serve to focus attention upon a few generalizations in regard to behavior which have implications for nursing care.

The patient with feelings of worthlessness is regressing to an earlier pattern of behavior because of his frustration in regard to a lost love object. His disappointments in his early phases of psychosexual development are again reflected in his present relationships with others. He resorts to his early patterns of incorporating and wishing to be devoured but usually expels anything that he does not wish to retain.

His desire to incorporate his environment makes him sensitive to environmental stimuli, and he is easily influenced or overwhelmed.

The hostility stemming from frustration during early experiences is directed inward, and the patient begins to feel guilty as his superego becomes very intense. The concomitant feeling of unworthiness gives rise to self-depreciating delusions, suicidal thoughts, and a desire for punishment. Such a patient is also a very dependent person, craving love and affection, but unfortunately unable to love others in a mature way. When the patient is "going into" or "coming out of" a depression his anxiety may be relieved by ritualistic patterns.

The acutely depressed patient manifests a slowing of all the bodily processes, and is apt to manifest poor skin turgor, dry skin and poor appetite and elimination. He is also likely to complain of tiredness, and will probably move, think and speak slowly. He is careless in matters of personal appearance and hygiene, and seems indifferent to the objects in his environment which formerly were of interest to him.

NURSE-PATIENT INTERACTION

An effective nurse-patient relationship with the type of patient we have just described will not be easily established. The nurse must have a genuine interest in the patient and must really want to help him. As the nurse empathizes with the patient, she will try to reflect a mood and attitude which is in harmony with his, in that it will not be overtly cheerful. At the same time she will try to be warm, calm, serious, kind and understanding. She should not argue with the patient when he tries to convince her of his unworthiness, but may respond by an understanding nod or comment such as, "You're feeling pretty bad today, aren't you?" Above all, she will not laugh or make light of his ideas by such comments as, "It'll all blow over by tomorrow," or "It'll all come out in the wash, and tomorrow is another day." The thought of beginning another day may be too much for the patient, and he may respond by carrying out his ideas of self-destruction. When he sees others who are cheerful, he may be overwhelmed because he feels that he will never again be that way. Thus, he reasons, why should he put forth the effort? Cheerfulness in contrast to his own depression may emphasize his own feelings of sadness.

The nurse should speak to the patient, and address him by name even though he does not respond. She should also gradually increase the time she spends with him, even though she does nothing more than sit beside him. In time, a rather dependent relationship may develop. If this occurs, the patient may begin to express some hostility toward the nurse. It will be important, in such instances, for the nurse to accept the patient's feelings and to refrain from criticizing him. It will be easier for the nurse to do this if she remembers that the patient is acting out his ambivalent feelings toward her, and is testing new responses to his old problems. In addition, the nurse may wish to point out slight improvements to the patient by such comments as, "You were able to drink all your fruit juice this morning." It may be too overwhelming to the patient to make such statements as "You're getting much better." He will probably not agree with you because he can find no improvement in his condition. He may reason that he doesn't deserve to feel better.

The nurse may try to encourage and reassure the patient by conversing with him on neutral topics. At first he may not respond, and if the nurse insists that he talk he may become irritable. The nurse may elicit some response from him each day by asking him questions to which he cannot respond by a mere yes or no answer. Gradually he will begin talking, and the nurse will then be an attentive listener. She will let the patient know that she is interested by an occasional nod or comment. At times he may wish to tell her too much. Then, it may be necessary for the nurse to tell the patient that he should save such information for the doctor. As the patient gets deeper insight into his problems through his psychotherapy, he will become less dependent in his relationship with the nurse. As he begins to take more interest in himself and those about him, the nurse will gradually withdraw her attention by standing by and acting as a catalyst in his relationships with others. When the patient is well, he will not need the nurse, and she can withdraw entirely from the situation.

Since the patient is reacting to a disappointment earlier in life, the nurse should be consistent in her relationship with the patient so that he will not again be disappointed. It is especially important that the nurse be truthful with the patient and refrain from making promises that cannot be fulfilled in the near future.

In the type of relationship described above, the nurse will work closely with the physician and other members of the psychiatric team so that all efforts will be directed toward the patient's recovery. The nurse will, of course, communicate her observations to all those concerned with the patient's care.

PREVENTING SELF-INJURY AND DESTRUCTION. Because of the patient's ideas of unworthiness, the nurse will observe him closely. It is important that she know his whereabouts, and know what he is doing at all times. He should not be left alone with articles that could be used for self-injury or destruction. The patient may try to leave the hospital in order to carry out his intentions, and will have to be watched closely in this respect. The nurse working with psychiatric patients will review first-aid measures to be taken in such instances. A physical approach may be necessary to restrain the individual, if the nurse should encounter him carrying out his destructive impulses. However, the nurse can often anticipate the patient's behavior in this respect and thereby prevent any occurrences of this nature.

Vigilance should not be relaxed as the patient seemingly improves. This period is one in which suicide is most apt to occur. As the patient's depression lifts, and he begins to gain more insight, his anxiety may increase temporarily. Then, too, he may be only masking his true feelings so that he will be given more leeway to carry out his former threats. The patient may also tend to look back, and think that he can no longer tolerate going forward on the long road to recovery.

MEETING THE OTHER REQUIREMENTS OF THE PATIENT.   The patient may wish to punish himself by not eating, and the problem of providing an adequate food and fluid intake may be a crucial one. The patient may reason that the food is too expensive, and that he is too unworthy to eat. Nevertheless, the nurse will always serve him his tray, and assume that he will eat. He may feel more like eating, however, if he is helped to improve his personal appearance, is assisted in brushing his teeth and in using a mouth rinse before the meal is served. Withholding his tray until he asks for it or threatening him with a tube feeding may only serve to convince him, more than ever, that he deserves to be punished. Every opportunity should be provided for him to be served the foods he likes. He should be given such assistance as buttering his bread, cutting his meat, and any other help indicated. A suggestion that he take a sip of milk or a bit of meat may help him to begin. He may be able to consume the major portion of his food if the nurse breaks down the task of eating into minute steps. Sometimes it will be necessary for her to place the container to his lips so that he may drink or place the solid food in his mouth with a spoon. If such assistance is necessary, it should be given in the absence of others. The nurse should be cautioned not to hold the patient's nose to make him swallow. Such action enhances the possibility of aspirational pneumonia or a lung abscess.

Keeping a record of the kind and amount of food eaten at each meal will often provide an index to whether the patient is receiving sufficient variety in his intake. Usually the patient will tolerate soft foods that are easily chewed and swallowed. Small amounts of food served more frequently may also be more appealing to him. The patient's weight loss and the condition of his skin will serve as fairly reliable criteria as to how insistent the nurse should be in regard to this problem. If all else fails, it may be necessary to tube-feed the patient. If the patient's illness is of long duration, he will probably be prone to secondary infections, and an adequate intake of fluid is essential. Sometimes just a reminder to take a drink from the fountain or serving high-caloric fluids between meals will be beneficial.

Some attempt should be made to keep a record of the patient's output. He will not always complain when he is uncomfortable because of the retention of urine or feces; if he has not voided a significant amount in eight hours, or has not had a bowel movement within three days, the physician should be notified. With the slowing down of bodily processes an impaction may result. It will be well for the nurse to remember that diarrhea is sometimes a symptom of an impaction. Some patients have complaints in regard to their digestive tracts, and the nurse should avoid stimulating the patient's concern by overemphasis of these aspects.

Since the circulation of the extremities may be impaired, the patient may feel cold. A sweater, shawl or extra blanket will often be appreciated. Passive exercise, as well as light massage, may also be helpful. Since the patient may be so depressed that he will remain in one position for long periods of time, it would be well for the nurse to suggest that he change his position, move to another chair, or elevate his feet on a stool.

The patient's skin may become dry and cracked but will usually become moist again when his fluid intake is adequate. Some type of lanolin preparation will serve to relieve the dry condition temporarily. It is especially important that the nurse call the physician's attention to any unfavorable skin conditions. In older patients particularly, the skin may break down or a secondary infection may occur.

More frequent rest periods may help the patient's feeling of tiredness, but care should be taken that he doesn't spend the major part of his time in bed. Since he is basically a dependent person he probably will need gentle but firm encouragement to be kept up and about.

We have implied that the acute patient will need some assistance with his personal appearance and hygiene. Since he moves slowly, the nurse should initiate these activities with him before other patients begin their routine. She may have to assemble clothing for him, and at first, she may have to dress him. Usually if he is handed one piece of clothing at a time, however, he will dress himself. Such comments as, "Now here's your stocking. Put on your stocking," may encourage him in this difficult task. It may also be necessary for the nurse to interest the patient in keeping his clothing in condition to wear. However, during his acute illness, it may be necessary to make arrangements for either his relatives or a commercial laundry service to do his laundry. Later he will be able to do these things for himself. It will be important for him to do a little toward these ends every day rather than to wait and do it all at once. Large tasks are often overwhelming to him, and he will be able to gain satisfaction from completing activities that are of short duration. Quite often the patient will feel better when his appearance is more acceptable to others. However, he will probably prefer to wear his ordinary clothing rather than his best apparel. As he becomes more active he should be encouraged to make more decisions in regard to the type and color of clothing he prefers. The patient will probably need assistance with his bath, and care should be taken that he is not left alone in the tub or shower. The nurse will be observant for attempts at drowning or scalding. If the patient prefers not to take a daily bath, the nurse should not insist, since her prodding may confirm a delusion that he is dirty.

Male patients may need to be shaved. Needless to say, they should not be left alone with a sharp razor. If possible, an electric razor should be provided. Women patients will need special assistance with their hair. Sending them to the beauty shop when they are severely depressed may make them feel unworthy, but as their depression becomes more superficial they will be stimulated by this activity.

PROVIDING A THERAPEUTIC ENVIRONMENT. It is preferable that the static environment of the depressed patient be a modest one with soft coloring. Luxuriously furnished suites that are too bright and gay usually leave the patient with a feeling of utter despair. Something that appears just a little more optimistic than the patient's mood may prove stimulating but not overly so. The nurse should also provide adequate ventilation free of drafts; because of the patient's retardation, a room temperature of about 74° F. will be more comfortable for him. Since noise will tend to irritate him, precautions should be taken to minimize it as much as possible.

The dynamic environment should be both nonoverwhelming and nonirritating. The patient will probably prefer a roommate who is not too chatty or boisterous, and one who is about his own age. Association with younger people tends to make him think about what he should have done or what he might have done before his illness. He will also probably prefer to remain in his room or some dark corner. The nurse should try to get him to sit in a quiet corner of the dayroom with a few other quiet patients, or she may sit with him. The patient may be introduced to a larger and more active group gradually. At first this introduction nay be done by moving his chair a little closer to the center of the activities. As the patient gradually begins to enjoy being a spectator, he may then be approached in regard to becoming a more active participant.

Activities. The patient may at first resist any attempts in helping him to socialize. The nurse may begin to initiate his interest by asking him to do small tasks in cooperation with her. Such projects as dusting the table tops or the window sills will probably not loom out of proportion. As he progresses, the nurse may interest him in doing something for others, such as making a gift for a close friend or relative. Later he will be able to participate with the nurse in simple games that do not require too much concentration. Games in which he can express his aggression outwardly are often helpful. He can gradually be brought into more active games, both indoor and outdoor, and may then enjoy going to a party as a spectator. Later he will be able to participate more actively. He will, however, be more apt to take part in activities if he does things for others rather than for himself.

Summary

The main characteristics in the behavior of the patient with feelings of worthlessness have been summarized within the chapter, and so further elaboration will be omitted here. The nurse's relationship with the patient was described as being a warm, calm, serious, and understanding one. The nurse will try to reflect a mood in a manner that is slightly more optimistic than that of the patient. As the patient becomes more aware of his ambivalent feelings, the nurse can expect that at times he may be openly hostile to her. The nurse may encourage him by pointing out very small and specific things that he has accomplished each day. She should be consistent, and try not to disappoint him by making promises that she cannot fulfill.

One of the nurse's main concerns will be the prevention of self-injury or destruction. Vigilance should not be relaxed even though the patient appears to be less depressed, since this period is one in which suicide is most likely to occur.

The patient's problems in regard to food and fluid intake, as well as those concerning elimination have been discussed. Factors in regard to both the static and dynamic environment have been elaborated, and the problems in regard to meeting personal and hygienic needs have been described.

Suitable activities are those that take into account the patient's slowness in regard to thought and movement, so that they will not be too overwhelming for him.

Bibliography

Abraham, Karl: *Selected Papers on Psychoanalysis*. London, Hogarth Press, 1927.
Beck, Aaron T.: "Thinking and Depression: I. Idiosyncratic Content and Cognitive Distortions." *Arch. Gen. Psychiat.*, *9*:324-333, 1963.
Beck, Aaron T.: "Thinking and Depression: II. Theory and Therapy." *Arch. Gen. Psychiat.*, *10*:561-571, 1964.
Bellak, Leopold, *et al.: Manic-Depressive Psychosis and Allied Conditions*. New York, Grune & Stratton, Inc., 1952.
Bychowski, Gustav: *Psychotherapy of Psychosis*. New York, Grune & Stratton, Inc., 1952.

Cameron, Norman: *The Psychology of Behavior Disorders.* Boston, Houghton Mifflin Co., 1947.
Campbell, John D.: *Everyday Psychiatry.* Philadelphia, J. B. Lippincott Co., 1949.
Custance, John: *Wisdom, Madness and Folly.* New York, Pellegrini & Cudahy, Inc., 1952.
Federn, Paul: *Ego Psychology and the Psychoses.* New York, Basic Books, Inc., 1952.
Fenichel, Otto: *The Psychoanalytical Theory of Neurosis.* New York, W. W. Norton & Co., Inc., 1945.
Gregory, Ian: *Fundamentals of Psychiatry.* Philadelphia, W. B. Saunders, 1968.
Kolb, Lawrence C.: *Noyes' Modern Clinical Psychiatry.* 7th ed., Philadelphia, W. B. Saunders, 1968.
Mikesell, W. A., ed.: *Modern Abnormal Psychology.* New York, Philosophical Library, Inc., 1950.
Redlich, Frederick C., and Freedman, Daniel X.: *The Theory and Practice of Psychiatry.* New York, Basic Books, Inc., 1966.

Suggestions for Further Reading

Ashford, Mary E.: "Home Care of Mentally Ill Patients." *Am. J. Nursing,* 57:206-207, February, 1957.
Aud, Frank J., Jr.: "The Anti-depressants." *Am. J. Nursing,* 65:67-84, June, 1965.
Beers, Clifford: *A Mind That Found Itself.* Garden City, Doubleday, Doran & Co., 1929.
Bidder, Geroge T.: "Are Drugs the Answer in Mental Depression?" *Am. J. Nursing,* 61:60-63, October, 1961.
Donner, Gail: "Treatment of a Delusional Patient." *Am. J. Nursing,* 69:2643-2644, December, 1969.
Freyhan, F. A.: "The Modern Treatment of Depressive Disorders." *Am. J. Psychiat.,* 116:1057-1064, 1960.
Gibson, John: "Involutional Melancholia." *Canadian Nurse,* 55:1028-1030, November, 1959.
Gibson, John: "The Manic-Depressive Psychosis." *Canadian Nurse,* 55:928-930, October, 1959.
Gibson, R. W., Cohen, M. B., and Cohen, R. A.: "On the Dynamics of the Manic-Depressive Personality." *Am. J. Psychiat.,* 115:1101-1107, June, 1959.
Greenblatt, Milton, Grosser, George H., and Wechsler, Henry: "Differential Response of Hospitalized Depressed Patients to Somatic Therapy." *Am. J. Psychiat.,* 120:935-943, April, 1964.
Kraines, S. H.: "The Physiologic Basis of the Manic-Depressive Illness: A Theory." *Am. J. Psychiat.,* 114:206-211, September, 1957.
Lurie, Max L., and Salzer, Harry M.: "Tranylcypromine (Parnate) in the Ambulatory Treatment of Depressed Patients." *Am. J. Psychiat.,* 118:152–155, August, 1961.
Neylar, Margaret Prowse: "The Depressed Patient." *Am. J. Nursing,* 61:77-78, July, 1961.
Ryklen, Marjorie R.: "The Nurse's Role in Preventing Suicide." *Nursing Outlook,* 6:377, July, 1958.
Schneidman, Edwin G.: "Preventing Suicide." *Am. J. Nursing,* 65:111-116, May, 1965.
Schwartz, Morris S., and Shockley, Emmy Lanning: *The Nurse and the Mental Patient.* New York, Russell Sage Foundation, 1956, pp. 113-148, 167-181.
Sorenson, Gladys: "Dependency—A Factor in Nursing Care." *Am. J. Nursing,* 66:1762-1763, August, 1966.
Thaler, Otto F.: "Grief and Depression." *Nursing Forum, V,* No. 2:8-22, 1966.
Ujhely, Gertrud B.: "Grief and Depression Implications for Preventive and Therapeutic Nursing Care." *Nursing Forum, V,* No. 2:23-35, 1966.
Wilson, David C.: "Group Psychotherapy and Manic-Depressive Psychosis." *Am. J. Psychiat.,* 110:911-915, June, 1954.

UNDERSTANDING THE ELATED PATIENT

It has been stated that the patient with feelings of worthlessness may, at times, experience the opposite mood, that of elation. In many respects the dynamics of elation and worthlessness are similar. The individual is basically dependent, ambivalent, narcissistic and ready to incorporate his environment. He, too, has a wish to be incorporated, and seems capable of spitting out the "bad" incorporated objects. When he can tolerate the feeling of worthlessness no longer, he uses the pattern of denial. By denying his problems he can also avoid anxiety, a feeling that is intolerable to him. Such a defense enables the patient to deny reality and thus relaxes his superego. He then regresses to a period of infancy, where at the breast he feels happy, blissful, and reborn. When he is interrupted by an object in his environment, he responds with irritability. He may also become profane in speech.

The elated individual has been described as one who is experiencing a sleep equivalent[1] in that he is able to carry out his wish-fulfilling fantasies. He loves the world, and tries to incorporate everything in his environment. He is likely to be meddlesome and domineering in re-

---

[1]Bertram D. Lewin: *The Psychoanalysis of Elation*. New York, W. W. Norton & Co., Inc., 1950, p. 101.

gard to the affairs of others. He seems to go from one pleasurable idea to another, and seems to discard the previous one for a more pleasurable one. He wants all objects in his environment to be as pretty and happy as he is; frequently he decorates himself and his environment to attain this end. His thoughts are rapid, and his speech goes at such a fast pace that he frequently skips words altogether. Thus, he may appear incomprehensible to the casual observer. His wit is keen, and his eyes "take in" everything. Although he can easily be distracted for a moment or so, his attention is difficult to hold. After being very circumstantial he goes back to the original topic until it is exhausted.

The individual's motor activity is accelerated, and he does not stay in one place very long. He is usually so busy with his various activities that he has no time to eat, and thus may present quite a problem in this respect. His skin is usually warm and dry, and he may have difficulty with elimination. Sleep is almost impossible because he is at such a high pitch emotionally.

SUMMARY OF CHARACTERISTICS

Before discussing the elated patient in detail, it may be well to summarize a few of the main characteristics of his behavior. The elated patient, like the individual with the feeling of worthlessness, is regressing to earlier patterns of behavior, and is basically ambivalent and dependent. He devours his environment through the process of incorporation, but yet yearns to be devoured. By denying reality he is able to avoid anxiety about his problems and therefore can feel elated. His superego relaxes, and permits him to carry out his wish-fulfilling fantasies in a playful way. His manner is sometimes obscene.

In the elated patient, thought and motor activities are accelerated to a high pitch. The patient appears distractable, and has a tendency toward a "flight of ideas." He is apt to be domineering, meddlesome and irritable, and may present many problems in regard to food and fluid intake, sleep, and elimination.

NURSE-PATIENT INTERACTION

Since the elated patient feels happy, he is likely to be domineering with the nurse. The patient may be irritable, if the nurse does not reflect his mood, since she is perceived as part of him. The nurse's attitude should be as permissive as the hospital environment permits. She will be warm and affectionate, but somewhat less optimistic than the patient. It is important that she not "laugh at" him, but occasionally "laughing with" him may make him less irritable at her intrusions. The nurse should avoid arguments with him and should not condemn him for his profanity and obscene actions. She will find that it is usually not necessary to answer his questions and accusations, since he will probably go ahead in his conversation without giving the nurse an opportunity to respond. If he expects and wants an answer, a short, truthful, and concise one will suffice. He may be impatient and may not wait for long explanations. He may make many demands that are not possible to fulfill, but when he makes a reasonable request it should be given every consideration.

At times it will be necessary for the nurse to be firm with the elated patient. For example, the patient may insist that he does not want his medication, and it may be necessary for the nurse to tell him gently but firmly that she expects him to take the medication at a given time.

It will also be necessary for the nurse to protect the patient against giving away his clothing and other possessions that he has with him. For this reason, too, his letters may be read by the physician before they are mailed to ensure that he is not giving away his property or property that he does not in reality own.

CREATING A THERAPEUTIC ENVIRONMENT.   Because the elated patient has incorporated so many objects in his environment, and because he is so full of energy and emotion, he needs a large space in which to move about. It is unfortunate that many hospitals are built with small rooms in which to seclude the elated patient from others. Often, however, the patient can be alone in a large space such as the gym, where he can romp and play with only the nurse to supervise his activities.

The elated patient will like very bright and gay furnishings, but these may tend to overstimulate him. Something that is colorful but soft, nonirritating, and not too stimulating may be effective. Since he seems to absorb almost everything in his environment, soothing music which is slow in tempo but rhythmical may help to retard his motor activity.

Because of the patient's excessive activity, the room should be free from drafts, and the temperature a little cooler than that which most patients prefer. The lighting should be soft and dim but not dreary. Loud and sudden noises tend to interrupt him and make him irritable. Therefore, these should be minimized.

Because the patient is meddlesome, domineering, and easily stimulated, an effective dynamic environment is somewhat difficult to provide in the average hospital. It is best, in the acute phase, that he have a room of his own, since he will prove very annoying to anyone else who is ill. Also, at times during the day, it may be necessary to exclude him from other patients. When most of the other patients are away from the unit, he can usually be taken into the dayroom. If the dayroom is large, he can be given something to do in one corner so as not to disturb the other patients. If an inside court or porch is provided, he will enjoy spending his time there when it is not in use by others. It is very important that he not be shut in a small room all day, even though he may have to be removed from the group for short periods. As the patient begins to quiet down, he can and should be gradually introduced to other patients.

Meeting the needs for restoration of energy. We have mentioned that the patient will usually have difficulty sleeping, and yet he needs his rest because of his increased activity. A warm bath before retiring may help the patient to relax. When the patient awakens during the night, the nurse may converse with or listen to him for a while. By making suggestions in a monotonous tone, the nurse may persuade the patient to sleep. Sedatives may be ordered, and the nurse will want to review the toxic effects of those commonly prescribed on the psychiatric unit. Certain types of sedatives may make the patient more active rather than drowsy; if the desired effects are not obtained, the physician should be notified. Short rest periods should also be provided during the day. Even though the patient may not sleep, he may be induced to occupy himself with some quiet activity that can be pursued while he is sitting down.

The patient may not wish to eat because he either is too busy playing or does not wish to have his happy state interrupted. He will be more likely to eat foods that he can carry about, for example, fruit, sandwiches, or cookies. High-caloric fluids should be offered at least every two hours, and should be served in a plastic or paper container since the patient may throw it. When the patient is in a very elated state, he should eat alone, since he is inclined to play and throw his food. In addition, he is easily distracted and stimulated; therefore, being with others may make it impossible for him to concentrate on eating.

If tube feedings should become necessary, it is best to tell the patient just prior to beginning the procedure. Long explanations and arguments will not help. In such instances additional help may be necessary to restrain him, but care should be taken that he is not injured. Pressure upon the abdomen, chest or neck should be avoided. Since the patient may injure someone accidentally by kicking, it is best to remove his shoes beforehand. It will also be necessary to restrain his arms, since he may displace the tube by pulling it, thus causing him to aspirate fluid.

A record of the food and fluid intake as well as the patient's output should be kept. The elated patient may also experience constipation because of loss of water through perspiration and because of his low fluid intake. Special care should be given to the skin, since it will probably be dry and cracked. The patient will also have to be watched for minor cuts and abrasions; he may injure himself accidentally in his antics. He will be particularly prone to secondary infections because of his increased activity and lack of rest. Because of his loss of body fluids he may have an elevated temperature; therefore, special mouth care may be indicated.

In regard to personal appearance the elated patient may tend to adorn himself with beads, flowers, brightly colored clothing or anything else that he preceives to be ornamental. At times he may strip off his clothing because of his belief that his body is beautiful. Inexpensive but durable and attractive clothing will be most suitable while he is in this state. He will probably not object to wearing moccasins if they do not look too much like bedroom slippers. If he has access to all his clothing, he will usually turn out to be the laughingstock of the ward, so it will be well for the nurse to select his clothing, and take it to him.

It may not be possible to shave male patients during an extremely acute phase of their illness. They may not hold still and may get cut with the razor. An electric razor will minimize this danger. The patient may even be able to use it himself under close supervision if his interest can be maintained for that length of time.

Women patients tend to wear too much make-up, and it is usually wise to provide them with only one type of cosmetic at a time. If the nurse chooses subdued shades of cosmetic for the patient, it will not look too ridiculous even though the patient uses it to excess. As the patient is able to participate in self-care, he should be encouraged to do so; however, some supervision is usually required even in milder states of elation.

Activities. Since the elated patient does not pursue any one activity for very long, it is important that his interest be directed toward projects that can be completed in a very short period of time. He usually likes to write and draw and, if provided with materials, may produce voluminous notes and pictures that will aid the psychiatrist in his therapy. Since the patient enjoys smearing, he will also probably like finger painting or clay modeling. Care should be taken that he pursues this activity in an environment where it will not matter if he adorns the wall, floor, and furnishings. The patient also likes to tear up things, and may enjoy tearing rags for rugs. Pounding metal may also be an outlet for his excessive energy. He will enjoy outdoor activities but he will need to be observed closely; he tends not to stay in any one place, and may attempt to leave the hospital grounds. As he gains satisfaction from completing small projects, he can gradually assume the responsibility for completing larger ones and begin participating with other patients. However, as his elation subsides he may still tend to overdo. Therefore, he will require supervision so that he will not dominate others. As he becomes better, he frequently becomes the group leader, and arranges activities for the ward. The nurse will want to encourage him in this respect so long as he does not become too demanding of other patients.

Summary

The main characteristics in the behavior of the elated patient have been summarized within the chapter, and so we shall omit further elaboration here.

The relationship with the elated patient was described as being one that is calm, firm, kind, warm and affectionate, but also one that portrays an attitude that is somewhat less optimistic than that of the patient. It is important to "laugh with" the patient rather than to "laugh at" him. If the nurse understands why the patient is behaving as he does, his accusations, profanity and obscenity will not be condemned.

The elated patient will need some protection from injuring himself because of the possibility of accidents during very elated periods. An environment that would be effective for the elated patient is a large spacious area, and one that has a minimum of irritating and stimulating objects.

In the restoration of energy, the patient's inability to sleep and his refusal to eat are important factors for the nurse to consider. As with the patient with feelings of worthlessness, the elated patient's intake and output should be closely observed.

In regard to activities, the patient will enjoy writing, painting and drawing as well as those in which he can pound and tear. As he becomes less elated he can begin to enter into group activities, but some supervision will be needed to protect the rights of others.

Bibliography

Abraham, Karl: *Selected Papers on Psychoanalysis.* London, Hogarth Press, 1927.
Bellak, Leopold, *et al.: Manic-Depressive Psychosis and Allied Conditions.* New York, Grune & Stratton, Inc., 1952.
Bevers, Stacie Virginia: "Music Therapy." *Am. J. Nursing, 69:*89-92, January, 1969.
Bychowski, Gustav: *Psychotherapy of Psychosis.* New York, Grune & Stratton, Inc., 1952.
Cameron, Norman: *The Psychology of Behavior Disorders.* Boston, Houghton Mifflin Co., 1947.
Campbell, John D.: *Everyday Psychiatry.* Philadelphia, J. B. Lippincott Co., 1949.
Custance, John: *Wisdom, Madness and Folly.* New York, Pellegrini & Cudahy, Inc., 1952.
Federn, Paul: *Ego Psychology and the Psychoses.* New York, Basic Books, Inc., 1952.
Fenichel, Otto: *The Psychoanalytical Theory of Neurosis.* New York, W. W. Norton & Co., Inc., 1945.
Gregory, Ian: *Fundamentals of Psychiatry.* Philadelphia, W. B. Saunders, 1968.
Kolb, Lawrence C.: *Noyes' Modern Clinical Psychiatry.* 7th ed., Philadelphia, W. B. Saunders, 1968.

Lewin, Bertram D.: *The Psychoanalysis of Elation.* New York, W. W. Norton & Co., Inc., 1950.
Mikesell, W. A., ed.: *Modern Abnormal Psychology.* New York, Philosophical Library, Inc., 1950.
Redlich, Frederick C., and Freedman, Daniel X.: *The Theory and Practice of Psychiatry.* New York, Basic Books, Inc., 1966.
Rhodes, Martha: "Nursing the Acutely Ill Psychiatric Patient." *Nursing Outlook, 14*:25-26, February, 1966.

Suggestions for Further Reading

Clack, Janice: "Nursing Intervention into the Aggressive Behavior of Patients." In Shirley F. Burd and Margaret A. Marshall, eds.: *Some Clinical Approaches to Psychiatric Nursing.* New York, Macmillan Co., 1963, pp. 199-205.
Fernandez, Theresa M.: "How to Deal With Overt Aggression." *Am. J. Nursing, 59*:658-660, May, 1959.
Gibson, John: "The Manic-Depressive Psychosis." *Canadian Nurse, 55*:928–930, October, 1959.
Gibson, R. W., Cohen, M. B., and Cohen, R. A.: "On the Dynamics of the Manic-Depressive Personality." *Am. J. Psychiat., 115*:1101-1107, June, 1959.
Henderson, Sir David, and Batchelor, Ivor R. C.: *Henderson and Gillespie's Textbook of Psychiatry,* 9th Ed., London, Oxford University Press, 1962, pp. 208-220, 240-249.
King, Joan M.: "Denial." *Am. J. Nursing, 66*:1010-1013, May, 1957.
Kirkpatrick, W. F.: "A Patient With Recurrent Mania." *Nursing Times, 59*:124-126, February 1, 1963.
Kolb, Lawrence C.: *Noyes' Modern Clinical Psychiatry,* 7th Ed., Philadelphia, W. B. Saunders Co., 1968.
Kraines, S. H.: "The Physiologic Basis of the Manic-Depressive Illness: A Theory." *Am. J. Psychiat., 114*:206-211, September, 1957.
Maloney, Elizabeth M., and Johanneson, Lucille: "How the Tranquilizers Affect Nursing Practice." *Am. J. Nursing, 57*:1144-1147, September, 1957.
Peplau, Hildegarde E.: *Interpersonal Relations in Nursing.* New York, G. P. Putnam's Sons, 1952, pp. 189-207.
Schwartz, Morris S., and Shockley, Emmy Lanning: *The Nurse and the Mental Patient.* New York, Russell Sage Foundation, 1956, pp. 21-89.
Speroff, B. J.: "Empathy Is Important in Nursing." *Nursing Outlook, 4*:326-328, June, 1956.
Wilson, David C.: "Group Psychotherapy and Manic-Depressive Psychosis." *Am. J. Psychiat., 110*:911-915, June, 1954.

Chapter 18 The Patient With Problems of Senescence

The older person has the same basic and acquired needs as all other people, and also has additional needs that are characteristic of his age. Some of these needs are often forgotten by those caring for the older person. It is particularly important that the older person have an opportunity to give love as well as receive it. He has also the need to be respected by others by virtue of maintaining respect for himself. He needs to be useful, to feel wanted, to accept and carry out responsibility, to have creative experiences, to have social participation with others in his community, to continue to strive toward reaching his potentials and also to identify his spiritual, religious and philosophical values.

THE TASKS OF THE AGED

All ages have their tasks of life and the older person has his tasks. These tasks or responsibilities of the aged are stated very concisely in the New York report on aging, and are as follows:

1. Keep oneself self-supporting as long as possible consonant with one's health.
2. Learn and carry out the sound principles of mental health and physical health.

3. Keep active, alert and useful as long as possible.
4. Develop his potential as an individual in his later years.
5. Cherish but not dominate his children or children's children.
6. Serve friends, neighbors and community to the best of his ability.
7. Transfer to others the wisdom the years have accumulated.
8. Adapt to new conditions and circumstances, with open mind.
9. Plan for his later years.
10. Avoid those characteristics of aging which alienate one's standing among friends, neighbors and the community, such as garrulousness, obstinacy, inflexibility, social withdrawal, grouchiness, despair.[1]

These new tasks in life are mastered by some without difficulty. Adolf Vischer a great man with a profound understanding of the aged, speaks as follows about the tasks of life:

But for not a few the passage into the higher stage of life is a serious crisis. In the first half of life the man is confronted with tasks connected with his profession, the married state, posterity, and all sorts of ties and relations. From the middle point of life the necessity of adapting himself to the inner self makes itself felt; he must turn toward the inner spiritual realities, hitherto but little regarded.[2]

SPECIAL REQUIREMENTS OF THE AGED

PROTECTION

Older people apparently are more cognizant of their limitations than younger people. They are less likely to be involved in serious accidents than younger persons, but they often need protection from dangers such as falls, infections and abuse by others. Low beds not only make it easier for the patient to get up, but also help to prevent serious injuries from falls. In some cases a railing extending about four inches upward from the mattress will be enough to keep the patient from rolling out of bed. If the patient is confused and if the railing is high, he may attempt to climb over it, and thereby fall an even greater distance. In cases of extreme confusion, it may be well to place one side of the bed against the wall and place a mattress on the floor, so that any fall will be cushioned and cause less injury to the patient.

Since older patients do not always see too well, and because they are apt to have some impairment of motor functions, it is important that stairways be walled off rather than open, that hand railings be

---

[1]New York State Joint Legislative Committee on Problems of the Aging: *Age Is No Barrier.* Legislative Document No. 35, 1952, p. 10.
[2]A. L. Vischer: *Old Age: Its Compensations and Rewards.* London, George Allen and Unwin, Ltd., 1947, p. 184.

provided in corridors and stairways, and that the lighting be especially good. If the patient walks outside in the winter, ice grippers on the soles of shoes may prevent sliding and falling. Windows should also be equipped with mechanical devices so that they can be opened and closed without having to lean out.

Bathrooms should be equipped with nonskid floors, square tubs with seats and hand grips, and should not provide excessively hot water; however, if all this is not possible, rubber bathmats on the bottom of the tub and on the floor next to the tub may prevent slipping. Supporting the patient with a dry towel between the nurse's hand and the patient's body may, when assisting the patient from the tub, also prevent him from slipping. If the tub is placed against the wall, or if the patient is unable to get into a tub without much assistance, placing him on a stool in a shower may take less effort and be much safer. Baths, because of danger of accidents and because they dry the skin, need not be given daily. Two or three times or even once a week may be sufficient. Because the patient may have some heart complication and because of danger of burns, the temperature of the water should be just a little above lukewarm. The room, however, should be free from drafts, and about 80° F.

If the older patient smokes, it is very important that he be supervised while smoking in bed because he may drop off to sleep before he is finished.

The older patient, if inclined to be confused at night, may have fewer illusions and fears if a night light is left on. It is especially important that bathrooms be well lighted during the night to prevent accidents.

The older patient may need protection from those who abuse him by either offering him "get-rich schemes" or "special bargains." It is also important from a legal standpoint that the nurse not influence or offer any comments that may influence the patient in making his will. Such action on the nurse's part may make the will invalid. If the patient asks her advice about wills, she should suggest that he obtain the services of an attorney. The patient's possessions need to be given special care to make sure that they are not appropriated by other patients who may hoard or by someone who may steal them.

REST AND EXERCISE

The older patient needs to be out of bed unless he is suffering from an illness that would contraindicate such a procedure. However, if he is placed in a chair with his legs dangling, this position may be worse than lying in bed. Too often the older person is placed in a chair early in the morning and forgotten until time to put him in bed in the evening. He needs to exercise his arms, legs, and hands, even though it is done passively. The physician or rehabilitation center can often prescribe the right kind of exercise to keep the joints mobile and to keep circulation unimpaired. If the patient does go to the physical therapy department, it is especially important for the nurse to carry out any recommendations made by them so that the patient can eventually care for himself.

A short rest in bed in the afternoon will often prevent the patient from becoming excessively tired. When getting the patient up after being in a prone position, the nurse should give him plenty of time to adjust to a sitting position, thereby preventing possible dizziness.

PRIVACY

Lack of privacy may be more degrading to the older person than to younger ones. A good many older individuals were reared in families that took a dim view of showing the body. They grew up in an age that placed high value on modesty. It was an age when all women wore long dresses. Older female patients may be very reluctant to let the younger physician or nurse view their bodies. This modesty sometimes accounts for the patient's reluctance to bathe. Sometimes it will help if the nurse lets the patient wear a hospital gown while taking a bath in the presence of the nurse or others. The wet gown can be easily removed, and a dry one can replace it without exposing the patient unnecessarily. It is especially important that the older patient's privacy be maintained during treatments and procedures, and that the nurse be present when the male physician examines the female patient.

The older, long-term patient will appreciate having a room of his own, or at least a cubicle, so that he can bring some of his own furniture and other personal possessions that will make him feel more at home. He will also appreciate short periods during the day when he can be alone with his activities or thoughts.

SKIN CARE

The older person may need special attention paid to his skin, especially if he does not maintain good bowel and bladder control. Since his skin is often thin, dry and scaly, it may be necessary to minimize bathing. When he is bathed, a soap with a cold cream or oil base may prove less irritating to the skin. It is important, too, that special care be given to skin surfaces that touch, and that all soap be carefully removed. Since alcohol tends to dry the skin, oil applied after the bath may prevent further drying and scaling. So as not to impair circulation, the patient's position should be changed every two hours even though he may be in a chair.

If the patient does not maintain good bowel and bladder control, he should be given special attention to keep him dry. Small, soft pads under the patient may be easily removed and Diaparene chloride may help to prevent odors and to make the urine less irritating to the skin. If the hours of the patient's bowel and bladder habits are recorded, the nurse may establish the patient's pattern and, therefore, assist him to the bathroom before a mishap occurs. If the patient's other needs are met, this habit of soiling is sometimes easier to control. The soiling in some cases may be a way of expressing hostility on the part of the patient.

Any dermatitis or break in the skin should be reported to the physician so that immediate treatment can be instituted. Regardless of how careful the nurse has been, decubitus ulcers do sometimes occur and the nurse need not feel guilty.

FOOT CARE

The older patient also may have considerable difficulty with his feet. Callous skin on the sole of the foot may often itch, burn and be quite painful. Toenails, too, may be thick, distorted, and ingrown. If the patient is not visited regularly by one who gives special care to the feet, it may be necessary for the nurse to soak the feet, remove the dry skin by friction with a towel and then apply oil to soften the skin. Toenails should be cut straight across. If there is a tendency for them to "ingrow," a very small piece of cotton, moistened with an antiseptic, tucked under the edge of the toenail may relieve pain. When walking, the patient should wear well-fitted, soft leather oxfords with low rubber heels to support his feet and to help maintain good body posture. When sitting in a chair, the patient should keep his feet elevated on a footstool to maintain good circulation.

FOOD INTAKE

Older people, for many reasons, are apt to have an unbalanced food intake if not closely supervised. For most people, eating is a social event, but, if the older person is living alone or is isolated in a hospital room, eating may not take on the significance that it once did; therefore, an opportunity to eat with others will perhaps stimulate his interest in food. With a decline in the sense of taste, it is particularly important that foods look especially attractive. The older person will also appreciate smaller servings at more frequent intervals.

Any difficulties with dentures should be corrected to make eating more pleasant for the older patient, as well as for those around him, and since the patient often takes naps frequently, the use of a mouth-wash before eating may make food more palatable.

It is often necessary, if the patient cannot see well, to point out to him what foods his tray contains. If he is unable to cut meat, he should be given assistance with it. It should be emphasized that, unless it is contraindicated by his illness, he should be taught to do these things for himself. It often takes much more time and a great deal of patience in the beginning of the teaching process. It will, however, save the nurse more time in the end and it will give the patient a sense of accomplishment.

The older person should be given plenty of time to eat. Often he tires easily and his movements are slower so that it takes him longer than the younger patient. Also, since he has a need to preserve his autonomy, the older person should be given as much choice as possible in regard to foods he likes and dislikes while still keeping within his prescribed diet regimen.

It is considered paramount that the older patient drink sufficient milk, even though it may be necessary for skim milk to be used. Because the blood maintains a certain calcium level at all times, other tissues of the body may be robbed in order to maintain this level.

If the patient is eating at home, and is somewhat incapacitated, a service such as "meals on wheels" may be available to provide hot meals for him. If the patient prepares his own meals, it is advisable for him to use an electric stove or hot plate rather than gas burners. He may forget and let foods boil over, extinguishing the flame, and thereby be asphyxiated.

The patient may need to be taught certain facts in relation to his diet and then supervised to make sure that he is able to carry them out. Often this information will be new to the patient, because most older patients had only grade school education at a time when very little was known about adequate food intake. Since he is more likely to be foreign born than younger patients, cultural food habits should also be explored.

If the patient is inclined to spill his food, he may need extra napkins. At any rate, he should be protected from going about with food smeared on his face and clothing.

GROUP ACTIVITIES

The older person needs opportunities to socialize with others. Often these activities can be used in such a way that they are useful to others as well as the patient. In small groups where the patient can exercise his autonomy, such as groups for self-government, the patient may be able to maintain a feeling of self-respect.

Whether at home or in an institution, the older person needs some contact with groups in the community. If at home, especially in rural areas, he may need transportation, and often volunteer groups can be of assistance in this respect.

Colleges and other schools in the community can often be encouraged to offer courses where the older person can continue to learn. It should be emphasized to the older patient that he can learn, and he must be expected to do so. Lack of motivation and interest are considered to be factors when he does not. The nurse can assist in exploring his interest with him, and perhaps motivate him to learn faster.

The patient may also be interested in participating in some of the hospital chores, which, if not too tiring, may be of help to the institution and also give the patient a feeling of usefulness. All tasks should be small enough so that they can easily be completed in a short period of time, thus giving the patient a feeling of accomplishment.

It is especially important for the older patient to pursue some hobby. If he already has one, then he should be encouraged to maintain those skills. Often he may learn a new hobby and, if it can bring him some income, it will add to his feeling of independence.

In some communities the aged are provided with sheltered workshops, rehabilitation centers, counseling and job placement centers, senior citizen groups and clubs such as the Golden Age Club. When the older person retires, he often has abilities that can be used in industry, or he can still supplement his income by caring for children or engaging in some other useful activity that is within his ability and which will contribute to society.

Some communities provide vacation services for the aged, such as camping and traveling. In some areas there are also facilities to take care of the aged while the older person's family takes a vacation. Frequently, too, older persons become foster grandparents to children in the community.

OTHER ASPECTS OF DAILY LIFE

One aspect of the patient's daily life in which almost every patient can exercise his autonomy is the opportunity to designate the clothing he wishes to wear on a given day. While this may seem a small thing for him to govern, it gives the patient a great deal of satisfaction in responding to, "What would you like to wear today?" or, "Would you like to wear your white shirt or your blue shirt?" The nurse can also do a great deal merely by providing the patient physical support while he dresses himself. When he can perform these activities, either shared with the nurse or alone, he will not be totally dependent upon her, and he can maintain more self-respect than if someone does it for him.

While the problem of lack of bowel and bladder control has been mentioned, it is equally important to observe the patient for constipation or retention of urine. Older patients may become impacted and diarrhea may only be a symptom. Nonsaline cathartics are often prescribed because the patient may have some tendency for retention of fluid in the tissues. Mineral oil is usually avoided since it absorbs vitamins from the body. In some cases an accurate record of fluid intake and output is necessary. Usually a urine output of 1000 cc. is indicative of adequate fluid intake.

In general, the more the nurse can do to keep the patient a functioning member of society, the less he will be apt to regress from mere disuse of biologic, psychologic, or social functions.

THE OLDER PATIENT WITH PSYCHIATRIC DISORDERS

The older patient tends to experience more stress than the younger patient and, because of his advancing age, is less able to deal with it. For this reason, older persons are considered among the high-risk group insofar as mental illness is concerned. The two psychiatric illnesses particularly common in the aged individual are cerebral atherosclerosis and senile psychosis. These conditions, however, are not manifested by all older persons.

Cerebral atherosclerosis is characterized by sclerosis and/or deposits of fat in the blood vessels of the brain. Although the illness may be seen earlier in life, it is most common between the ages of 50 and 65. The patient, prior to the acute onset, may complain of dizziness, fatigue, headache, inability to concentrate, drowsiness, numbness of the extremities and discomfort in the neck. Often the attack begins by a sudden state of confusion or excitement, with clouding of consciousness, restlessness and incoherence. There is often impairment of attention and memory. At night the patient may be very bewildered and may manifest both delusions and hallucinations. The patient's behavior also is often characterized by an emotional lability. He may laugh inappropriately and, just a few moments later, cry for no apparent reason. The disease also may be insidious, with a more gradual manifestation of the above symptoms. The patient may have periods of remission when he manifests few symptoms of the illness. The patient may be hostile or depressed or may manifest an exaggeration of any of the patterns of defense. The illness is more common in men than women. The patient is usually aware of his mental state, and this knowledge is often quite disturbing to him.

The nurse will try to discover the periods in which the patient is more amenable, and use these to her advantage in ministering to him. It will be especially important for the nurse to protect the patient from suicide, since its occurrence is not rare. Diets to influence lipid metabolism are still controversial. Quite often, however, nicotinic acid is used to improve circulation. Chlorpromazine may sometimes be used in reducing nocturnal symptoms, but, because of a possible hypotensive reaction to the drug, it is usually given orally. Barbiturates are not usually administered, since they tend to aggravate confusion. Aminophylline, four grains given four times per day, may be prescribed by the physician to relieve dizziness, headache, insomnia, and confusion. Hydrotherapy at short intervals and psychotherapy are also common treatments.

Since the patient may be very forgetful, it may be necessary for the nurse to repeat instructions to the patient on innumerable occasions. It will often be necessary to repeat her name to the patient every time she approaches him. In some cases, since the patient seems so aware of his loss of memory, he may find it helpful to carry a pad and pencil about so that he can write reminders to himself.

A very rigid schedule for the patient's activities of daily living may help to keep him oriented during periods when he is inclined to be confused. Such little things as always putting his glasses and other articles in the same place may also help to keep him oriented. The patient should be encouraged to participate in both individual and group activities; however, he should not tire or overexert himself.

The patient should be watched for signs of infection so that immediate treatment can be instituted. During periods of infection, the patient's mental state usually becomes exaggerated and management may be exceedingly difficult. It should be noted, however, that older patients may have a rather serious illness and may not appear sick.

Signs and symptoms of "strokes" should also be observed and reported promptly, since the physician may wish to prescribe anticoagulants such as Dicumarol or heparin. If the patient has impaired function of his extremities after a cerebral accident, passive exercises should be instituted almost immediately at the physician's direction. In cases of aphasia, speech therapy is usually considered.

Since little is known about the treatment and prevention of atherosclerosis, a number of medications and treatments may be tried to alleviate the patient's symptoms. Often such drugs and treatment are on a research basis, and the accuracy of the nurse in noting cardinal signs and symptoms as well as other aspects of the patient's behavior may be crucial.

The nursing care, in general, will be dependent upon the dynamics involved, the symptoms manifested, the treatment prescribed, as well as the general requirements essential in the care of the older person.

Senile psychosis, another illness found in some older people, is usually gradual in its onset. Although in some cases there are changes in the brain, these do not always correlate with the individual's psychologic functioning. Quite often the person who develops senile psychosis is one whose earlier life has been characterized by rigid and static habits with few established patterns of effective adjustment. The illness is more commonly found in women than in men, and is not particularly marked until after the age of 60. The patient usually has a gradual decline in memory, his vocabulary becomes disorganized, and descriptive phrases may be substituted for names of persons or objects. The patient is often disoriented as to time, place and person, and he may wander out of his room and onto the street. He often confuses days with nights and dreams with reality. The patient may also have suspicious, self-accusatory, and hypochondriac delusions. Often the patient is physically feeble and uncertain on his feet.

Impulsiveness, irritability, and depression are also common symptoms. The patient's judgment may be markedly impaired, and he may need protection so that he does not marry impulsively, commit criminal sexual acts, or make foolish financial ventures.

Carelessness in personal appearance and toilet habits, the hoarding of apparently meaningless objects, delusions of theft, blunting of affect, repetitive acts, and a tendency to isolation may also occur. Unlike the patient with cerebral atherosclerosis, the patient with senile psychosis is usually unaware of his mental condition, and he does not seem to have periods of remission.

If there is early recognition of the illness and the patient can be influenced to take a more active interest in life, further mental deterioration may be prevented.

Mild hypnotics such as paraldehyde are often prescribed for restlessness, and, in confused states, vitamin therapy and nicotinic acid are frequently used. Tension and hyperactivity are often counteracted by the tranquilizing drugs such as reserpine, chlorpromazine and Miltown. Glutamic acid is also sometimes prescribed, and is thought to be effective in making the patients less isolated and more inclined to participate with others socially. If the patient is receiving antipyretics, analgesics, or opiates, he should be observed for signs of cyanosis and depression of the respiratory centers; the older person is more apt to react adversely to these drugs. Other treatments sometimes prescribed are electroshock and hydrotherapy.

The whereabouts of the patient should be known at all times, since he may attempt suicide or wander away in his confusion. Like the patient with cerebral atherosclerosis, the nursing care is dependent upon the same factors as mentioned earlier.

Summary

Health problems of the older patient have been elaborated, and nursing care in relation to protection, rest and exercise, privacy, skin care, foot care, food intake, group activities and other aspects of daily life have been discussed.

Just as all ages have their tasks of life, the older person has his tasks. The older person has many responsibilities or tasks which society impo̒ses upon him at the period in life when he is apt to be least able to cope with them.

In addition to the problems that accompany the aging process, psychiatric disorders may be manifested, commonly in the form of cerebral atherosclerosis and senile psychosis.

We see that cerebral atherosclerosis is often acute in onset, with periods of remission. There may be confusion, impairment of attention and memory, and emotional lability.

Senile psychosis is usually gradual in onset, and is without periods of remission. There is a gradual decline in memory and a disorientation of time, place, and person. The patient also may have suspicious, self-accusatory, and hypochondriac delusions. While cerebral arteriosclerosis is more common in men than women, senile psychosis is more commonly found in women than in men.

Nursing care of the older patient with psychiatric disorders is dependent upon the dynamics involved, the symptoms manifested, the treatment prescribed, as well as the care necessary for the older patient in general.

Bibliography

Agate, John N.: *Medicine in Old Age.* Philadelphia, J. B. Lippincott Co., 1966.

Bloom, Bernard L.: "The Ecology of Psychiatric Hospitalizations for Acute and Chronic Brain Syndrome." *J. Geront.,* 24:48-54, January, 1969.

Busse, Ewald: "Advances in Medical Science." *Gerontologist,* 8:129-30, Summer, 1968.

Cautela, Joseph R.: "A Classical Conditioning Approach to the Development and Modification of Behavior in the Aged." *Gerontologist,* 9:109-113, Part I, Summer, 1969.

Ciompi, L.: *Geronto-Psychiatric Literature in the Postwar Period.* National Institutes of Health, Washington, D.C., U.S. Government Printing Office. (Translated from Fortschr. Neurol. Psychiat. (Stüttgart), 34(2):49-159, 1966.)

Corsellis, J. A. N.: *Mental Illness and the Aging Brain.* Maudsley Monograph No. 9, London, Oxford University Press, 1962.

Cowdry, E. V. (ed.): *The Care of the Geriatric Patient.* St. Louis, C. V. Mosby Co., 1968.

Epstein, L. J. and Simon, A.: "Organic Brain Syndrome." *Geriatrics,* 22:145-150, 1967.

Evans, Frances Monet Carter: "Visiting Older People: A Learning Experience." *Nursing Outlook,* 17:20-22, March, 1969.

Ferraro, Armando: "Psychoses with Cerebral Arteriosclerosis." *In* Silvana Arieti, ed.: *American Handbook of Psychiatry.* Vol. II. New York, Basic Books, Inc., 1959, pp. 1078-1108.

Ferraro, Armando: "Senile Psychoses." *In* Silvano Arieti, ed.: *American Handbook of Psychiatry.* Vol. II. New York, Basic Books, Inc., 1959, pp. 1021-1043.

Howell, Sandra C., and Loet, Martin: "Nutrition and Aging, A Monograph for Practition-
ers." Vol. 9, Part II, Autumn, 1969.
Kinoy, Susan K.: "Home Health Services for the Elderly." *Nursing Outlook, 17*:59-64,
September, 1969.
Kolb, Lawrence C.: *Noyes' Modern Clinical Psychiatry.* 7th Ed., Philadelphia, W. B. Saunders,
1968.
Lawton, Alfred H.: "Characteristics of the Geriatric Person." *Gerontologist, 8*:120-123,
Summer, 1968.
Lissitz, Samuel: "The Challenge of the Senile Aged." *Gerontologist, 9*:114-119, Part I,
Summer, 1969.
New York State Joint Legislative Committee on Problems of the Aging: *Age is No Barrier.*
Legislative Document No. 35, 1952.
Potter, Minerva C.: "The Nurse as Community Crises Counselor." *Nursing Outlook,
17*:39-42, September, 1969.
Riley, Matilda White, and Fonner, Anne: *Aging and Society.* New York, Russell Sage
Foundation, 1968.
Simon, Alexander: *"The Geriatric Mentally Ill."* *Gerontologist, 8*:7-15, Part II, Spring, 1968.
Stone, Virginia: "Give the Older Person Time." *Am. J. Nursing, 69*:2124-2127, October,
1969.
Thomas, Isabelle E., Flowers, Peggy, and Varner, Lois J.: "A Project Called Well-Being."
Am. J. Nursing, 69:1260-1263, June, 1969.
Vischer, A. L.: *Old Age: Its Rewards and Compensations.* London, George Allen and Unwin,
Ltd., 1947.
Watson, Charles G., and Fulton, John R.: "Treatment Potential of the Psychiatric-Medi-
cally Infirm. II. Psychiatric Symptomatology." 23:226-230, April, 1968.
Wolff, Kurt: *Geriatric Psychiatry.* Springfield, Illinois, Charles C Thomas, 1963.
Zeman, Frederic D.: "Neuropsychiatric Symptoms of Somatic Disorders in the Aged."
Gerontologist, 9:219-220, Part I, Autumn, 1969.

Suggestions for Further Reading

Brudno, Joseph J., and Seltzer, Herbert: "Re-Socialization Therapy Through Group
Process with Senile Patients in a Geriatric Hospital." *Gerontologist, 8*:211-214, Part I,
Autumn, 1968.
Burnside, Irene M.: "Group Work Among the Aged." *Nursing Outlook, 17*:68-71, June,
1969.
Carey, Robert G.: "The Aging Skin." *Am. J. Nursing, 63*:110-112, June, 1963.
Gibson, John: "Mental Diseases of Old Age." *Canadian Nurse, 56*:604-605, June, 1960.
Hulicka, Irene M.: "Fostering Self-Respect in Aged Patients." *Am. J. Nursing, 64*:84-89,
March, 1964.
Kinoy, Susan: "Home Health Services for the Elderly." *Nursing Outlook, 17*:59-62, Sep-
tember, 1969.
Larson, Laura: "How to Select A Nursing Home." *Am. J. Nursing, 69*:1034-1037, May,
1969.
Lawton, M. Powell, and Brody, Elaine: "Assessment of Older People: Self-Maintaining
and Instrumental Activities of Daily Living." *Gerontologist, 9*:179-186, Part I, Au-
tumn, 1969.
McCown, Pauline, and Wurm, Elizabeth: "Orienting the Disoriented." *Am. J. Nursing,
65*:118-119, April, 1965.
Mead, Margaret: "The Right to Die." *Nursing Outlook, 16*:20-21, October, 1968.
Miller, Barbara: "Assisting Aphasic Patients with Speech Rehabilitation."*Am. J. Nursing,
69*:983-985, May, 1969.
Panicci, Carol, et al.: "Expanded Speech and Self-Pacing in Communication with the
Aged." In *ANA Clinical Sessions,* New York, Appleton-Century-Crofts, 1968, pp.
95-101.
Sollar, Genevieve R.: "The Aging Patient." *Am. J. Nursing, 62*:114-117, November, 1962.

Stafford, Nova Harris: "Bowel Hygiene of Aged Patients." *Am. J. Nursing, 63*:102-103, September, 1963.

Stone, Virginia: "Give the Older Person Time." *Am. J. Nursing, 69*:2124-2127, October, 1969.

Stroker, M.: "Prognosis for Psychiatric Illness in the Aged." *Am. J. Psychiat., 119*:1069-1075, May, 1963.

Thomas, Isabelle E., Flowers, Peggy, and Varner, Lois J.: "A Project Called Well-Being." *Am. J. Nursing, 69*:1260-1263, June, 1969.

Wayne, George J.: "The Psychiatric Problems of the Elderly Patient." *Mental Hygiene, 44*:257-268, April, 1960.

Weinstock, Comilda, and Bennett, Ruth: "Problems in Communication to Nurses Among Residents of a Radically Heterogeneous Nursing Home." *Gerontologist, 8*:72-75, Summer, 1968.

Chapter 19   The Patient with Insatiable Longings

Insatiable longings are comparable to vague yearnings or gnawing sensations that keep one in a constant state of anticipation which is never fulfilled and which cannot be fulfilled in the ordinary way. The individual with insatiable longings is vulnerable to addiction or "being taken over by" some substance or activity. People may become addicted to almost anything—morphine, phenobarbital, cocaine, marijuana, alcohol, food and even hobbies. The number of individuals who are addicted to drugs and alcohol is increasing daily and poses a serious public health problem in the United States.

UNDERSTANDING THE ADDICTED PATIENT

The patient who becomes addicted has little tolerance for feelings of depression, anxiety and frustration and, therefore, resorts to taking into his body something that will give him temporary relief. He is primarily a narcissistic individual who is still in the infantile oral stage, hunger-gratification. He is so dependent upon oral satisfaction that all else yields to this need. He derives his pleasures chiefly through tactile sensations in the oral area and other cutaneous tissues. Because of his narcissism, dependency and desire for gratification without giving anything in return, he has little capacity for loving others in a mature way. In his relationships with others he is not openly dependent but manifests what is called a concealed taking relationship. The person who is the object of his relationship exists only to provide for his needs.

As he becomes older, he is terrified of loneliness; therefore, he is overly eager to please others. At the same time he is unable to accept criticism from anyone without resentment. He thrives upon a great deal of praise and reacts with disappointment if he doesn't receive enough recognition. Jellinek refers to a basic sense of estrangement from people—a feeling of being an outsider, of not belonging.[1] Since he has set for himself almost unattainable goals, he may be somewhat of a perfectionist. He believes he must surpass everyone in order to gain the recognition he desires. Often he has mood swings, vacillating between elation and depression. Underlying his facade of joviality and gaiety is a basic sense of hopelessness and futility.

When his ego becomes intolerant of pain and anxiety, and fails to master guilt, he regresses to his infantile pattern of satisfying his oral needs, and his addiction becomes a substitute for a love relationship.[2] Through the effects of toxic substances, he is able to deny reality and to achieve his goals through fantasy. In fantasy his obstacles become minute and his high ideals and goals seem more attainable. The addicted individual needs outside assistance in order to oppose the strictness of his superego.

The consumption of harmful drugs reflects the addicted individual's masochism and desire for punishment. By such methods he may eventually destroy his body, but, in so doing, he also harms those who are close to him. As he begins taking larger doses more frequently, his periods of elation become shorter and his post-elated depressions become longer until finally he is a picture of total dejection. During these periods, he becomes aware of what he is doing to himself and others, but this thought is so unbearable that he again resorts to drugs. By deceiving himself, which is another of his characteristic traits, he is able to tell himself that he can get along without alcohol, but this, of course, is impossible.

The inability to express aggression seems to be characteristic of many individuals who become addicts. In situations which tend to evoke their aggressive feelings, they experience extreme anxiety. By resorting to narcotics this individual is able to withdraw passively to a level where he experiences a minimum of anxiety and trouble. In this way, he attains an optimum level of equilibrium with an overall state of satisfaction; he feels contented, with no existing needs requiring satis-

---

[1]E. M. Jellinek: "Phases of Alcohol Addiction." *Quart. J. Stud. Alcohol, 13:*673, 1952.
[2]Gustav Bychowski: *Psychotherapy of Psychosis.* New York, Grune & Stratton, Inc., 1952, p. 306.

faction. In many respects his condition is comparable to the infant who experiences a "state of bliss" after he has been bathed and his stomach is full of warm milk.

Anderson, in his book *The Other Side of the Bottle,* describes a certain type of alcoholic who has a feeling of conversion as he "hits the bottom." This feeling, he says, occurs as an awakening, and at that moment the individual is "ripe" for treatment. The understanding of the alcoholic individual displayed by this author is as yet unsurpassed; his book is recommended as indispensable reading to supplement the material presented in this chapter.[3]

NURSING CARE OF PATIENTS IN ACUTE STATES

The initial treatment of most addicted individuals usually requires hospitalization in order to provide for any untoward symptoms that may develop and to limit the accessibility of the needed drug or alcohol. Since the patient is usually disheveled, the nurse will provide a bath, special mouth care, and other measures to increase his comfort. She should also observe his head for pediculi and his skin for infections, since he may have spent some time in the gutter or in a flophouse. She will also be alert to ensure that drugs or alcohol are not concealed in his personal effects.

The usual addicted individual is considered a social outcast and is forced to live a marginal existence. The drug addict very often becomes involved in criminal activities in order to pay the high price of his illegal narcotics. His over-all standard of living results in social deterioration, and, if barbiturates or alcohol are involved, physiologic impairment and cerebral deterioration may also occur. It is imperative that the nurse know how she feels about "addicts," because she will be able to provide the supportive care that is so essential only if she is free from a critical, punitive and/or vindictive attitude.

The individual who has become addicted to drugs, with the exception of cocaine and marijuana, has developed a new physiologic dependency, and if the drug is withheld he experiences what is called the abstinence syndrome. At first the patient begins to yawn and sneeze, his pupils become dilated, his small muscles begin to twitch and he gradually develops regular muscle spasms. He experiences both fear and anxiety as these body changes continue. As his body supply of the drug becomes more depleted, he begins to perspire profusely, his temperature and blood pressure shoot up, he becomes nauseated and

---

[3]Dwight Anderson: *The Other Side of the Bottle.* New York, A. A. Wyn, Inc., 1950.

may vomit, his muscle twitching becomes much more exaggerated and may lead to convulsions. He rapidly becomes extremely dehydrated and, if effective measures are not instituted, death may occur.

Because of the severity of the addicted individual's reaction to withholding his narcotics, most physicians prefer a method of gradual withdrawal. The two most common methods involve morphine or methadone, a synthetic opiate, with the drug being reduced slowly over a period of days. The morphine method is more rapid, but the patient still experiences fairly severe withdrawal symptoms. After the patient's physiologic dependency on the narcotic has been resolved, he is ready for some form of psychotherapy so that he can re-establish his place in society. The benzodiazepine derivatives, chlordiazepoxide (Librium), diazepam (Valium), and oxazepam (Serax), are now being used intramuscularly during the acute phase of alcoholism and are producing much better responses than did promazine.

Insulin and hydrotherapy are sometimes found to be effective treatment in the acute states, and the physician may prescribe them. The nurse will find in Chapter 11 a discussion of the nursing care required for the patient during insulin or hydrotherapy.

The physician may order a lavage and gavage, and the nurse will make preparations for these procedures. Since the patient's blood may contain highly concentrated toxic substances, extra fluids may be ordered. Vitamins will also probably be given, since the patient's food intake has usually been inadequate.

The patient will usually be restless and will manifest considerable motor activity. Paraldehyde or some other sedative may be prescribed. The patient will also experience hallucinations and illusions, and because of these he will be in an intense state of fear. Since he tends to misinterpret his environment, the nurse will remove all objects in the room except those that are absolutely essential. For the same reason, it is important that his room be kept well lighted. It is necessary for the nurse to remain with the patient during this period of fearfulness, since he may try to leap out the window or harm himself in some other way in order to "get away from the animals." Since the patient is often suspicious, the nurse will not stimulate this tendency by whispering or talking in a low voice.

As the patient begins to respond to his treatment, the nurse may find that his oral needs can be satisfied somewhat by giving him orange juice, milk or other fluids by mouth. She should anticipate that the patient will be very dependent upon her, but, as the psychotherapy with the physician progresses, the patient should become more independent and interested in doing something for others. Giving the patient advice or a lecture will not only be of no avail but may arouse resentment, since he cannot tolerate criticism. It is helpful for the nurse to remember that the addicted patient's behavior is the best response that he is capable of making in his present circumstances as he perceives the situation.

Hospitals that care for alcoholics are beginning to seek the help of Alcoholics Anonymous. If the hospital policies permit, the nurse should welcome the assistance of members of this organization who call on the patient. She will often find that they can give the alcoholic patient the understanding and help he needs to proceed in his treatment.

The general nursing care of all addicted patients is similar to the above but may differ slightly because of the particular drug or substance involved.

NURSING CARE OF PATIENTS IN CHRONIC STATES

In chronic states of alcoholic addiction, the patient usually has some neurologic involvement. The specific type of nursing care indicated will depend upon the extent of the damage to the nervous tissue.

When there is a peripheral nerve involvement, the patient will experience a numbness or pain in his extremities. In such instances, it is important for the nurse to take special precautions to prevent burns by hot water bottles or showers or other hot applications, since the patient will not always be aware of the degree of heat his skin can tolerate. If swelling of the extremities occurs, the nurse may elevate them or give a light massage, if not contraindicated. Since these patients are prone to foot drop or wrist drop, the nurse will protect the involved extremities with cradles and by holding them in the correct position with the use of sand bags. The nurse will be alert to the condition of the patient's skin and give special care as indicated.

If the patient's personality has deteriorated – that is, if sufficient cerebral damage has occurred – the nurse should anticipate that he may have little concept of ethical and moral values. She will, of necessity, serve as his superego and will have to make minor decisions for him and protect his rights. The patient may also need assistance in maintaining his personal appearance and in carrying out his personal hygiene. A review of Chapter 10 will be helpful to the nurse in meeting the patient's needs in this respect.

The nurse should also anticipate that the patient may be confused and disoriented as to time, place and person. It may be necessary to help him to recall these simple facts several times each day. Since he may experience hallucinations or illusions, it is important for the nurse to call him by name as she approaches him. If the nurse touches him without warning, he may be startled and become abusive before he is fully aware of what he is doing.

If the patient is in the older age group, it will be helpful to review material on geriatric nursing and to make applications as indicated. Every effort should be made to help the patient become interested in a hobby or some activity so that he will have an outlet from which he can gain satisfaction when he returns home.

Summary

The person with insatiable longings has been described as one who is unable to tolerate frustration and who turns to drugs or alcohol in an attempt to gain temporary relief. He is a narcissistic individual who has regressed to his earlier pattern of hunger-gratification wherein he derives pleasure. He is also a dependent person who thrives on praise and recognition.

The nursing care for the addicted patient has been elaborated by discussing his care in both the acute and chronic stages. In the acute stage it was emphasized that the nurse should remain with the patient during his intense state of fear and that she keep the room well lighted to lessen the patient's tendency to misinterpret environmental stimuli. The nursing care in the chronic stages will vary according to the involvement of the nervous system. If personality deterioration has occurred, the nurse will anticipate that the patient has little concept of ethical and moral values and may experience periods of confusion; she will, therefore, set up some external structure and also serve as his external superego. If the patient is in the older age group, the nurse will apply pertinent principles of geriatric nursing in caring for him.

Bibliography

Anderson, Dwight: *The Other Side of the Bottle*, New York, A. A. Wyn, Inc., 1950.
Bychowski, Gustav: *Psychotherapy of Psychosis.* New York, Grune & Stratton, Inc., 1952.
Campbell, John D.: *Everyday Psychiatry.* Philadelphia, J. B. Lippincott Co., 1949.
Chafetz, Morris, Blane, Howard, and Hill, Marjorie, eds.: *Frontiers of Alcoholism.* New York, Science House, 1970.
Fenichel, Otto: *The Psychoanalytical Theory of Neurosis.* New York, W. W. Norton & Co., Inc., 1945.
Hirsch, Joseph: *The Problem Drinker.* New York, Duell, Sloan & Pearce, Inc., 1949.
Jellinek, E. M.: "Phases of Alcohol Addiction." *Quart. J. Stud. Alcohol, 13*:673, 1952.
Knight, Robert: "The Psychoanalytic Treatment of Chronic Addiction to Alcohol in a Sanatorium." *J.A.M.A., 3*:1443–1448, Oct. 15, 1938.
Kolb, L.: "Drug Addiction and Its Relation to Crime." *Ment. Hyg., 9*:74, 1935.
Lolli, G.: "Alcoholism as a Disorder of the Love Disposition." *Quart. J. Stud. Alcohol, 17*:96, 1956.
Mueller, Edward E.: "Group Therapy with Alcoholics in a Hospital Setting." *Dis. Nerv. System, 10*:298-303, 1949.

Nyswander, M.: "Withdrawal Treatment of Drug Addiction." *New England J. Med.,* *242*:120–128, 1950.

Nyswander, M.: "The Treatment of Drug Addicts as Voluntary Out-Patients." *Am. J. Orthopsychiat., 28*:714, 1958.

O'Connor, William A.: *Psychiatry.* Baltimore, Williams & Wilkins Co., 1948.

Rado, Sandor: "Narcotic Bondage." *Am. J. Psychiat., 114*:165, 1957.

Reichard, J. D.: "Narcotic Drug Addiction, A Symptom of Human Adjustment." *Dis. Nerv. System, 4*:275–287, 1943.

Simmel, E.: "Alcoholism and Addiction." *Psychoanalyt. Quart., 17*:6–31, 1948.

Williams, E. Y.: "The Anxiety Syndrome in Alcoholism." *Psychiatric Quart., 24*:782–787, 1950.

Wilson, Ruth: "An Evaluation of Treatment Methods in Alcoholism Therapy." *Ment. Hyg., 35*:260–290, 1951.

Suggestions for Further Reading

Abrams, Stanley: "An Evaluation of Hypnosis in the Treatment of Alcoholics." *Am. J. Psychiat., 120*:1160–1165, June, 1964.

Alpert, Murray, and Silvers, Kenneth: "Perceptual Characteristics Distinguishing Auditory Hallucinations in Schizoprenia and Acute Alcoholic Psychoses." *Am. J. Psychiat., 127*:298–303, 1970.

Anderson, Dwight: *The Other Side of the Bottle.* New York, A. A. Wyn, Inc., 1950.

Arieti, Sylvano, ed.: *American Handbook of Psychiatry.* New York, Basic Books, Inc., 1959, Vol. I, pp. 614–643.

Block, Samuel, Owens, Kenneth, and Wolff, Ronald R.: "Patterns of Drug Use: A Study of 5,482 Subjects." *Am. J. Psychiat., 127*:420–423, 1970.

Brown, Mary Louise: "Helping the Alcoholic Patient." *Am. J. Nursing, 58*:381–382, 1958.

Cameron, Dale C.: "Addiction-Current Issues." *Am. J. Psychiat., 120*:313–319, October, 1963.

Chafetz, Morris: "The Prevention of Alcoholism." *Internat. J. Psychiat., 9*:329–348, 1970-71.

Cherkas, Marshall S.: "Synanon Foundation – A Radical Approach to the Problem of Addiction." *Am. J. Psychiat., 121*:1065–1068, May, 1965.

Cohen, Felix: "Personality Changes Among Members of Alcoholics Anonymous." *Ment. Hyg., 46*:427–437, July, 1962.

De Lint, Jan E. E.: "Alcoholism, Birth Rank and Parental Deprivation." *Am. J. Psychiat., 120*:1062–1065, May, 1964.

Freedman, Alfred M.: "Action Research in a Treatment Center." *Am. J. Nursing, 63*:57–60, July, 1963.

Gelber, Ida: "The Addict and His Drugs." *Am. J. Nursing, 63*:52–56, July, 1963.

Golder, Grace M.: "The Alcoholic, His Family and His Nurse." *Nursing Outlook, 3*:528, 1955.

Golder, Grace M.: "The Nurse and the Alcoholic Patient." *Am. J. Nursing, 56*:436, 1956.

Hart, William T.: "A Comparison of Promazine and Paraldehyde in 175 Cases of Alcohol Withdrawal." *Am. J. Psychiat., 118*:323–327, October, 1961.

Hart, William T.: "The Treatment of Alcoholism in a Comprehensive Community Mental Health Center." *Am. J. Psychiat., 126*:1275–1281, 1970.

Hirsch, Joseph: "Alcohol Education – Its Needs and Challenges." *Am. J. Pub. Health, 39*:649–653, 1949.

Holehouse, Edna: "The Alcoholic in Industry." *Am. J. Nursing, 59*:206–207, 1959.

Karpman, Benjamin: *"The Alcoholic Woman."* Washington, D.C., Lineacre Press, 1948.

LaLancette, Therese M.: "The Alcoholic Patient." *Nursing Outlook, 10*:636–638, November, 1960.

Lewis, John A.: "Alcoholism." *Am. J. Nursing, 56*:433, 1956.

Lolli, Giorgio: "Alcoholic Addiction." *Am. J. Nursing, 48*:505–507, 1948.

McCarty, Raymond G.: "Alcoholism," *Am. J. Nursing, 59*:203–205, 1959.

Moroz, Roman, and Rechter, Emanuel: "Management of Patients with Impending and Full-Blown Delirium Tremors." *Psychiatric Quart., 38*:619–626, October, 1964.

Noyes, Arthur P., and Kolb, Lawrence C.: *Modern Clinical Psychiatry.* Philadelphia, W. B. Saunders Co., 1958, pp. 191-211, 564-573.

Ostrow, Seymour: "The Medico-Legal Conflict." *Am. J. Nursing, 63*:67-71, July, 1963.

Ouiros, Alyce: "Adjusting Nursing Techniques to the Treatment of Alcoholic Patients." *Nursing Outlook, 5*:276, 1957.

Parry, Allen A.: "Alcoholism." *Am. J. Nursing, 65*:111-113, March, 1965.

Pescar, M. J., and Walker, Prudence K.: "The Treatment of Drug Addiction," *Am. J. Nursing, 51*:611, 1951.

Podolsky, Edward: "The Inadequate Chronic Alcoholic Personality." *Ment. Hyg., 46*:103-106, January. 1962.

Rohde, Ildaura Murillo: "The Addict as an Inpatient." *Am. J. Nursing, 63*:61-66, July, 1963.

Sarvajic, Joan: "Chronic Alcoholism." *Nursing World, 131*:21-22, August, 1957.

Sarvajic, Joan: "The Treatment of Chronic Alcoholism." *Nursing World, 131*:23-24, September-October, 1957.

Selzer, Melvin L., Payne, Charles E., Gifford, Jean D., and Kelly, William L.: "Alcoholism, Mental Illness, and the 'Drunk Driver.' " *Am. J. Psychiat., 120*:326-331, October, 1963.

Tamerin, John S., and Mendelson, Jack A.: "The Psychodynamics of Chronic Inebriation." *Am. J. Psychiat., 125*:886-899, 1969.

Walton, H.: "Group Methods in Hospital Organization and Patient Treatment as Applied in the Psychiatric Treatment of Alcoholism." *Am. J. Psychiat., 118*:410-418, November, 1961.

Wikler, Abraham: "Diagnosis and Treatment of Drug Dependence of the Barbiturate Type." *Am. J. Psychiat., 125*:758-765, 1968.

Chapter 20 The Patient with Antisocial Feelings

Antisocial feelings are most frequently found in patients exhibiting sociopathic behavior. By sociopathic behavior we mean that which is antisocial in that it is overtly and aggressively directed against society. It is also that which society protests and does not tolerate or condone. We should be careful not to confuse it with asocial behavior, which refers to that manifested by the patient who does not spontaneously mix with others. Sociopathic behavior is seen most consistently in the patient with sociopathic personality, which is also known as psychopathic personality and a host of other diagnostic classifications.

UNDERSTANDING THE SOCIOPATHIC INDIVIDUAL

To the casual observer the sociopathic individual appears charming, intelligent and well adjusted. As we become better acquainted with him, however, we realize that his behavior is only a mask which reveals a different profile under even slight provocation. We soon learn that what we thought was a vast store of knowledge is only fragments of superficial information. The individual seems to use his energy to collect a peculiar array of encyclopedic facts that he does not understand or use except in his attempts to impress others through conversation. Seldom does he converse at length with others who are authorities on the topic under discussion. He often appears to master superficial social situations with a charm that makes others envious. However, if frustrating situations occur, such as being involved in a heated argument, he may become incensed or outraged. He is often filled with anxiety but is able, under pleasant circumstances, to mask it with a charming smile. This individual cannot tolerate anxiety for any length of time, and frequently resorts to unusual ways to alleviate his feelings, such as forging checks and stealing. The sociopathic individual seems unable to activate his potential energy toward establishing any strong and consistent bond between himself and reality. His anxiety seems to be released and superficially attached to the first object he perceives in his environment.

Inconsistency is another characteristic of the sociopathic individual. He may go to church in the morning and by evening he may be participating in lewd sexual practices. He may help a blind person across the street upon occasion, but at another time he may knock him down in his hurry to get somewhere. He may go to work regularly for a few days or a few months, and then disappear, without an explanation to his employer or members of his family. Usually he changes positions frequently: these may vary from those that are somewhat "shady" in nature to those that are respectable. He can sell himself readily and even though his references are poor, he can talk himself into almost any type of position. At first he is usually well liked by his associates. Then, as his responsibilities increase and he has to produce, he becomes critical of his superiors and soon departs for greener pastures.

As we have implied, this type of individual is often untruthful and insincere. It is not unusual for him to tell a fantastic story even though he knows the truth will come out within the next few hours. If he is reproached, he is often indignant and gives almost fantastic excuses and rationalizations for his actions. At other times he may apologize profusely and make convincing promises. Rarely does he carry out such promises. He is almost uncanny in his ability to activate feelings in others that he seemingly does not feel himself.

According to Cleckley,[1] he seems unable to experience feelings of shame and guilt; however, this theory is refuted by Greenacre and others. At least, he does not seem to learn from his past experiences. Even though he may be punished for his behavior and is intellectually able to express what is "right" and what is "wrong," he does not seem able to carry out these concepts in real life situations.

Greenacre[2] describes the individual as behaving as though he will

---

[1]Hervey Cleckley: *The Mask of Sanity.* St. Louis, C. V. Mosby Co., 1950, p. 364.
[2]Phyllis Greenacre: *Trauma, Growth and Personality.* New York, W. W. Norton & Co., Inc., 1952, p. 167.

THE PATIENT WITH ANTISOCIAL FEELINGS

somehow be absolved and be saved from the consequences of his acts. She also mentions the "unplannedness" and lack of deliberation in regard to his actions. In actual situations his judgment seems poor in that he seems to do whatever he perceives to be the easiest at a given moment. He is able to say what one "ought to do" in a specific situation but he is unable to do it.

The sociopathic individual is also unable to express very much affect. Cleckley[3] describes the affect of a sociopathic individual as a readiness of expression rather than a feeling with depth and strength. He is often witty in social gatherings, but does not usually provoke humor of any depth. He is superficial in his relationships with others and is unable to form close attachments for any period of time. It has been said that he has an incapacity for love and true affection. In many respects he does not even seem to love himself, although he is often described as being both narcissistic and egocentric.

Such an individual has little insight into why he acts as he does, although he is able to fool many by his superficial knowledge of psychiatry and psychology. It is usually difficult for people who do not know him well to fix blame upon him. He is so evasive and ready to explain the circumstances, which are often colored by his rationalizations, that the real truth is difficult to sift out.

The sex life of the sociopathic individual is usually sordid. Overt homosexual practices and other perverse sexual activities are not unusual. Genital sensations in sexual relations do not appear to be as pleasant to him as sensations in other areas.[4] Since he abhors monotony, his perverse sexual acts seem to provide a change of pace from his daily life routine. In addition, he frequently resorts to alcohol and drugs for pleasure of short duration.

Unless the sociopathic individual has another concomitant psychiatric disorder, or is under the influence of drugs or alcohol, he does not experience delusions and hallucinations. Although he may often talk of suicide when he is in a "jam," it is seldom that his threats are carried out. Why, then, does this individual behave as he does? Are the assumptions in regard to behavior made in the first chapter unfounded?

It is not unusual to find that the sociopathic individual comes from a family that is both prominent and respected in the community. The father is usually described as an awe-inspiring, righteous and stern individual who is an authority in his occupation or profession and is absorbed with it; whereas the mother is often described as overindulgent and protective of such a person during childhood. The mother's attachment and her reluctance to let such a child give up his infantile

---

[3]Hervey Cleckley: *The Mask of Sanity*. St. Louis, C. V. Mosby Co., 1950, p. 372.
[4]*Ibid.*, p. 390.

ways, and the child's fear of the father, account for the close attachment to the mother. As the child becomes older, however, he often hurts all members of his family by his acts, which are unintelligible and embarrassing to them. He seems to take delight in causing the family grief. They usually try everything and may finally "wash their hands" of him altogether.

Family conflicts often occur in regard to attitudes and ideals. In trying to "keep up with the Joneses" or in maintaining a position of respect in the community, the family frequently builds up a wall which is a façade. The family is often embarrassed for others to know its true circumstances, even though there is little of which to be ashamed. Often the mother and father have arguments in regard to what the patient ought to do, and there is much discussion in his presence. As he becomes older there is usually disagreement as to what occupation he should follow and where he should go to school. The individual soon becomes more concerned with what he ought to do rather than what he is actually doing. He becomes more interested in impressing others than in coping with real situations. It is no wonder that his ideals are high but are remote from reality.

When the individual is small, his parents seem to enjoy "showing him off" for the sake of narcissistic reflections of themselves. Later in life, because of the father's prominence, the patient is described as the father's son or daughter but seldom is reference made to the individual's own attainment.

Because of the mother's narcissistic attachment, this type of child is never able to control his infantile aggression. His ego is described as being weak and his perception of reality peculiar. The superego, too, is said to be underdeveloped. Greenacre expresses the theory that the individual feels guilt and that he resorts to his unusual behavior in order to be punished. The dynamics of the personality of the sociopathic individual do not seem to be fully understood, which probably accounts for the little success in treatment.

Legally, the individual with sociopathic behavior is held responsible for his acts. There are no provisions made for his hospitalization except in instances where he can afford to enter a private hospital. In other circumstances, he may be sent to a state hospital for a short period for diagnosis but not for treatment. Often he ends up in jail, where treatment is not available; when he has served his sentence he is again at large. His behavior is differentiated from that of the usual criminal in that the criminal is more consistent in obtaining what he wants. The criminal's acts, although not condoned by society, are more logical; the criminal spares himself but not others, and his crimes may be those that require a major prison sentence. On the other hand, the sociopathic individual's criminal acts usually are punishable only by minor prison sentences. As we can readily see, there is a great cultural lag in regard to the care of the individual with sociopathic personality.

NURSE-PATIENT INTERACTION

It is unfortunate that so little is known in regard to successful treatment and care of the individual with antisocial feelings. However, in the light of present knowledge, the nurse may serve as a superego figure for the patient. Her attitude should be kind, matter-of-fact and firm, unless the psychiatrist specifies otherwise. At first the patient will probably turn on his charm, and may possibly try to ingratiate the nurse to him. The nurse should also anticipate that when she is near the patient will probably carry out routines with what appears to be little difficulty.

The student nurse may wonder why he is in the hospital and at first think of this individual as a "model patient." The patient, however, is somewhat of an opportunist and may soon attempt to become overly familiar with the nurse. He may begin first with flattery and will be quick to pick up her first name. He may soon be asking favors which may deviate only slightly from the usual routines. As he seemingly gains the confidence of the nursing staff, he may gradually begin to take advantage of his opportunities. He may suddenly leave the hospital when, for example, he is helping the nurse do some chore just outside the doors. On the other hand, he may take advantage by securing narcotics or sedatives if the opportunity arises. He may not hesitate to ask the nurse to go out with him socially if he has outside privileges or if he is discharged. The nurse will have to guard carefully against his using her. It will appear that the nurse-patient relationship has been established readily. Since the sociopathic individual has great difficulty in establishing a lasting relationship with anyone it is likely that his apparent attachment to her is only superficial. If the patient is under intensive therapy, an older, more experienced nurse may be able to work with him more effectively.

The nurse may have to be firm in her insistence that the patient conform to hospital rules, regulations and routines. The patient may be somewhat sullen or outraged or he may invite her sympathy. It will also be important for the nurse to perform consistently in regard to the effects of others working with the patient. Consistency in this latter respect may eventually serve to strengthen his superego. The nurse, however, will have to be careful that she is not overly strict with him and should consult the patient's physician if doubt occurs as to whether she should be insistent in regard to very trivial aspects of the routines.

Group Activities. In addition to taking into account the general factors mentioned in Chapter 25, the nurse may find the following suggestions helpful. The patient's group activities should be planned to provide more variety and also more physical activity than that of the usual patient, so that the hospital routine will not seem so monotonous. Although he will no doubt be able to participate with the group, the nurse may find it necessary to intervene if the patient becomes too "bossy" or is using other patients to accomplish his own ends. Other patients may tire of his charm and his "big talk" and may need assistance in getting out from under his domination.

Other Aspects of Nursing Care.   Unless the patient's illness is complicated by other factors, it is not anticipated that he will need assistance with carrying out his personal hygiene. Nor will problems in regard to intake and elimination be anticipated.

The nurse should observe the patient especially after visitors leave, or after he returns from outside privileges, since he may secure alcohol, drugs or some weapon that can be used to help him escape.

The sociopathic individual often upsets the nonspecific emotional atmosphere of the ward. It will not be easy for the nurse to put her finger on the specific instances that incite the difficulty, but if she observes carefully she may find that this patient is agitating other patients, playing the doctor against the nurse, or one nurse against another nurse. Because he is very ingenious, the patient is able to cause considerable disagreement among the hospital personnel as well as the patient group.

The first step for the nurse is to gain the patient's confidence, since in his previous relationships he has been unable to trust anyone. As time goes on, it may be that the patient can be helped to see that his behavior is self-defeating and that new patterns of behavior will be more rewarding.

In England and in a few places in the United States, treating the sociopathic individual in a therapeutic community has met with some degree of success. The nursing care in such cases should be evolved through a positive nurse-doctor-patient relationship, and would depend upon the goals of treatment, with cognizance of social-environmental factors.

It should be emphasized that the sociopathic individual is a very sick person, although his condition may improve for a short period of time. With more research and concentration upon the problem, more effective methods will probably be discovered in regard to both treatment and nursing care.

Summary

Patients with sociopathic behavior were described as having both a defective ego and superego. They are characterized by a superficial charm that is captivating, but upon further observation they are found to be insincere and unreliable. Cleckley describes the individual as being unable to experience guilt, while Greenacre and others believe that his inconsistent antisocial behavior is an expression of guilt and his need for punishment.

It was also emphasized that, since he has little capacity for love and affection, a lasting and effective nurse-patient relationship will be difficult to establish. It was also pointed out that the nurse should maintain a firm, matter-of-fact and consistent attitude with him. With further research, more success may be achieved in the treatment and care of the sociopathic individual. Recently, treating the patient in a therapeutic community has met with some degree of success.

Bibliography

Arieti, Silvano, ed.: *American Handbook of Psychiatry.* Basic Books Inc., 1959 and 1966.

Bromberg, W.: "Psychopathic Personality Concept Evaluated and Re-evaluated." *Archives of General Psychiatry, 17:*641–645, 1967.

Caldwell, John M.: "Neurotic Components in Psychopathic Behavior." *J. Nerv. & Ment. Dis., 99:*134-148, 1944.

Campbell, John D.: *Everyday Psychiatry.* Philadelphia, J. B. Lippincott Co., 1949.

Cleckley, Hervey: *The Mask of Sanity.* St. Louis, C. V. Mosby Co., 1950.

Cruvant, Bernard A., and Yochelson, Leon: "The Psychiatrist and the Psychotic Psychopath: A Study of Interpersonal Relationships." *Am. J. Psychiat., 106:*594-598, 1953.

Greenacre, Phyllis: *Trauma, Growth and Personality.* New York, W. W. Norton & Co., Inc., 1952.

Gregory, Ian: *Fundamentals of Psychiatry.* Philadelphia, W. B. Saunders Co., 1968.

Jones, Maxwell: *Therapeutic Community.* New York, Basic Books, Inc., 1953.

Kolb, Lawrence C.: *Noyes' Modern Clinical Psychiatry.* 7th ed., Philadelphia, W. B. Saunders Co., 1968.

Lindner, Robert: *Rebel Without a Cause.* New York, Grune & Stratton, Inc., 1944.

Menninger, Karl A.: "Recognizing and Renaming 'Psychopathic Personalities.'" *Bull. Menninger Clin., 5:*150-156, 1941.

Partridge, G. E.: "Current Conceptions of Psychopathic Personality." *Am. J. Psychiat., 84:*53-99, 1930.

Redlick, Fredrick C., and Freedman, Daniel X.: *The Theory and Practice of Psychiatry.* New York, Basic Books, Inc., 1966.

Simon, Benjamin, Halzberg, Jules D., and Fisher, Joan: "A Study of Judgment in Psychopathic Personality." *Psychiatric Quart., 25:*132-150, 1951.

Suggestions for Further Reading

Bilber, Irving: "Homosexuality." *Am. J. Nursing, 69:*2637–2641, 1969.

Bromberg, Walter: "The Treatability of the Psychopath." *Am. J. Psychiat., 110:*604-608, February, 1954.

Cleckley, Hervey: *The Mask of Sanity.* St. Louis, C. V. Mosby Co., 1950.

Cruvant, Bernard A., and Yochelson, Leon: "The Psychiatrist and the Psychotic Psychopath: A Study of Interpersonal Relationships." *Am. J. Psychiat., 106:*594-598, 1953.

Greenacre, Phyllis: *Trauma, Growth and Personality.* New York, W. W. Norton & Co., Inc., 1952.

Jones, Maxwell: *The Therapeutic Community.* New York, Basic Books, Inc., 1953.

Layton, Sr. Mary Michele: "Behavior Therapy and Its Implications for Psychiatric Nursing." *Perspectives in Psychiatric Care,* IV, 2, 1966.

Lindner, Robert: *Rebel Without a Cause.* New York, Grune & Stratton, Inc., 1944.

Menninger, Karl A.: "Recognizing and Renaming 'Psychopathic Personalities.' " *Bull. Menninger Clin.,* 5:150–156, 1941.

Peplau, Hildegarde E.: *Interpersonal Relations in Nursing.* New York, G. P. Putnam's Sons, 1952, pp. 161–187.

Render, Helena Willis, and Weiss, Olga M.: *Nurse-Patient Relationships in Psychiatry,* 2nd Ed., New York, McGraw-Hill Book Co., Inc., 1959, pp. 141–142.

Whitaker, C.: "Family Treatment of a Psychopathic Personality." *Comprehensive Psychiatry,* VII, 5:397–402, 1966.

Chapter 21   The Psychosocial Milieu of the Mental Hospital

The recognition of the increased numbers of persons who have been disabled because of psychiatric disorders has resulted in new efforts in arriving at a solution to the problem of treatment. By 1950 approximately 55 per cent of patient days in all hospitals were spent by psychiatric patients.[1] Many such patients became "chronic," and remained institutionalized for long periods of time. Are these patients the result of our modern culture? What has been overlooked in psychiatric institutions that may contribute to the problem of chronicity? Recently, social scientists have observed the way psychiatric institutions operate and thus influence the social behavior of the people within. While such research is new, and the conclusions cannot be extended to cover every situation, a new approach to the treatment of hospitalized mental patients is being made in the form of milieu therapy. This new effort does not take the place of other therapies but serves to increase their effectiveness.

A therapeutic environment, sometimes termed therapeutic milieu, may be visualized as one in which positive resources within the patient and his surroundings are mobilized to effect behavioral change in a prescribed direction. For the sake of convenience and clarity, the envi-

---

[1] Joseph W. Eaton and Robert J. Weil: *Culture and Mental Disease.* Chicago, Free Press of Glencoe, 1955, p. 17.

ronment will be considered as consisting of two major aspects, the static and the dynamic.

DIMENSIONS OF THE HOSPITAL ENVIRONMENT

Static Environment.   The static environment refers to the physical properties of the hospital, as well as the formal social structure often represented by the organizational chain of command. While the physical structure of the hospital is not a psychosocial component in and of itself, it is linked, extricably, with psychosocial factors. The size of a room, for example, may hinder or promote informal gatherings. This aspect of the environment may act as a stimulus to "set off" reactions in both groups and individuals. In this respect it is similar to a catalyst. Even though the static environment may influence others, its nature does not usually change because of such influence. In other words, it is that part of the environment which is inanimate. Factors in this environment are heat, light, sound, hospital architecture, furniture, formal social structure and the like.

The nurse has a definite role in manipulating the physical properties of the ward structure. There is much she can do in order to establish and maintain an effective static environment. A room too warm or too cold can often act as a contributory factor in increasing the irritability of patients. Irritability set off in one or two patients may initate a chain of circumstances that tend to create a negative environment for the entire ward. The nurse may be able to do very little about changing the size of a room, but with some creative ability and interest, she can use what is available to make the room appear either larger or smaller, more inviting or homelike. The nurse may be able to do something "to" this environment, but she can do little "with" the static environment.

Dynamic Environment.   The dynamic environment is defined as that aspect of the patient's situation which changes constantly because of interpersonal interchange. This part of the environment is made up of various individuals who interact in some manner with the patient. These individuals may be other patients or members of the hospital staff. When the nurse interacts with the patient, if only to say "Good morning," she influences his reaction, and in turn the patient influences her in some manner. It can thus be seen that the dynamic environment probably will not be the same in any two instances. The skilled nurse can intentionally influence this environment in order to assist in bringing about certain changes in the patient's behavior. In such instances the nurse usually makes some type of plan in advance.

The patient may also be influenced by that part of the dynamic environment which cannot readily be identified and which is not intentionally structured by those on the ward. This aspect is sometimes referred to as the nonspecific emotional tone of the ward. All nurses have probably observed, at some time or other, wards where the general atmosphere was very tense and unpleasant or, on the other hand, very congenial and pleasant. We may have realized at a given time that we were comfortable or uncomfortable, but seldom did we ask ourselves what was going on or why. This nonspecific atmosphere is usually given impetus by the nurse in charge of the ward. It is she who has much to do with whether the atmosphere is conducive to establishing effective nurse-patient interaction. A knowledge of the characteristics of a therapeutic environment may be a criterion for her effective action, and help provide a framework within which the nurse can function.

CHARACTERISTICS OF A THERAPEUTIC ENVIRONMENT

It Provides for Immediate Needs of the Patient. By immediate needs we mean those that are essential in the day-to-day living of the patient—food, fluids, toilet articles, rest, wearing apparel, safety, and toilet facilities. At first glance it seems superfluous to mention these, but often hospitals are constructed and nursing routines and procedures implemented with little thought of these aspects of the environment. Placing the patient in a situation not too unfamiliar is often an important factor in determining whether the newly admitted patient remains in the hospital or leaves during the first 24 hours.

It Provides for Hygienic Care. In a hygienic environment the surroundings and equipment are relatively or reasonably clean. In the hospital it may be necessary to use more stringent methods than one would use in the home, since hospital wards are usually constructed to house more people than the home and pathogenic organisms are usually more prevalent. On the other hand, some nurses may go to an extreme, and many spend all their time cleaning and sterilizing so that other needs of the patient are given little consideration. In either extreme the nurse may well ask herself whether she is meeting her own needs or those of the patients.

It Provides for Protection. The patient's environment should provide optimal safety. It should, except in prescribed instances, protect him from injury or self-mutilation, from harming others and from anxieties of his former everyday environment. The hospital environment should also protect him from indiscriminate confessions that he may feel compelled to make and from making any major decisions that are above his current level of responsibility. The hospitalized patient must also be protected from cross infections and other somatic disorders, since he may not always be sufficiently alert to these developments.

IT IS ACCEPTING.   An accepting environment is *not* one in which a person's actions are judged as being either good or bad, or right or wrong. It is, however, one where the patient is respected as an individual with certain rights, needs and opinions.

There should be a common understanding among the staff members of an accepting environment and of the fact that any individual's behavior is merely a reflection of his needs, his past and his present situation; therefore, to gain any understanding of the patient as a person it will be necessary to accept him as he is, regardless of personal standards.

IT IS DEMOCRATIC.   Any accepting situation must, to some extent, be democratic. The degree to which democratic principles will be followed will depend upon the level on which the people in the environment are functioning. There are, however, many ways to minimize the feeling of restriction. Democracy is sometimes thought of as freedom granted in relation to the amount of responsibility assumed. In this respect, considerable flexibility will be necessary. An environment can be somewhat restrictive and still be considered democratic. A democratic environment, therefore, will provide fewer restrictions and more freedom of choice as the patient again becomes able to assume increasing responsibility for his behavior.

IT TAKES INTO ACCOUNT THE PATIENT'S ECONOMIC STATUS, AS WELL AS HIS MEMBERSHIP IN A GIVEN CULTURAL GROUP.   The environment of the patient should be somewhat similar to the one from which he came. For example, a very plush static environment may make a patient from a poverty area uncomfortable. That is not to say, however, that the static environment should be totally depleted. There is a static environment which is minimal for therapeutic nursing. In addition, the dynamic environment should include those individuals with whom the patient can interact comfortably.

IT PROVIDES A TESTING GROUND FOR THE ESTABLISHMENT OF NEW PATTERNS OF BEHAVIOR.   In the course of getting well it is assumed that the patient will develop new ways of reacting to life situations. At first he may be groping for other ways of adjusting and, in doing this, he may try many things before he finds an effective way to deal with his problems. When the patient discovers that some methods work better than others in handling his difficulties, he may be encouraged to try these before leaving the hospital. In some instances, while the patient is searching for new patterns of adjustment, he may manifest destructive or assaultive tendencies. The hospital, therefore, must serve as a testing ground for all patterns of behavior, even though there may be some which would not be acceptable to the patient's former community.

IT PROVIDES FOR LINKAGES WITH THE COMMUNITY.   If the patient is to return to the community, opportunities for interaction should be provided so that he will not be cut off from the outside world. At first, it may be necessary to bring the community to the patient by such means as visitors, volunteers, mass communication media and the like. Later, opportunities for the patient to go into the community and to participate in community activities may be increased.

INDIVIDUAL VERSUS GROUP NEEDS

There are naturally many individual differences in regard to both needs and requirements in any given situation. What might be therapeutic for one patient might be entirely inappropriate for another, and what might be helpful to the patient at one time might be enitrely unsuitable for him at another. Consequently, both the group and the individual must be considered in any attempt to provide a milieu that will be most beneficial to all concerned.

In the matter of placement of patients, for example, both the individual and the group may be made to suffer unnecessarily if too much attention is given to individual needs. If there are two patients who are fearful that they will be harmed, and each is quite mistrustful of the other, it would be hoping for the impossible to expect them to sleep in proximity. We would instead anticipate that each would have to remain awake to watch the other. This action would, in turn, have a disturbing influence on the group as a whole.

The welfare of the group should not be imperiled for the benefit of any individual. On examination of instances where such has occurred, it has usually been found that the individual was not yet ready for group living and that the experience was detrimental to him as well as the group.

As would be expected in any group of people who live so closely together and share as many experiences as the usual group of psychiatric patients, there will be indications of leadership within the group. This leadership may be either negative or positive, but if adequate supervision is provided so that complete domination or subordination is minimized, the group interaction may be a beneficial experience for everyone.

THE SOCIAL STRUCTURE OF MENTAL HOSPITALS

Formal Structure.   Several researchers have pointed out the sharply defined status hierarchy that exists in the hospital. At the top of the hierarchy are the senior physicians, then the residents or interns, next the nurses, the attendants and, at the bottom, the patient. Within the nursing group there are also status hierarchies, beginning with the nursing director, followed by the supervisor, the head nurse, the staff nurse and the student. To complicate the picture even more there is sometimes the student's supervisor, such as the clinical instructor.

A rather unique aspect in hospital organization is that each of the above role groups is "mobility-blocked."[2] In the hospital one cannot advance, as in other organizations, from being an attendant to being a nurse and, perhaps later, to being a physician without a long formalized training period at each status level. Each of these role groups has developed a different set of values and perceptions of the hospital.[3] When groups of people in the same setting have different values, ideologies and perceptions of how things are, conflict is not unusual.

Another characteristic of the formal social structure of the hospital is multiple subordination—that is, each person performing tasks of the organization is subject to a number of bosses.[4] For example, the nurse may be given orders by the clinical director, the resident, the hospital administrator, the nursing supervisor and perhaps others. If the directions given to the nurse by those above her are incompatible, there is conflict for the nurse. If the conflict is not resolved, the nurse may perhaps leave the institution or, for example, seek refuge behind a desk full of charts.

The structure of hospitals is often characterized by a long chain of formal channels of communication, making it impossible to get speedy action on situations at hand. Thus, there is a tendency to jump the channels to get to one who will take action.[5] There are also informal channels of communication, like those developed over a cup of coffee or in the cafeteria. The formal structure is at times a barrier to freely expressed communication, and the informal channels of communication are sometimes hidden; however, it is through these informal channels that emotions about situations are quickly transmitted. These sometimes bring about "mood sweeps" through the entire institution.[6]

---

[2]The term "blocked nobility," according to Caudill, was first mentioned by Smith.

[3]William Caudill: *The Psychiatric Hospital as a Small Society.* Cambridge, Mass., Harvard University Press, 1958, p. 7.

[4]Jules Henry: "The Formal Structure of a Psychiatric Hospital." *Psychiatry, 17:*139–151, 1954.

[5]*Ibid.*

[6]William Caudill: *The Psychiatric Hospital as a Small Society.* Cambridge, Mass., Harvard University Press, 1958, p. 10.

The sharpness of role boundaries is another characteristic of the formal social structure of the psychiatric hospital. As Caudill expresses it, one must always act as a nurse, or as a doctor. One "cannot act solely as Dr. Ryan, or Miss Nugent."[7] To enact the role of physician with conformity may not be so difficult as enacting the role of nurse with conformity, since this role is less well defined. Even though a role may be taken by a number of people, each with different personalities, Caudill states that there is a link between personal motivation and social role.[8] While there may be particular motivation to enact a role in a certain way, the hospital exerts pressure for conformity. Perhaps the hospital insists on conformity because the turnover rate of personnel is so great that conformity of role makes replacement easier. Some hospitals seem to replace personnel, especially those in low status positions, almost like parts in a machine.

Informal Structure. When the upper echelon is autocratic, barriers in communication usually exist. Communication is often rechanneled through informal situations, which may be the only means of communication. Informal communication has advantages, but if it is one of the few means of communication, the same thing is not communicated to all those concerned with the problems at hand. When administrators do not listen to problems, do not get all the information, or do not have the active participation of those most directly concerned with the problems, there is usually either a hostile or an apathetic feeling on the part of the staff and the patients. When those concerned with the care of large numbers of patients are not actively included in conferences about problems, they are apt to feel that they are not important in carrying out solutions to the problems. If one is not important in carrying out solutions, his job does not seem very crucial, and his attitudes may be antitherapeutic.[9]

In several cases where conferences have been instituted to include nurses and attendants, these groups have made few comments. In general, the persons who talked most were at the top of the hierarchy, and those who talked least were at the lower end of the hierarchy.

Since doctors and nurses are members of different role groups, each of which have different values and perceptions of ward life, there is apt to be tension around situations that involve patients or will eventually involve them. These emotions, in turn, may be transmitted to patients. When disagreements between physicians and nurses occur, and are not satisfactorily "aired" and resolved, patients are apt to withdraw and regress. At times, as indicated by Caudill,[10] a collective

---

[7]*Ibid.*, p. 9.

[8]*Ibid.*, p. 9.

[9]M. Greenblatt, Daniel J. Levinson and Richard H. Williams, ed.: *The Patient and the Mental Hospital.* Chicago, Free Press of Glencoe, 1957, p. 614.

[10]William Caudill: *The Psychiatric Hospital as a Small Society.* Cambridge, Mass., Harvard University Press, 1958, p. 88.

disturbance occurs in which all the patients' behavior on several different wards becomes more exaggerated or deviant at the same time.

Sabshin states that sometimes doctors and nurses tend to identify with certain forms of treatment, and are opposed to other forms.[11] When the nurse and doctor involved with a patient happen to have opposing views, then the treatment may not have its maximum effect. For example, a nurse who believes that psychotherapy is detrimental to a given patient may comment to the patient that he is making little progress. The patient, in turn, may become dissatisfied or discouraged by the treatment, and regress to some of his former patterns of behavior. The physician, however, may consider psychotherapy as the only treatment of value for the patient, and not be concerned with what goes on the rest of the day. He may expect the nurse to be a constantly giving figure with all patients; however, few people are able to be an all-giving figure all of the time.

Caudill states that the patient's role in the hospital is the least defined role of all.[12] The patient may be subject to the expectations of other patients, the nursing group, the administration, the physician and others. In some cases, the expectations of these different role groups are in conflict with one another. More research is needed in this area.

LINKAGES BETWEEN HOSPITAL AND COMMUNITY

Greenblatt refers to the fact that patient care and the sociotherapeutics of the hospital environment cannot reach levels higher than those that the staff attitude can support. He also makes it clear that the hospital cannot develop beyond the tolerance of the community.[13]

A revolutionary change in the attitudes and functions of personnel implies . . . a lowering of communication barriers, de-emphasis on hierarchy, elevation of status and non-medical personnel to positions paralleling their importance to patients, and an increase in role flexibility with the possibility of utilizing people in roles other than those for which they were specifically trained; greater freedom of expression, greater acceptance of the ideas and behavior of personnel, increased sensitivity to the latent social and recreational talents of all, from casual conversation to ballet dancing.[14]

---

[11]Melvin Sabshin: "Nurse-Doctor-Patient Relationships." *Am. J. Nursing*, 57:190, 1957.

[12]William Caudill: *The Psychiatric Hospital as a Small Society.* Cambridge, Mass., Harvard University Press, 1958, p. 11.

[13]M. Greenblatt, et al.: *The Patient and the Mental Hospital.* Chicago, Free Press of Glencoe, 1957, p. 612.

[14]*Ibid.*, p. 615.

It has also been suggested that patients take a more active part in the therapeutic process, and patient government groups have been established in some hospitals. A therapeutic community within the hospital was pioneered by Jones in England. Here, the community was the doctor, and all persons within the community, including patients, gave and received treatment. The ideology was characterized by four basic ideas: democratization, permissiveness, communalism (staff and patients shared facilities) and reality confrontation.

Within the United States, the therapeutic community with the above ideology did not meet with much success. Psychiatric training for the staff became irrelevant, and in the long run patients did not seem to improve. Perrow points out that, in this case, ideology was mistaken for a new technology. According to Perrow, a change in ideology should not have brought about a change in the organizational structure.[15]

Caudill suggests, too, that patients be grouped so that they can give support to one another.[16] Another innovation has been to pair staff members who are congenial with one another, as, for example, nurses, physicians and attendants. This idea might even be carried further in relation to assigning a particular group of staff members to care for a certain group of patients who seem to feel more secure with this group.

The addition of a clinical anthropologist or sociologist has been suggested by some so that when disturbances first begin they can be recognized, and appropriate action taken. Others have also suggested a ward socialization index to be filled out by nurses in order to test the effect of certain ward management procedures, as well as to serve as a basis for promoting socialization of patients in group activities.

The idea has also been proposed that, after the establishment of therapeutic environments for patients, the community be invited to participate. As the fears about mental patients are lessened, the community will be less resistant to the reintegration the patient into his former home environment.

Greenblatt summarizes criteria for staff action as follows:

(a) Actions and activities designed to develop therapeutic potential of the staff so as to (b) remove restrictive and punitive barriers that exist between staff and patients, (c) develop the social environment as a therapeutic force, (d) obtain participation of patients in the therapeutic process, and (e) help in

---

[15]Charles E. Perrow: "Hospitals: Technology, Structure and Goals." *In* March, James, G. (ed.): *Handbook of Organizations.* Chicago, Rand McNally and Company, 1965, pp. 910-971.

[16]William Caudill: *The Psychiatric Hospital as a Small Society.* Cambridge, Mass., Harvard University Press, 1958, p. 320.

merging of the inner and outer community with the dual goals of education of citizens for participation in mental health work and facilitation of ex-patients in the community.[17]

Summary

The therapeutic environment has been discussed from both the static and dynamic points of view. We find that the static environment is not reciprocally influenced by interpersonal relationships since it has an inanimate quality. The nurse, therefore, functions in manipulating this aspect of the environment by doing something "to" it rather than "with" it. The dynamic environment, on the other hand, is the animate aspect of the environment, which has a reciprocal quality in that it constantly changes because of interpersonal action.

A therapeutic environment is characterized by an accepting, protective and permissive atmosphere that provides a testing ground for the establishment of new patterns of behavior. Furthermore, provision is made for the immediate needs of the patient and optimal hygienic care in general. In addition, the therapeutic environment takes into account the patient's socioeconomic status and his membership in a given cultural group. The therapeutic environment also provides for linkages between the hospital and the community from which the patient came. Characteristics of the formal structure of psychiatric hospitals have been mentioned in relation to formal organization and formal channels of communication. Status hierarchies, role boundaries and nurse-doctor relationships, which either directly or indirectly affect the behavior of the patients, were described. Linkages between the hospital environment and the community were stressed.

Bibliography

Arafeh, Mehadin, et al.: "Linking Hospital and Community Care for Psychiatric Patients." Am. J. Nursing, 63:1050-1056, May, 1963.

Belnap, Ivan: Human Problems of a State Mental Hospital. New York, McGraw-Hill Book Co., Inc., 1956.

Burling, T., Lentz, E. M., and Wilson, R. N.: The Give and Take in Hospitals. New York, G. P. Putnam's Sons, 1956.

Cameron, Norman: The Psychology of Behavior Disorders. Boston, Houghton Mifflin Co., Inc., 1947.

Caudill, William: "Perspectives on Administration in Psychiatric Hospitals." Administrative Sc. Quart., 1:155-170, 1956.

Caudill, William: The Psychiatric Hospital as a Small Society. Cambridge, Mass., Harvard University Press, 1958.

---

[17]M. Greenblatt, et al.: The Patient and the Mental Hospital. Chicago, Free Press of Glencoe, 1957, p. 612.

Denber, Herman, C. B., ed.: *Research Conference on Therapeutic Community.* Springfield, Illinois, Charles C Thomas, 1960.

Devereux, George, and Weiner, F. R.: "The Occupational Status of Nurses." *Am. Soc. Rev., 15:*628-634, 1950.

Eaton, Joseph W., and Weil, Robert J.: *Culture and Mental Disorders.* Chicago, Free Press of Glencoe, 1955.

Freeman, H. E., and Reeder, L. G.: "Medical Sociology: A Review of the Literature." *Am. Soc. Rev., 22:*73-81, 1957.

Georgopoulos, Basil S.: "The Hospital System and Nursing: Some Basic Problems and Issues." *Nursing Forum,* V, *3:*8-35, 1966.

Goffman, Erving: "Characteristics of Total Institutions." *Symposium on Preventive and Social Psychiatry,* Washington, D.C., Walter Reed Army Institute of Research, Walter Reed Army Medical Center, 1957, pp. 43-84.

Greenblatt, Milton, Levinson, Daniel J., and Williams, Richard H., eds.: *The Patient and the Mental Hospital.* Chicago, Free Press of Glencoe, 1957.

Greenblatt, Milton, York, R. H., and Brown, E. L.: *From Custodial to Therapeutic Patient Care in Mental Hospitals.* New York, Russell Sage Foundation, 1955.

Henry, Jules: "The Formal Structure of a Psychiatric Hospital." *Psychiatry, 17:*139-151, 1954.

Herz, Marvin J., *et al.:* "Problems of Role Definitions in the Therapeutic Community." *Arch. Gen. Psych., 14:*27-276, March, 1966.

Holmes, Marguerite J., and Werner, Jean A.: *Psychiatric Nursing in a Therapeutic Community.* New York, The Macmillan Co., 1966.

Hyde, R. W., and Solomon, H. C.: "Patient Government: A New Form of Group Therapy." *Digest of Neurology and Psychiatry, 18:*207-218, April, 1950.

Jones, Maxwell: *The Therapeutic Community.* New York, Basic Books, Inc., 1953.

Michler, E. G., and Tropp, A.: "Status and Interaction in a Psychiatric Hospital." *Human Relations, 9:*187-205, 1956.

Perrow, Charles E.: "Hospitals: Technology, Structure and Goals." *In* March, James G. (ed.): *Handbook of Organizations.* Chicago, Rand McNally and Co., 1965, pp. 910-971.

Sabshin, Melvin: "Nurse-Doctor-Patient Relationships." *Am. J. Nursing, 57:*188-192, February, 1957.

Stanton, Alfred H., and Schwartz, Morris S.: *The Mental Hospital.* New York, Basic Books, Inc., 1954.

Wessen, Albert, ed.: *Psychiatric Hospital as a Social System.* Springfield, Illinois, Charles C Thomas, 1964.

Suggestions for Further Reading

Briggs, Dennis Lynn: "Social Psychiatry in Great Britain." *Am. J. Nursing, 59:*215-220, February, 1959.

Briggs, Dennis Lynn, and Wardell, Marion F.: "A Locked Ward Was Opened." *Am. J. Nursing, 61:*102-105, September, 1961.

Carleton, Estella I., and Johnson, Joan Canatsy: "A Therapeutic Milieu For Borderline Patients." *Am. J. Nursing, 61:*64-67, January, 1961.

Clark, D. H., Hooper, D. F., and Oram, E. G.: "Creating a Therapeutic Community in a Psychiatric Ward." *Human Relations, 15:*123-147, May, 1962.

DeWitt, Henrietta B.: "What Hospitalization Means to the Mental Patient, the Community and the Hospital Social Worker." *Ment. Hyg., 31:*266-295, 1947.

Findley, Annie P.: "They're Learning to Live Again." *Am. J. Nursing, 61:*84-86, June, 1961.

Fuentes, Claude E.: "The First Open Psychiatric Unit in a General Hospital in Puerto Rico." *Am. J. Psychiat., 131:*473-475, November, 1964.

Gilbert, Doris C., and Levinson, Daniel J.: "Ideology, Personality, and Institutional Policy in the Mental Hospital." *In* Neil J. and William T. Smelser (eds.): *Personality and Social Systems.* New York, John Wiley & Sons, Inc., 1963, pp. 619-629.

Gilbert, Doris C., and Wells, Fred L.: "A Ward Socialization Index." *Am. J. Nursing, 57:*59-61, January, 1957.

Holmes, Marguerite J., and Werner, Jean A.: *Psychiatric Nursing in a Therapeutic Community.* New York, The Macmillan Co., 1966.

Hooper, D. F.: "Changing the Milieu in a Psychiatric Ward." *Human Relations, 15*:111–122, May, 1962.

Hyde, Robert W., and Coggan, Norma E.: "When Nurses Have Guilt Feelings." *Am. J. Nursing, 58*:233–236, February, 1958.

Jacoby, Marks George, and McLamb, Eileen C.: "Adjusting to Permissiveness in a State Hospital." *Am. J. Nursing, 59*:1742–1743, December, 1959.

Jones, Maxwell: "The Concept of a Therapeutic Community." *Am. J. Psychiat., 112*:647–650, February, 1956.

Kennard, Edward A.: "Major Patterns of the Mental Hospital." *In* Marvin K. Opler (ed.): *Culture and Mental Health,* New York, The Macmillan Co., 1959, pp. 391–409.

Lamb, Josephine T.: "Freedom for Patients in Mental Hospitals." *Am. J. Nursing, 58*: 358–360, March, 1958.

LeBar, Frank M.: "Some Implications of Ward Structure for Enculturation of Patients." *In* Albert F. Wessen (ed.): *The Psychiatric Hospital as a Social System.* Springfield, Illinois, Charles C Thomas, 1964, pp. 5–19.

Morimoto, Francoise R.: "The Socializing Role of Psychiatric Ward Personnel." *Am. J. Nursing, 54*:53–55, January, 1954.

Pearlin, Leonard I., and Rosenberg, Morris: "Nurse-Patient Social Distance in a Mental Hospital." *Am. Soc. Rev., 27*:56–65, February, 1962.

Perrucci, Robert: "Social Distance Strategies and Intra-Organizational Stratification: A Study of the Status System on a Psychiatric Ward." *Am. Soc. Rev., 28*:951–962, December, 1963.

Ruhlman, Rose G., and Ishiyoma, Toaru: "Remedy for the Forgotten Back Ward." *Am. J. Nursing, 64*:109–111, July, 1964.

Sabshin, Melvin: "Nurse-Doctor-Patient Relationships in Psychiatry." *Am. J. Nursing, 57*:188–192, February, 1957.

Schaefer, Aileen: "Participants—Not Patients." *Am. J. Nursing, 65*:94–95, February, 1965.

Siegel, Nathaniel H.: "What Is a Therapeutic Community?" *Nursing Outlook, 12*:49–51, May, 1964.

Simpson, George, and Kline, Nathan S.: "A New Type of Psychiatric Ward." *Am. J. Psychiat., 119*:511–514, December, 1962.

Smith, Colin M., and McKay, Lois L.: "The Open Psychiatric Ward and Its Vicissitudes." *Am. J. Psychiat., 121*:763–767, February, 1965.

Thrasher, Jean H., and Smith, Harvey L.: "Interactional Contexts of Psychiatric Patients. Social Roles and Organizational Implications." *Psychiatry, 27*:389–398, November, 1964.

Von Mering, Otto: "Beyond the Legend of Chronicity." *Nursing Outlook, 6*:290–293, May, 1958.

Wallace, Anthony F. C., and Rashkis, Harold A.: "The Relation of Staff Consensus to Patient Disturbance on Mental Hospital Wards." *In* Neil J. and William T. Smelser (eds.): *Personality and Social Systems.* New York, John Wiley & Sons, Inc., 1963, pp. 630–636.

Chapter 22 Socio-environmental Nursing in a Deprived Milieu: A Special Case

Nursing care is associated with many factors in both the animate and inanimate environment. Some environments are said to be enriched, in that they exhibit a high degree of tolerance for adequate and humane care and are affluent with respect to material resources. Other environments are said to be deprived, since they tend to deal harshly with human beings and are poverty-stricken with respect to material resources.

We shall turn now to a discussion of the deprived environment of aged persons and later to a discussion of the nurse's intervention in the processes between aged patients and their environment. The aged patient has been used to exemplify the culturally deprived individual since such cases are fairly prevalent. Actually, any patient of any age group, with any type of health problem, may be found in deprived situations. Specific understanding and skills are essential in working with these people. With the present national interest in this group, the nurse may be able to formulate some generalizations that are helpful in other situations.

Women from middle-class families make up the majority of the nurse population. Often the nurse in the middle socioeconomic group is unsuccessful in implementing plans for patient care because she expects patients from enriched environments and patients from culturally deprived environments to conform to her own middle-class stand-

279

ards. Because there are still many psychiatric patients in culturally deprived environments, the description that follows may give the nurse some understanding of these patients.

CHARACTERISTICS OF A DEPRIVED ENVIRONMENT[1]

A deprived environment, often typical in institutions providing care for the indigent aged, is but a reflection of society's attitude toward older persons. When the aged person is institutionalized in buildings that are run down and often ready for destruction, the patients are impressed with the fact that they, too, are considered ready to be junked soon by their social system. When the staff, often poorly trained, further reinforces this feeling of worthlessness, an attitude of hopelessness seems to pervade the atmosphere.

MATERIAL ENVIRONMENT

The material environment in such institutions is usually lacking in space and is characterized by long rows of beds so situated that both the patients' and the personnel's freedom of mobility is restricted. Walls are sometimes dingy and in need of paint, and lighting is usually inadequate. Fire and other material hazards remain uncorrected.

PERSONNEL

Members of the nursing staff, frequently few in number, tend to deal harshly with the patients, for there seems little satisfaction in caring for those cast from society because they are believed worthless. Medical personnel, too, tend to entrust some of their responsibilities to nurses who, in turn, delegate the unwanted tasks to the aides who are on the low-status end of the hierarchial structure. What emphasis there is on patient care seems centered on high-visibility functions carried out without skill and discrimination. Treated as an inanimate object of our material culture, the patient is apparently assumed to be immune to infection and void of feelings and emotions.

The institutionalization of the aged person with indigency and

---

[1]Some of this material evolved from a seminar co-sponsored by Martha M. Brown and Jules Henry, anthropologist, at Washington University School of Nursing. Graduate nursing students participating were: Carolyn Baker, Patricia Brown, Marion Chamberlain, Betty Finger, Dorothy Hutter, Mary Kathryn Langdon, Jean Lagerstrom, Irene Pollert, Anna Shannon, Ruth Wallis and the late Mary Willoughby.

chronic illness in a deprived environment forces the patient lacking in outside ties to become dependent upon the personnel almost exclusively for his acceptance as a person. When this unmet requirement is coupled with lack of protection, a feeling of defenselessness and distrust is created in the patient, who first becomes hostile and then apathetic to his predicament. For a while at least there seems to be a negative solidarity among the patients that is based upon their unmet needs.

Confronted with the numerous demands and requests of patients, the personnel manifest an attitude of indifference as a defense. Serving as hostility targets for the patients, the aides receive little satisfaction in ministering to "mean old people," and so they seek to enhance their position by forcing the patients to beg for scarce articles or to be humiliated into offering meager tips for such favored services as an extra glass of milk. In such instances where there is a scarcity of creature comforts, such as linen, soap and washcloths, the personnel, apparently to save time in rummaging through junk-laden shelves or to later enhance their prestige, tend to hoard and to protect the few scarce material objects found in the social system.

MASS COMMUNICATION OBJECTS

Communication with the outside world is not encouraged, and this fact is often exemplified by the lack of reading materials, properly fitted visual and hearing aids, radios, televisions, visitors or volunteers. When mass communication objects such as radio or television are employed, the programs are usually geared to the interests of the staff rather than to those of the patients.

LACK OF PROTECTION AND RESPECT

Lack of mutual respect between the staff and the patients is frequently reinforced by being "called to" in a manner such as "Hey, Pop" or "Hey, you." It is not uncommon for the patient's "worthlessness" to be discussed in his presence by such statements as "He won't do a thing for himself" or "He's as helpless as a baby."

Patients seem further isolated from the staff and from each other in that they tend to use incontinence and untidiness in their personal attire and habits as a hostile defense. While the patient may have some organic basis for this physiologic dysfunction, it should also be remembered that it can be used as an effective weapon against the personnel, causing them disgust and extra work.

In a deprived environment characterized by lack of protection of its charges, there is little privacy. Even in dying the patient is in trouble with the staff. He may be put in a room where others, in trouble, too, because they are blind, mentally retarded or argue with the staff, are apparently asked to view their impending fate. Someone, waiting impatiently for death to become complete, is likely to ask, "Ain't he dead yet?"

Lack of protection is seen also in the pilfering of the patient's meager material possessions such as eyeglasses, dentures, letters, soap, fruit, and the like. While this practice is often committed by other patients who are in the habit of hoarding, there is social solidarity among the patients in the belief that the members of the staff have stolen these valued articles from the patient's already shrunken world of material objects.

Malnutrition, another area in which lack of protection is exemplified, is often not only characterized by the assembly line haste in the returning of uneaten trays of food but also in the quality and quantity of food served. Food high in carbohydrate but lacking in other essential values is comparatively cheap, and is characteristic of what the economy has provided. Contraband food, sometimes brought from the outside by patients who are more mobile, is often high in sodium or some other quality contraindicated in the effective treatment of patients with certain conditions. While some staff members tend to ignore such practices, and others tend to forbid it, seldom is an adequate explanation made to the patients. Not knowing the danger in this continued practice, the patient wanting the "forbidden fruit" interprets the action of those who restrict it as being malicious and vindictive behavior. The practice of tipping, as mentioned earlier in relation to extra milk, is not only appalling but also amazing in that these supposedly demented people can yet count out the exact amount of small change, frequently pennies, for what they have specifically requested.

ADAPTIVE RADIATION OF PATIENTS

A striking characteristic, even in institutions imposing their depravation on patients, is the phenomenon to which the writer refers as "adaptive radiation." To each new stranger venturing through the wards, the older patient seems literally to extend his hands, offer a faint smile, and make simple requests which he has previously made again and again without avail. It is believed that one could argue that, as long as a cell is alive, it will make many adaptations to its situation before it dies. The plant bending toward the light is an example of an occurrence of this phenomenon seen by the botanist. It is quite astonishing that older persons, the one group least adept at making changes, are not only required by society to do so but can make, in some fashion, numerous adaptive responses to their constant decline in power and status in a distorted environment.

Almost ceaseless, in a deprived institutional setting, is the sighted aged patient's ability to watch. Watching is not only the first step in socialization but also one of the last in becoming completely withdrawn from reality. Watching out the window, for the older person sheltered in a hostile atmosphere, offers the opportunity to turn away from the ward world while at the same time it provides a chance for contact with the world outside.

A WORLD OF BLANKETS AND BIBLES

In an institution that offers little in the way of creative comforts, a blanket and Bible often are the only objects offering security to the older patient. Not only is the blanket used as a protection from the cold but it is also employed as a facility for watching. Huddled beneath the blanket the older patient can peek at what is going on about him and even hoard contraband information to be used later, strategically, against his opponents.

Excluding stimuli from the outer environment is another use of the blanket, for it may serve to conserve energy or as a retreat from reality. The use of the blanket, for the apathetic patient, may be his only method of communication with others. Beneath it, he may be in a fitful sleep, in misery with pain or discomfort, or resigned to the role-lessness that society has ascribed to him.

The ownership of a Bible is one of the few rights permitted in a deprived environment, as well as one of the few personal objects not regarded as contraband. The older patient in a deprived environment is usually very possessive of his blanket and his Bible, and may, in some cases, carry them around with him so that he can keep a watchful eye on them. The Bible is not only symbolic of the patient's religious views but serves as a useful container for precious letters, locks of hair from loved ones and other remnants from the patient's former life. The Bible also offers to an older patient one of the few opportunities to exercise his autonomy, for he can govern as well as maintain full rights in its use. It also provides for privacy in that those who are harshest in their treatment of the aged do not dare open it, for even they are not, as the older person discovers, that heartless.

THE INTERVENTION OF THE NURSE

Although the nurse may be limited to some extent by the degree of tolerance that an institution has for the therapeutic care of the aged, she can intervene in the procedures in such a manner that she will help to reverse certain trends and direct them toward a more positive role for the aged, indigent, institutionalized patient.

The aged person needs opportunities that will make it possible for him to communicate effectively with others; however, one should be reminded that it takes time for the older person to hear what is said to him and it takes time for him to respond to those around him. When one approaches the bedside of the aged patient and speaks, there will be a silence while the patient "tunes in" on the sound from his environment, while he brings into focus the "form" in front of him, and while he decides whether the person approaching him has good intentions. It may be necessary to recall bits of conversation, and to repeat one's name when first approaching the patient.

When several different people, not known to the patient through any degree of sustained contact, make an approach to him several different times in a 24-hour period, the patient may become confused. The same person caring for the patient at the same time each day seems to maximize effective communication with the patient. The patient seems to look forward, for example, to the period of from 1 to 2:00 P.M. when his nurse will be available to him. The constancy of time seems to keep him oriented, and he will learn to store up information that he wishes to give the nurse, questions he wants answered, and technical care he wants to receive from her. The writers do not wish to imply, however, that the patient does not receive care during other periods of the day. Other care, except in unforeseen emergency circumstances, may be given by the nursing assistant under the supervision of the nurse.

Any change in the pattern of care necessitates careful explanation to the patient, since the abrupt absence of the nurse may be quite disturbing to him.

The writer has made a few comments, reflections and speculations through the case analysis of a very limited number of older patients[2] in a deprived environment similar to the one described. While the observations were not checked for bias or for reliability in the coding of data, they may serve to illustrate that the older patient can perform positively with skilled nursing care. Perhaps, too, these comments will offer some clues for an experiment more rigidly controlled.

---

[2]The data were provided by participant observations over a six-week period by the following graduate nursing students who were awarded special research fellowships from the United States Public Health Service: Carolyn Baker, Patricia Brown, Marion Chamberlain, Betty Finger, Mary Kathryn Langdon, Jean Lagerstrom, Irene Pollert, Anna Shannon and Ruth Wallis. Two other students, the late Mary Willoughby, who received a fellowship from the National League for Nursing, and Dorothy Hutter, who received a part-time research fellowship made possible through a grant from the United States Public Health Service, also participated.

TRENDS ASSOCIATED WITH PATIENT MOBILITY

It appeared that the nurse with a more mobile patient had more opportunity to introduce communications about outside events, since the patient who could get around was more interested in maintaining a larger world than the patient confined to bed. Mobile patients had more sustained conversations about the outside world, while less mobile patients tended to change the topic of conversation to some comment about themselves or their immediate environment. The degree of mobility of the older patient may be an indicator in the evaluation of the effectiveness of nurse-patient interaction.

TRENDS IN VISIBILITY OF SERVICE[3]

During the six-week period the nurse gave approximately two times more low-visibility service than high-visibility service. High-visibility service, wh'l not developing so rapidly as low-visibility service, did show an increase in the six-week period of time. As time went on, the patient seemed more accepting of high-visibility service and gradually gave the nurse freedom to add more such service and also participated more in his technical care in relation to the daily activities of living. It seemed, therefore, that the giving of high-visibility service offered the nurse a unique bridge to understanding the patient and thereby served as an approach to increased communication, a low-visibility service.

The high frequency of patient "chat" in the beginning of the interaction seemed to reflect the patient's need for communication with others.

TRENDS IN COMMUNICATION ABOUT THE PAST

It seemed that, as the patient's needs were more adequately met, he offered less conversation about the past, since reminiscing on the part of the older patient seemed at a minimum when compared with other patients receiving the care standard in the institution. When reminiscing did occur, it tended to be in the meaningful context of current activities—that is, it did not appear as a one-way process, with the patient relating the same story over and over. Also, it was interesting to note that when the patient talked about the past, either he had been requested to do so or it was implied by the nurse that he should do so.

---

[3]Definitions of high- and low-visibility service are to be found in Chapter 1.

TRENDS IN PATIENT COMPLAINTS

The older patient in a deprived environment seems to capitalize on his biologic dysfunctions. Since he does not relate to the economy as a man with a job, it may be that his numerous chronic complaints serve as substitutes for these lost symbols. There may also be a relationship between the extent to which the patient emphasizes his physical complaints, and the value placed on them by others in his immediate environment. As the nurse listened to the complaints and then initiated his interest in other aspects of his environment, the patient's complaints about his biologic dysfunctions and his environment tended either to stop or to diminish.

TRENDS IN PATIENT APATHY AND HOSTILITY

In general, the older patient in a deprived environment seemed to manifest an attitude of either apathy or hostility; men appeared more apathetic while women seemed more hostile. The male patients seemed more indifferent to their situation and seemed to have less hope than the female patients, who tended to rebel against the situation and to be discontent with the "status quo."

The men, while at first apathetic, soon began to express their hostility, and the nurse appeared to serve as a specific target for hostile reactions. The women, on the other hand, seemed to "take it out" on one another. It may be that being ministered to is more accepted by women than men; the older male patient seems to resent being dependent upon the nurse.

In the beginning of the nurse-patient interaction the hostility expressed by the older patient seemed diffuse, but, as time passed, it became more differentiated. At first, patients had a tendency to make reference to a vague "they" — " 'They' won't let you do that." Later, the patients made such comments as "Miss R. doesn't like for patients to do that."

The almost complete lack of hostility expressed by the patient toward his family and outside friends may indicate what a small place the outside world plays in the patient's life and, conversely, how large a place the institutional setting has in his life. However, it should be mentioned that most of the patients had few living relatives, and it seems unlikely in our culture that they would express open hostility toward the dead.

In general, the more mobile the patient, the more hostility he seemed to express. Increased mobility seemed to bring more human contact with others and, therefore, evoked more hostility. The less mobile patients refrained from openly expressed hostility not only because they seemed to have less human contact with others but also because they were more dependent upon others for care and, therefore, seemed more hesitant to express their hostility to one who could withhold such care.

While, in general, the patients' expression of hostility seemed to decrease after the intervention of the nurse, the hostility of those patients receiving special care increased toward those patients receiving the care standard in the institution.

It is also interesting to note that, as the nurses gave patients more opportunity to make both positive and negative responses, the patients' hostility toward the environment seemed to diminish and they began to exercise more autonomy in their activities of daily living.

TRENDS IN NONVERBAL COMMUNICATION

The patients' "signal behavior" to the nurse, as manifested by nonverbal signs, gestures and facial expressions, seemed to develop more slowly than verbal communications. It appeared that, as "signal behavior" was developed and recognized by the nurse, there was less need for verbal communication, which developed more rapidly, and showed more fluctuation than nonverbal communication. One might speculate that the nonverbal exchanges between the nurse and older patient may be more significant than is now realized.

TRENDS IN SUGGESTIONS

Although the proportion of patient suggestions were lowest as compared with the initiating of requests and the giving of information, there was a significant increase over a period of time. It appeared that, as the patient acquired more information, he became increasingly more interested in making suggestions to the nurse not only in relation to his own care but also in relation to the institution as a whole.

TRENDS IN REQUESTS

An inspection of the patients' requests reveals a few interesting trends. In comparing the requests for high- and low-visibility service, patient requests to the nurse for low-visibility service out-numbered patient requests to the nurse for high-visibility care by a ratio of 3:1. The patients' reluctance to request high-visibility service may reflect the fact that one learns early in life not to request material objects and services if he is unable to pay for them.

In regard to requests for information, the nurse, in the beginning of the interaction, requested more than the patient. After a period of time, however, the patients' requests for information exceeded those made by the nurse. However, near the end of the six-week period, requests for information from the patient and the nurse seemed evenly distributed. The nurse, during the entire period, gave three times more information than the patient requested. It may be that the patient's requests for information increased because he felt more freedom to ask a giving person. The patient seemed to rely on the nurse who came at a certain time, and soon learned to use this time advantageously.

As the patient's interests expanded to include the nurse, the patient began to request more information about the personal life of the nurse as examplified by such questions as, "Do you go to school?" "Are you married?" Near the end of the six-week period, patient requests for information had expanded to include more about events and persons in the outside world and less requests in relation to himself.

TRENDS IN PATIENT RESPONSES TO REQUESTS

The patient gave about twice as many positive responses as negative responses to the nurses' requests. Negative responses, while fairly low in frequency, did increase slightly during the six-week period. It may be that, in a deprived environment, the patient may tend to withhold negative responses because of the fear of the environment's hostile reaction; however, the fact that both positive and negative responses increased may indicate that the patient, after a time, felt greater freedom in saying "Yes" and "No" to the nurse.

While the nurses caring for the few selected patients tended to maximize nursing care, they, too, seemed to fluctuate in their feelings about the care of the older patient. Sometimes they seemed overwhelmed by what apparently needed to be done in the situation as a whole; they seemed to feel guilty about not giving care to all patients. On the other hand, they learned to see and feel satisfaction from minute changes in progress of a few patients. One of the greatest hindrances, however, to maximizing positive nurse-patient interaction was the low degree of the institutional tolerance for therapeutic care. It would seem that, if nursing is to be maximized, some change must take place not only in the institution's tolerance but also in the larger social system of which it is only a part. A brief mention of the plans implemented in a few communities is made in the following section.

COMMUNITY ACTION

If attitudes in regard to our aged are to be changed, a program of educating the public is necessary before a community can take specific steps in initiating changes in its policies and facilities for the care of older persons. The nurse, as a member of the health team and as a member of the community, is in a more strategic positon to help in changing attitudes of others if she is aware of the proposals for improvement made by other community groups.

It has been suggested that counseling and placement centers be made available for the aged so that their abilities can be assessed and they can be gainfully employed as useful members of society. It is believed that retirement plans should not be based on chronologic age but upon the individual's capacities. Perhaps industry can institute more gradual retirement plans for employees. With the redesigning of many jobs, industry can utilize the abilities of many older workers effectively. In some cases, the older person with experience may serve as teacher or senior consultant to less experienced individuals. Placement agencies often have a difficult job in convincing employers that older persons can contribute; however, with an increasing number of persons of nonproductive age, it will be necessary for our economy to take some kind of action. So few cannot support so many.

Housing for the older citizens is another need in most communities. It has been emphasized that diversity in housing is very important if it is to meet the needs of socioeconomic groups with varying degrees of capacity. There is need for low rent, safety-designed, efficiency apartments; retirement homes; small apartments in retirement homes; small apartments with general supervision of the occupants by a manager; family style homes for four to eight persons; nursing homes; day centers; "half-way" homes for those convalescing from illness; facilities that provide care for those who need a minimum of psychiatric treatment; geriatric units in general hospitals; and also facilities that will provide short-term care for older persons while younger members of their families are on vacation.

Most older persons like to live some place where they can have quiet, privacy and independence but also be near transportation, shopping centers, churches, family and friends.

The older person can often maintain independence if he has shopping service, homemaker service and home care plans for chronic illness. "Meals on wheels" service can often provide the patient with hot food that meets his nutritional requirements.

The older person too often needs more financial assistance than he now has. His savings, once thought to be adequate, may not last very long with the increased costs of living and medical care.

For the aged, some communities have also organized vacation services, camping, sheltered workshops, retraining centers, clubs and services to meet special needs such as those concerned with dental, foot, optical and hearing impairment.

There is a great need for research and for more training for those who work with older persons, as well as for an increase in the number of persons in this field. The aforementioned plans initiated in certain communities are but a few of the community possibilities for meeting needs of the older person.

Our aged are our treasure. Depository of our wisdom, storehouse of our know-how, guardian of our honored traditions, stabilizers of our economy, who through young and middle years helped make America great, our senior citizens of today are our prized gems whose lustre, dimmed by years of neglect, is being restored to its true brilliance.[4]

The above discussion assumes that man is a completely rational being; however, in some communities nurses and other health workers find that man does not always act in a completely rational manner. Not all behavior is rational and can be accounted for by learning theory. Maier states that the consequences of action are not a factor in the selection of behavior under frustration.[5] Behavior is not always instigated by motivation, but in some cases may be instigated by frustration and, as such, is not rational. Motivational behavior is goal-orientated, flexible and adaptative; however, in contrast, frustration-instigated behavior appears senseless when viewed as if it were motivated. Maier classifies responses to frustration as: (1) fixation, (2) regression, (3) aggression and (4) resignation.[6]

Health and welfare workers in the southern Appalachians have met with failure in some of their attempts to help these people, who have a long history of frustration. The student will find the articles at the end of the chapter which deal with responses to frustration to be of considerable help if she has a special interest in understanding and helping "hard-core" poverty groups, the elderly and other such minority groups who have experienced considerable frustration.

Summary

The deprived environment in an institution for the aged has been characterized as one in which there is a lack of material needs, an

---

[4]New York State Joint Legislative Committee on Problems of the Aging: *Age Is No Barrier.* Legislative Document No. 35, 1952, p. 4.
[5]Norman R. Maier: *Frustration.* New York, McGraw-Hill, 1949, p. 93.
[6]*Ibid., p. 94.*

inadequate nursing staff, a lack of persons with whom to communicate, lack of protection, lack of respect, and lack of creature comforts.

Nurses were introduced into a deprived environment, where they attempted to give nursing care without altering other aspects of the patients' environment. Patient response indicated that something could be done for them.

Trends in the nurse-patient interaction have been discussed in relation to patient mobility, communication about the past, visibility of service, patient complaints, patient apathy and hostility, nonverbal communication, suggestions, requests and patient responses to requests. Community action designed to help older people has been discussed.

Bibliography

Brown, Martha M., and Henry, Jules: *The Depersonalization of Older Patients: A Research Project Report.* (Mimeographed) Saint Louis, Missouri: Washington University School of Nursing, 1958.

Coe, Rodney M.: "Self-Conception and Institutionalization." *In* Arnold M. Rose and Warren A. Peterson (eds.): Older People and Their Social World. Philadelphia, F. A. Davis Co., 1965. pp. 225-243.

Gornick, Marian E., Freedman, Helen B., and Gorten, Martin K. "The Use of Medical Services as Demanded by the Urban Poor." *Am. J. Pub. Health,* 59:1302-1311, 1969.

Hochstim, Joseph R., Athanasopoulos, Demetrios, and Larkins, John H.: "Poverty Area the Microscope." *Am. J. Pub. Health,* 58:1815-1827, October, 1968.

Prock, Valencia N.: "Effects of Institutionalization: A Comparison of Community, Waiting List, and Institutionalized Aged Persons." *Am. J. Pub. Health,* 59:1837-1844, October, 1969.

Stanley, Manfred: "Nature, Culture and Scarcity." *American Sociological Review,* 33:855-869, December, 1968.

Weiss, James M. A., ed., Brown, Martha M., Brown, Patricia R., Glidewell, John C., and Hunt, Raymond G.: *Nurses, Patients and Social Systems.* Columbia, Missouri, University of Missouri Press, 1968.

Weller, Jack E.: *Yesterday's People.* Lexington: The University of Kentucky Press, 1965.

Suggestions for Further Reading

Ball, Richard A.: "A Poverty Case: The Analgesic Subculture of Southern Appalachians." *American Sociological Review,* 33:885-893, December, 1968.

Clifford, Maurice C.: "Health and the Urban Poor." *Nursing Outlook,* 17:62-63, December, 1969.

Dumas, Rhetaugh G.: "This I Believe . . . About Nursing and the Poor." *Nursing Outlook,* 17:47-49, September, 1969.

English, Joseph T.: "The Dimensions of Poverty." *Am. J. Nursing,* 69:2424-2428, November, 1969.

Geiger, H. Jack: "The Endlessly Revolving Door." *Am. J. Nursing,* 69:2436-2445, November, 1969.

Leo, Patricia, and Rosen, George: "A Bookshelf on Poverty and Health." *Am. J. Pub. Health,* 59:591-607, April, 1969.

Loeb, Bertram: "United Funds, Health, and the Urban Crises." *Nursing Outlook,* 17:36-38, September, 1969.

Mahoney, Margaret E.. "Momentum for Change." *Am. J. Nursing, 69*:2446-2454, November, 1969.

McNerney, Walter J.: "Changing the Health Care System." *Am. J. Nursing, 69*:2428-2435, November, 1969.

Mumford, Emily: "Poverty and Health." *Nursing Outlook, 17*:32-35, September, 1969.

Robertson, Helene R.: "Removing Barriers to Health Care." *Nursing Outlook, 17*:43-46, September, 1969.

Standeven, Muriel: "What the Poor Dislike About Community Health Nurses." *Nursing Outlook, 17*.72-75, September, 1969.

Velazquez, Janet M.: "Alienation." *Am. J. Nursing, 69*.301-304, February, 1969

Part Four   Psychiatric-
Mental Health Nursing in
Community Settings

Chapter 23   Beliefs and Practices of the Past

If changes are to be initiated either in hospitals or in the community, the cultural beliefs about health and illness held by people involved in effecting the innovation must be known. Therefore, a history of society's attitudes and beliefs about mental illness may be helpful in understanding why certain practices were retained and why some innovations were accepted, as well as why others failed.

EARLY DEVELOPMENTS

Although little is known about the attitude of primitive man toward psychiatric disorders, it seems likely that he regarded them with mysticism. In Biblical days there was some recognition of the problem, as illustrated in the descriptions of madness, but little thought was given to the idea that such individuals were ill.

The Greeks were the first to recognize that aberrations in behavior were diseases. Hippocrates, the father of medicine, rescued the study of psychiatry, and placed psychiatric disorders side by side with other diseases. Although he contributed much to clinical descriptions and the classification of psychiatric disorders, he used the older methods of treatment, such as blood-letting. It was left for Plato to suggest that such patients should be watched over by relatives. Later Asclepiades postulated that mental diseases were due to emotional disturbances. He, like Plato, emphasized that patients should be treated humanely.

WITCHCRAFT AND MYSTICISM

With the decline of Greek and Roman influences, mysticism and superstition flourished. Sprenger and Kraemer, two theologians, wrote a book entitled *Malleus Malificarum,* which advocated that witches be punished and burned. Here, criteria were developed to determine whether or not an individual practiced witchcraft. These criteria were descriptions of symptomatology, and therefore contributed to the study of psychiatry. People of this age feared psychiatric disorders, and believed that the evil spirits had to be driven from the bodies of those inflicted before the bodies were burned. This practice was continued for several centuries, and it was not until the Renaissance that a Spanish philosopher, Juan Luis Vives, postulated some of the concepts that became a forerunner for the work of Freud.

SEPARATION OF PSYCHIATRY FROM THEOLOGY

Johann Weyer, a physician in the sixteenth century, devoted his life to treating psychiatric patients in a humane manner. He was the first to divorce psychiatry from theology. He set psychiatry aside as a branch of medicine, but unfortunately, his work was not well known in his time.

SEVENTEENTH AND EIGHTEENTH CENTURIES

In the seventeenth century the new discoveries and methods of research in the field of physical sciences were brought to bear upon psychiatry. This approach resulted in a mechanistic study of the mind, and tended to retard the progress of psychiatry during this period. Before 1800 there were relatively few hospitals devoted to the care of psychiatric patients. The first of these institutions was established in Florence, Italy, in 1389, and in 1409 the Spaniards built an "asylum for the insane" at Valencia. In America, as late as 1736, the only institution care provided was in the dungeons of the poorhouses, workhouses and houses of correction. The first hospital to make provisions for such patients in America was the Blockley Hospital (later called the Philadelphia General Hospital), which was founded in 1731. The first state hospital in America was established in 1773 in Williamsburg, Virginia.

The eighteenth century brought American independence and the French Revolution. In this spirited age Pinel, a French physician, suggested that the psychiatric patients in a Paris hospital be released from their chains. It was under his leadership that psychiatric hospitals became a center for both the study and treatment of patients. William Tuke, a Quaker but not a physician, independently proceeded in England along the same lines as Pinel. Also in the eighteenth century, Benjamin Rush, a well-known Philadelphia physician, became the first American teacher of a well-organized course in psychiatry. He wrote the first treatise on the subject in America, and it was the only American work of this kind for the next seventy years. In addition, Rush became involved in the humanitarian movement for improving the care of the mentally ill. He was later known as "the father of American psychiatry."

NINETEENTH CENTURY

Much discussion of nonrestraint methods ensued during the nineteenth century, and psychiatrists spent a great part of their time in organizing hospitals for the humane treatment of their patients. The emphasis on nonrestraint meant that the patients were to be viewed as human beings with a personality that had to be given some consideration by those who cared for them. The psychiatric patient was no longer to be ignored, and this created the problem of securing individuals who could care for them. In the early 1800's, the nursing personnel consisted of either patients or persons serving prison sentences.

In some parts of Europe and America, however, such patients were often cared for by the sisters of Catholic nursing orders. In Germany, perhaps in part because of the opposition to Catholicism, the sisters were considered incompetent to care for the "insane." The Sisterhood of St. Vincent de Paul supplied many of the psychiatric nurses of this period. These sisters were required to serve a three-month probationary period after spending two years as a novitiate. In this order, also, there were two levels of nursing, and this division was somewhat comparable to that of the attendants and professional nurses of today.

William and Samuel Tuke in England, Kirkbride in America, and others were asking for better preparation of the psychiatric nursing staffs. Again the question of female nurses caring for male patients arose, and Isaac Ray helped to promote their employment in America. It was noticed that patients became quieter, and that marked changes took place with the advent of female nurses. It was noted, also, that on wards where female nurses were employed the mortality rate was lower. However, the question of female nurses was still being debated in 1900.

Later in the nineteenth century there was a move to extend nursing care over the twenty-four-hour period. At first, night watchmen were employed, and it was emphasized that they should sleep lightly. Kirkbride, in 1854, suggested that both night and day attendants be employed. At Columbus State Hospital in Ohio a night attendant was employed for the suicidal patients, and by the end of the century the practice was fairly widespread. The attendant-patient ratio soon improved from 1:50 to 1:15, and in a few instances it was raised to 1:9 and 1:6.

At this time salaries for female nurses and attendants were much lower than those for male employees. Female psychiatric nurses received $25 per month, while male psychiatric nurses were paid $4 and $5 per day. The hours of employment consisted of a fourteen-hour day and a six-and-one-half-day week. It was not until 1907 that the eight-hour day day was inaugurated in Kalamazoo State Hospital in Michigan.

Although formal classes were held for attendants, instruction for psychiatric nurses did not develop until about 1880. At McLean Hospital, Massachusetts, the first training school for nurses in a psychiatric hospital was established. A few years later this school arranged for an affiliation with Massachusetts General Hospital.

Finally, it was suggested that nurses be freed from cleaning chores so that standards for nursing functions could be elevated. In 1908 the State of New York make it compulsory for every state hospital to employ a superintendent of nurses. The role of the nurse, however, was chiefly custodial in nature.

The trend toward state care of the mentally ill in the United States was reinforced in 1890 by the passage of the New York State Care Act. This trend may be traced to 1751, when the state of Pennsylvania made appropriations for the erection of the Pennsylvania Hospital in Philadelphia, and later Virginia made appropriations for a state hospital in Williamsburg. Soon, because of overcrowded conditions, it became necessary for certain states to build more hospitals. During this period, also, Dorothea Lynde Dix, a retired schoolteacher from Boston, began her crusade in both America and England for improvement in the care of the mentally ill.

This period was also known as the era of systems, and much thought was given to classification and nomenclature. Kraepelin, a German psychiatrist, contributed much toward developing a systematic terminology so that the field could establish its own body of knowledge.

PSYCHOANALYTIC THEORIES AND THEIR DEVELOPMENT

During the same century Mesmer, a physician from Austria, began his study of neurosis. He believed that these disorders were caused by a disturbance in the balance of a "magnetic fluid" in the body. He attempted to restore this balance by use of a magnetic wand, and his methods flourished despite the criticism of the medical world. In 1842 James Baird, an English surgeon, became interested in the technique and used it as an anesthetic during surgical procedures. It was Baird who introduced the word hypnosis in place of mesmerism. The scientific world resented Mesmer's introduction of mysticism into scientific endeavors; in addition, he was not well liked as a person. Nonetheless, Mesmer focused attention upon psychodynamics and brought psychotherapy for the first time to the attention of many.

At about the same time that Mesmer flourished, two French schools were established, one in Nancy and the other at the Salpêtrière in Paris. Liébeault, in Nancy, proposed that suggestibility was characteristic not only of the person with hysteria but also of all individuals. His views were in opposition to those of Charcot at the Salpêtrière, who was more conservative. Although Charcot's theoretical contributions were not too enlightening, he had a great influence on psychiatry. He was a great teacher, and scholars from the world over came to hear him. His clinic soon became the world center for postgraduate study. Janet also studied hysteria and introduced the term "unconscious." However, it was left to Freud to develop the theories further.

Freud, a neurologist, became interested in the study of neurotic individuals. He studied for a short time at Nancy and then returned to Vienna to work with Joseph Breuer, who devised the method of catharsis. Freud and Breuer published their joint work on hysteria in 1895. Later hypnosis fell into disuse. Freud, too, discarded the practice. He then developed other psychoanalytic concepts such as repression, resistance and the unconscious. On his own, Freud postulated many of the basic assumptions in psychoanalysis as they are used today. While most eminent authorities considered his new approach ridiculous, Freud began to gather a few followers, and the International Psychoanalytical Association was established in 1910.

In the early part of the twentieth century, several of Freud's colleagues resigned from the ssociation, but Freud continued his work revis ng his old concepts and postulat'ng new ones. He was given little recognition during his lifetime, and was finally driven from Austria to England by the Nazis. In the meantime Jung, Adler, Stekel and others developed their own schools of thought, and various deviations from orthodox psychoanalysis occurred.

Freud's contributions found more acceptance in America than anywhere else, and soon several psychoanalytic institutes were established as centers for study. During World War II, physicians in the armed services were called upon to give immediate care to many patients, and through the use of narcosynthesis they were able to get the patient to reveal his innermost views. The results of this method convinced many people of the soundness of Freud's work.

Psychoanalytic theories began to creep into the classes of young physicians, social workers, clinical psychologists and anthropologists as well as into nursing. The concepts taught in schools of nursing have gradually become less descriptive and more dynamic.

EARLY TWENTIETH CENTURY PROGRESS IN AMERICA

As progress was made in research, chiefly under the impetus of Adolf Meyer, the field of psychiatry became less isolated. Dr. Meyer evolved the school of psychobiology and became known as the father of dynamic psychiatry in America. It was Meyer who enlisted the assistance of social workers. Simultaneously, the profession turned toward psychologic theories. With the assistance of social workers, the "aftercare" movement began. A great need arose for adequate research and education, and an institution for these purposes was established at the University of Michigan in 1901. Gradually other institutes of this nature developed. General hospitals also became interested in the care of psychiatric patients, and in 1902 a pavilion in Albany Hospital was designated for their care.

At about the same time, there was a crusade on many fronts to fight disease, and this movement paved the way for Clifford Beers and his mental hygiene movement. Beers, a manic-depressive, spent several years in various types of psychiatric institutions. Appalled by the conditions, he was determined to do something about the care and treatment of psychiatric patients. In 1908 he published *A Mind That Found Itself*, which describes his experiences during his hospitalization. Much public interest was aroused, and in 1909 the National Committee for Mental Hygiene was organized. Very soon after Beers's publication and the advent of social workers, a trend appeared toward the individualization of patient care.

Although previous interest had been shown in work with children, the movement toward child guidance did not emerge until 1922. By 1946, there were 285 such clinics for children in the United States. At about this time, too, Sullivan contributed much to the field of American psychiatry. It has been said that if Freud had not postulated the concepts of psychoanalysis, Sullivan was the only American psychiatrist capable of doing so.

The depression that began in 1929 resulted in a curtailment of state budgets for the psychiatric hospitals, and the standards for patient care were lowered. Overcrowding existed and patients received little care. The family care plan, although not new, was again revived to help relieve the situation.

About 1930 more interest was shown in occupational therapy, and a formulation of principles was evolved at this time by Dr. Hermann Simon. In 1937 a study was made of state hospitals, and deplorable conditions were revealed. With the advent of World War II, psychiatric institutions were depleted of their staffs, and in 1946 the American Psychiatric Association looked frankly at the situation. A system of inspection and rating was formulated and a set of standards evolved. These standards have done much to elevate the quality of patient care. Even today, however, many state hospitals have not attained these goals, but they are seriously striving to improve the standards of care.

As the need for funds for research and education increased, the national government became interested and the National Mental Health Act was passed in 1946. The act provides for grants to be given to universities for the purpose of research and for education of physicians, clinical psychologists, social workers and nurses. With the funds made available through grants from the United States Public Health Service, the concerted efforts of various disciplines interested in the psychiatric patient have contributed much toward the solution of one of the nation's major health problems. The years to come should bring even greater strides in the advancement of psychiatry and its allied fields.

LEGAL PRACTICES IN PSYCHIATRY

Partly because of the mysticism surrounding psychiatry and the false belief that the mentally ill have sinned, legal procedures in regard to psychiatric patients often have a criminal flavor and lack awareness of medical and social facts. However, since not all patients recognize that they are ill, states have devised legal ways of retaining them either for their own protection or for the protection of others.

Each state has its own legal procedures, which vary widely, for admitting and releasing state hospital patients. The student of nursing will undoubtedly be introduced to procedures specific to her own state by the instructor.

Commitment procedures in early American history were relatively simple, but about 1860 there were many complaints in regard to "railroading" of persons of sound mind into hospitals for the mentally ill. At about this time several states set up legal procedures to safeguard the rights of citizens. Such legal terminology as "insanity," "insane asylum," "parole" and others appeared in legislative documents. These terms were used, and still are in a few states, until as late as 1947, when ten states made changes in their statutes.

A report to the 1950 Governors' Conference on Mental Health Programs[1] listed the following principles for legislation governing hospitalization for the mentally ill:

> Hospitalization proceedings should involve a maximum reliance on medical opinion . . .
> Hospitalization procedures should be free of the characteristics of criminal proceedings. . . .
> There should be provision for temporary involuntary hospitalization without the necessity of court proceedings. . . .
> Opportunity for prompt recourse to judicial proceedings should be provided in connection with all involuntary proceedings, and ultimate responsibility for indeterminate hospitalization should rest with a judicial body. . . .
> Provisions should be made for continuing review of the mental condition of hospitalized patients and for conditional release and discharge as warranted by their condition. . . .
> Patients while in a hospital should be protected in the enjoyment of personal rights to the extent consistent with required treatment and detention. . . .
> Private mental institutions should be brought under unified administrative supervision at the state level.

In progressive states current legislation relevant to hospitalized patients reflects less regimentation—patients can enter the hospital voluntarily and have more freedom during their stay. The authorization of increased community services through state and federal legislation has enabled some patients to receive treatment earlier. If hospitalization is necessary, patients may receive aftercare service so that *long* hospitalization is unnecessary. For further elaboration on the evolution of community practices, refer to Chapter 24.

Summary

Historical developments and trends in psychiatry and psychiatric care have been described. Primitive man most likely regarded psychiatric disorders with mysticism. The Greeks were the first to recognize that aberrations in behavior were diseases, but with the decline of Greek and Roman influence, mysticism and superstition again flourished. Individuals who were thought to practice witchcraft were punished and burned. This practice continued for several centuries.

---

[1]Report to the Governors' Conference: *The Mental Health Programs of the Forty-eight States.* Chicago, Council of State Governments, 1950, pp. 66-69.

In the sixteenth century Johann Weyer was the first to divorce psychiatry from theology. The seventeenth century brought new discoveries and methods of research in the field of physical sciences, which were brought to bear also upon psychiatry. During the eighteenth century, Pinel, a French physician, freed psychiatric patients from their chains. The nineteenth century brought emphasis on nonrestraint, and patients began to be viewed as human beings.

Theories of Freud, Meyer, Sullivan and others evolved in the twentieth century. More recently consideration has been given to prevention of psychiatric disorders through work in mental hygiene, child guidance and therapy, and the appropriation of funds for research and education.

Legal procedures in regard to psychiatric patients have been discussed and certain legislation concerning the mentally ill patient in the hospital and community has been presented.

Bibliography

American Psychiatric Association: *One Hundred Years of American Psychiatry.* New York, Columbia University Press, 1944.

Bond, Earl D.: *Dr. Kirkbride and His Mental Hospital.* Philadelphia, J. B. Lippincott Co., 1947.

Boring, Edwin G.: *A History of Experimental Psychology.* New York, D. Appleton-Century Co , 1929.

Brand, Jeann L.: "The United States: A Historical Perspective." *In* Richard H. Williams and Lucy D. Ozarin (eds): *Com·un'ty Mental Health.* San Francisco, Jossey-Bass, Inc., 1968, pp. 18-43.

"Coping with Society." *The Wall Street Journal.* Midwest Ed., *1*:190, July 10, 1970, p. 1.

Davidson, Henry A.: "The Commitment Procedures and Their Legal Implications." In Silvano Arieti, ed.: *American Handbook of Psychiatry,* Vol. II. New York, Basic Books, Inc., 1959, pp. 1902-1922.

Deutsch, Albert: *The Mentally Ill in America.* New York, Columbia University Press, 1949.

Evans, Frances: *Role of the Community Mental Health Nurse.* New York, The Macmillan Co., 1968.

Felix, Robert H.: "Evolution of Community Health Concepts." *The American Journal of Psychiatry, 113*:673-679, February, 1957.

Heidbreder, Edna: *Seven Psychologies.* New York, D. Appleton-Century Co., 1933.

Kenefick, Donald P.: "The Past in the Present." *Ment. Hyg., 53*:472-476, July, 1969.

Mikesell, W. H., ed.: *Modern Abnormal Psychology.* New York, Philosophical Library, Inc., 1950.

Overholser, Winifred: "Major Principles of Forensic Psychiatry." In Silvano Arieti, ed.: *American Handbook of Psychiatry.* Vol. II. New York, Basic Books, Inc., 1959, pp. 1887-1901.

Overholser, Winifred: *The Psychiatrist and the Law.* New York, Harcourt, Brace and Co., 1953.

Report to the Governors' Conference: *The Mental Health Programs of the Forty-eight States.* Chicago, Council of State Governments, 1950.

Santos, Elvin H., and Stainbrook, Edward: "A History of Psychiatric Nursing in the Nineteenth Century." *J. Hist. Med. & Allied Sc.,* 4:48-74, 1949.

Williams, Richard, and Ozarin, Lucy D., eds.: *Community Mental Health.* San Francisco, Jossey-Bass Inc., 1968.

Zillboorg, Gregory, and Henry, George W.: *A History of Medical Psychology.* New York, W. W. Norton & Co., Inc., 1941.

Suggestions for Further Reading

Ackerknecht, E. H.: *A Short History of Psychiatry.* New York, Hafner Publishing Co., 1959.

Cowen, Emory L., Gardner, Elmer A., and Zax, Melvin: *Emergent Approaches to Mental Health Problems.* New York, Appleton-Century-Crofts, 1967.

Deutsch, Albert: "Dorothea Lynde Dix: Apostle of the Insane." *Am. J. Nursing,* 36:987-997, 1936.

Evans, Frances: *Role of the Nurse in Community Mental Health.* New York, The Macmillan Co., 1968.

Felix, Robert H.: "The National Mental Health Act—How It Can Operate to Meet a National Problem." *Ment. Hyg., 31*:363-374, 1947.

Gottlieb, Jacques S., and Tourney, Garfield: "Commitment Procedures and the Advancement of Psychiatric Knowledge." *Am. J. Psychiat., 115*:109-113, August, 1958.

Henderson, Sir David, and Batchelor, Ivor R. C.: *Henderson and Gillespie's Textbook of Psychiatry,* 9th Ed., London, Oxford University Press, 1962, pp. 1-15.

Lambertsen, Eleanor C.: *Education for Nursing Leadership.* Philadelphia, J. B. Lippincott Co., 1958, pp. 6-44.

Lowry, James V.: "How the National Mental Health Act Works." *Ment. Hyg., 33*:30-39, 1949.

Murray, Henry A.: "Historical Trends in Personality Research." In Henry P. David and J. C. Brengelmann, eds.: *Perspectives in Personality Research.* New York, Springer Publishing Co., Inc., 1960, pp. 3-39.

Noyes, Arthur P., and Kolb, Lawrence C.: *Modern Clinical Psychiatry,* 6th Ed., Philadelphia, W. B. Saunders Co., 1963, pp. 1-57 and 556-567.

Overholser, Winifred: "Commitment of the Mentally Ill." *Am. J. Nursing, 54*:190-192, February, 1954.

Santos, Elvin H., and Stainbrook, Edward: "A History of Psychiatric Nursing in the Nineteenth Century." *J. Hist. Med. & Allied Sc., 4*:48-74, 1949.

Schneck, J. M.: *A History of Psychiatry.* Springfield, Ill., Charles C Thomas, Publisher, 1960.

Shalit, Pearl R.: "The Nurse and the National Mental Health Act." *Am. J. Nursing, 50*:94-96, 1950.

Thompson, Clara: "The Different Schools of Psychoanalysis." *Am. J. Nursing, 57*:1304-1307, October, 1957.

Veith, Ilza: "Psychiatric Nosology: From Hippocrates to Kraepelin." *Am. J. Psychiat., 114*:385-391, November, 1957.

EVOLUTION OF CONCEPTS AND
PRACTICES IN COMMUNITY SERVICES

While a few innovations in community care of the mentally ill occurred in the United States in the early 1900's, Europe made considerable headway in treating the patient in his own locale. In 1930 the Mental Health Treatment Act, passed in Britain, authorized arrangements for voluntary treatment, outpatient service and aftercare to patients in their home communities. The National Health Service Act, passed in 1946 in England and Wales, united mental health services under a central authority. It later became an integral part of the comprehensive national health services. Also, England, by 1950, had made extensive use of day hospitals for psychiatric patients. This innovation was first introduced in Moscow in 1933. Another European innovation was initiated in Amsterdam in 1936. Here, a 24-hour emergency service for patients being treated out of the hospital was developed.

International Developments. The World Federation of Mental Health was organized by Rees in 1948. The general focus of its aims was on creating an atmosphere conducive to the progress of mental health for all people and all nations.

Another significant force in the development in community services was the World Health Organization's appointment of an Expert Committee on Mental Health. This committee first convened in 1949. The World Health Organization ranked the field of mental health as fifth among its priorities. The early sixties brought the establishment of the World Psychiatric Association (1961) and the First International Congress of Social Psychiatry (1964).

In the United States.   Psychopharmacology, introduced in 1952, made possible more fully the extension of community services to psychiatric patients. The pill-oriented society of today has made tranquilizing drugs well-accepted. The tranquilizers, in turn, have made psychiatric therapy possible, thus making the hospital more open to the community. The interest in physiochemical therapy in relation to the control of mental illness was not new. Hydrotherapy was used in very early times, while fever, insulin, metrazol shock and electroshock therapies, as well as frontal lobotomy, were introduced between 1917 and 1936.

Also in the United States, during the 1950's, several events took place which were forerunners of community mental health services on a large scale. There were several privately financed conferences held on community mental health services. The cost to states for financing large state mental institutions was becoming prohibitive, so alternative methods to custodial care for patients were offered through community care. In 1954, New York passed a community mental health act. Indiana, Connecticut, California, Minnesota, New Jersey, Vermont, Maine, South Dakota and Wisconsin soon followed, passing similar acts.

On the national scene, the federal government, authorized by the passage of the 1946 Mental Health Act, established the National Institute of Mental Health in 1949. Several demonstration and research projects with respect to social psychiatry were funded by the National Institute of Mental Health. In 1954, Stanton and Schwartz published their study, entitled *The Mental Hospital;* and in 1957, Greenblatt, Levinson and Williams published their study, *The Patient and the Mental Hospital.* In 1955, the Mental Health Study Act was passed. This act provided for the appointment of a Joint Commission on Mental Illness and Health to study and make recommendations for a national mental health program. Closely following this was the passage of Title V of the Health Amendment Act, in 1956. This legislation authorized the funding of mental health project grants for researching improved methods of treatment and rehabilitation of psychiatric patients.

The Joint Commission on Mental Illness and Health completed their report in 1961. This report emphasized the need for new community methods of care. By 1963, the Community Mental Health Centers Act was passed. This legislation authorized help in financing construction of centers for community mental health. In 1965, Public Law 89-105 was passed by Congress. This law provided for grants to assist in staffing new community mental health centers for a three-year period.

One of the greatest barriers to community mental health service, yet to be overcome, is the problem of interdisciplinary barriers. These barriers exist, not only between psychiatry and other behavioral sciences but also between psychiatry and the disciplines concerned with biological and physical sciences. There still exists, to some extent, the belief that there is a single cause for disease and that if the old medical model of the closed hospital system is followed in the treatment of mental illness the disease will dissipate. This model tended to ignore the patients' environment and the disciplines concerned with it.

Nursing, as a discipline, has been criticized by some in that it is geographically oriented within the hospital. That is, nurses tend to care for patients located in a given room or wing of a hospital. Actually, however, most members of health professions were formerly oriented to either the hospital or the community, and neither knew much about the other. The enculturation process of becoming a physician or a nurse or some other health service worker took many years to learn. The cumulative effects of the process will not be discarded easily. However, community mental health service has made it necessary for more decision-making to be done by the person "on the spot," regardless of his specific role. Some role-blurring, role conflict and role overload have taken place, not only among the professionals but among those for whom their help is intended. Until role expectations become clear, considerable strain for those in community mental health fields can be expected.

Readmission rates to mental institutions in the early 1970's are beginning to increase. While some patients have received adequate aftercare, many have been abandoned, with nowhere to turn. The best "mix" for delivering and financing comprehensive mental health service is yet to be developed, although much headway has been made in the overall problem.

DIMENSIONS OF COMMUNITY MENTAL HEALTH PRACTICES

Although there is some overlap of the two terms therapeutic community and community mental health care, there is a distinction between them which merits discussion. The idea implied by *therapeutic community* is that the patient is separated from society during the treatment phase. The patient is secluded so far as most of society is concerned, and is in a closed social system. That is, the hospital as a social system is not open to the mainstream of society. *Community care,* on the other hand, implies that there is exposure to society, with the patient remaining in the community during treatment. The overlap between the two terms occurs because the word community is difficult to define. Susser defines the term as follows: "A community . . . is an aggregate of people who have collective social ties by virtue of their shared locale for residence, for services and for work."[1]

Community care is a term used to refer to that given outside the hospital. It aims, according to Susser, "to expand the activities and obligations of the patient to a level at which they approximate the complex set of roles that fully functioning individuals assume in everyday life."[2] The individual learns the content of role behavior as he lives in a culture. Susser further states that "through participation a person comes to recognize the values of the culture as they are expressed in the norms and sanctions attached to its multiple social roles."[3] While this type of therapy has many values, there is a risk that it may make it necessary for the patient to conform to the moralities of the therapist.[4]

The patient's socialization in the community may be facilitated by drugs that may influence his receptivity. Organic capacities of the patient, however, operate to set limits on the socialization process. The learning which takes place in such a process may be of several kinds: (1) learning through direct conscious effort; (2) conditioned learning; (3) learning that is introspective in nature, i.e., learning insight into the self; or (4) learning to learn.

With new concept of community health care, a plethora of new approaches in prevention, treatment and rehabilitation are being made. Among the indirect services are comprehensive health planning, new organizational patterns within community mental health centers, socio-environmental therapy and new residential arrangements, as exemplified by partial hospitalization for adults. Among the direct services are such innovations as brief psychotherapies, family therapy, suicide prevention programs, priority services for children in child guidance units and new approaches in school systems.

---

[1]Mervyn Susser: *Community Psychiatry: Epidemiologic and Social Themes.* New York, Random House, 1968, p. 7.

[2]*Ibid.,* pp. 16–17.

[3]*Ibid.,* p. 18.

[4]*Ibid.*

THRUSTS TOWARD MENTAL HEALTH:
RESEARCH, PREVENTION AND
MANPOWER

EPIDEMIOLOGY OF MENTAL ILLNESS

Sata states: "The purpose of understanding the nature, distribution, and cause of disease is to develop measures to control, ameliorate and eventually prevent disease.[5] A study of the epidemiology of mental illness, according to Sata, involves several factors: (1) study of the population; (2) identification of high-risk groups; and (3) the development of methods to diminish morbidity. Systems analysis is a method which has considerable merit for such a study. The method utilizes indirect resources to bring about modification and alterations in a system in which there are large numbers of individuals.[6]

Before planning and research takes place, the development of a psychiatric case register is recommended. The utilization of such a register, while important for programs in research, health planning and evaluation, does violate human rights by invasion of privacy; however, as populations increase, rights of the individual may have to be sacrificed to some extent. This type of register provides data for longitudinal, comparative, retrospective and predictive studies.

The Inner City Community Mental Health Center Program in Baltimore serves as an outstanding example of an epidemiologic approach. Here, epidemiologic methods were used in establishing service components to such groups as children, southern migrants, fatherless families and alcoholics. The acceptance of the service was enhanced by involvement of community members during the planning process. A neighborhood advisory group was one organization that was involved.

PREVENTION

The field of public health recognizes three types of prevention: primary, secondary and tertiary. In *primary prevention,* diseases and disorders are eradicated, whereas in *secondary prevention,* the disease or condition is ameliorated through early detection and treatment. *Tertiary prevention,* on the other hand, serves to limit irreversible conditions and

---

[5]Lindbergh S. Sata: "Epidemiology: Prerequisite for Planning." *In* Leopold Bellak and Harvey H. Barten: *Progress in Community Mental Health.* New York, Grune and Stratton, 1969, p. 24.
[6]*Ibid.,* p. 25.

disease and to institute methods of rehabilitation. Precise methods of treatment and prevention require some knowledge of the causes of disease; however, sometimes methods of treatment and prevention are found to be effective in cases where causes are unknown. A well known example is the prevention of cholera as described by Snow.

An example of primary prevention that has implications for the nurse is crisis intervention. A brief résumé is presented here. The student will find an elaboration of content in the "Suggestions for Further Reading" at the end of the chapter.

Crisis Intervention and Primary Prevention.   According to Caplan a state of tension occurs in the individual just prior to the solution of a problem. Usually he is able to use habitual mechanisms and reactions in problem solving situations, and thus maintain his equilibrium. Caplan suggests that an imbalance occurs between the difficulty of the problem and the available resources for the problem's solution. The type of crisis intervention used by a professional, Caplan proposes, will be congruent with the profession's basically defined functions.[7] It is during the disequilibrium of a crisis period that the client may be helped by the professional to make choices from various available resources. It is this new coping response to the situation which has far-reaching effects on the future mental health of the individual.[8]

Treatment and Secondary Prevention.   One example of secondary prevention with which the student is familiar is electroshock therapy. This treatment may be administered to a patient with a brief episode of acute depression. This type of therapy serves to ameliorate the illness.

Hope Therapy and Rehabilitation.   An example of tertiary prevention is the use of "hope therapy," instituted in a community that has been deprived over a long period of time. Here, the nurse may find that positive expectations are a motivating force in social change. When one has positive expectations about the behavior of another, a ray of hope is sometimes generated. If the goal of expectation is not set too high, an individual may be motivated to attain it.

Stotland discusses six hypotheses for which supportive evidence relevant to the expectation of goals is cited. The community mental health nurse may find these helpful in guiding action programs relevant to disadvantaged people.

These hypotheses follow:

1. The greater the expectation of attaining a goal, the more likely the individual will act to attain it.
2. The more important a goal is, the more likely is the individual to attend selectively to aspects of the environment relevant to attaining it.

---

[7]Gerald Caplan: *Principles of Preventive Psychiatry.* New York, Basic Books, Inc., 1964, p. 39.

[8]*Ibid.,* p. 50.

3. Increased importance of the goal leads to more overt action to attain it.
4. Increased importance of goal attainment leads to more thought about *how* to attain the goal.
5. Increased expectation of goal attainment leads to more thought about how to attain the goal.
6. Increased expectation of goal attainment leads to more selective attention to aspects of the environment relevant to attaining the goal.[9]

Stotland's conceptualization relevant to hope and community action appears a useful one for the solution of problems. The author gives pertinent examples of the therapy of hope as applied to specific groups of mental patients.[10]

Sometimes practitioners feel handicapped and overwhelmed by a lack of knowledge in the etiological field; however, if one looks at past accomplishments, one sees that considerable headway has been made. Among diseases with known etiology are mental disorders caused by poisons, fetal infection, brain damage during childhood, certain genetic diseases, nutritional deficiencies as well as mental illness due to certain head injuries and general systemic diseases.

MANPOWER IN THE MENTAL HEALTH FIELDS

Mental health manpower is a crucial resource in the resolution and/or control of problems in the field of community mental health and illness. Therefore, it is necessary to have some knowledge with respect to the assessment and effective utilization of manpower within a given community.

Manpower Studies—Shortage Estimates. Although there is need for additional types of manpower studies, most studies in the field are concerned primarily with shortages. Shortages are determined in several ways. One method consists of comparing existing facts about quantity and quality of manpower with a predetermined minimum standard, i.e., a minimum standard set by the American Psychiatric Association. Another method is to estimate the need based upon the findings of a particular study. For example, the Surgeon General's Consultant Group on Nursing estimated the 1970 nursing manpower needs by basing their estimates upon a study which indicated that patient satisfaction was highest when at least 50 per cent of direct care was given by professional nurses.[11] A third approach is the use of data pertaining to the number of unfilled, budgeted positions. In general,

---

[9]Ezra Stotland: *The Psychology of Hope.* San Francisco, Jossey-Bass Inc., 1969, p. 17.
[10]*Ibid.*, pp. 206-242.
[11]Faye G. Abdellah and Eugene Levine: "Effect of Nursing Staffing on Satisfaction with Nursing Care." Hospital Monograph Series No. 4, Chicago, *The American Hospital Association,* 1958.

the three above approaches are those used by non-economists, and describe a gap between the existing situation and what ought to be.

Economists, on the other hand, view the situation quite differently. Hiestand states that, from this point of view, "a shortage indicates some discrepancy between the actual level of manpower supply and that which is possible, given the existing structure and level of demand for services and manpower in health and in all other fields."[12] Hiestand explains that the difference between what is possible and what actually exists occurs in two ways. One way is concerned with a gap between supply and demand due to a change in conditions where there has been insufficient time for reallocation through the market.[13]

The second type of shortage described by economists is due to deficiencies or imperfections in the market system, such as institutional limitations to manpower flow. Estimates of the *need* for manpower, rather than the *demand* for manpower, are helpful; however, Hiestand believes they are somewhat inadequate because most estimates of shortages are based on some apparently arbitrary relations between the population and the various manpower groups."[14] Little account is taken of age distribution, the natural, economic and technical environment, public practices and the like.

There seems sufficient evidence, in an economic sense, to say that a shortage of physicians exists. When demand is great, the market is willing to pay a high price. The income of physicians has been consistently higher than that of other health professionals. Few physicians leave the field and there are few student vacancies in medical schools. No such evidence exists insofar as nurses are concerned. Only about one-half of the nurses who have been educated are currently employed, and not all nursing schools operate to full capacity. In addition, nurses' salaries have not increased as rapidly as those in other largely female occupations during shortage situations.[15]

The above discussion of methods of estimating manpower shortages will, in part, explain why there is considerable variation in estimates made by investigators. The nurse in community mental health may have need of such information in interpreting data relevant to manpower in her particular locale.

Status of Manpower Groups.   In Chapter 1, high- and low-visibility functions of the nurse were discussed. The criteria elaborated there are applicable to the status of health professionals in general. Since the mind is not visible, as is the body, those whose work has the mind as a

---

[12]Dale Hiestand: "Research into Manpower for Health Service." *In* the *Milbank Memorial Fund Quarterly,* Part II, Vol. XLIV, October, 1966, p. 153.
[13]*Ibid.*
[14]*Ibid.,* p. 154.
[15]*Ibid.,* p. 156.

focus do not usually command as much prestige in our society: for example, the surgeon, whose work is highly visible is much admired. The low-visibility of practices related to the field of psychiatry sometimes makes it appear, in the eyes of the public, as a sort of mysticism that may be quackery. It is unfortunate that more progress has not been made in the epidemiology of mental illness, since a fairly rapid eradication of syndromes would perhaps make the work more visible.

Ewalt has pointed out that the problem of increasing our manpower pools in the mental health fields is "one of creating more interest in working with people rather than with things."[16] Currently the greatest manpower shortage is among teachers—especially in the fields of high school mathematics and science.[17] In general, American society tends to reward in a monetary manner those engaged in high-visibility functions. Professions draw their members from college graduates who place high values on a materialistic technology. There is, fortunately, a tendency for the new generation of college students to concern themselves less with the materialistic and more with humanistic concerns. It may be that this reversal will do much to offset the crisis in education described by Albee.

Career Opportunities. Career opportunities for new types of personnel within the mental health manpower field are rapidly increasing. Then too, patients, their families and members of the community in general are beginning to be given more responsibility as "care-givers" within the field of mental health and illness. Traditional roles of members in the major health professions are beginning to blur. Hopefully, in the years to come these will blend into a wide spectrum of occupational groups within the manpower field.

Many innovations are occurring in both the staffing and utilization patterns with respect to the role of the mental health-psychiatric nurse in the community. In community mental health care, the nurse will find some knowledge about group techniques helpful. A discussion of the nurse's role in this respect will be found in Chapter 25. The student may also find a more detailed discussion of specific innovations in the list of "Suggestions for Further Reading" at the end of this chapter.

Summary

The evolution of concepts and practices in community services has been discussed for both Europe and the United States. Important

---

[16]Jack R. Ewalt, *in* Albee, George W.: *Mental Health Manpower, A Report to the Staff Director, Jack R. Ewalt.* Joint Commission on Mental Illness, Monograph Series No. 3, New York, Basic Books, Inc., 1959, p. xxix.
[17]*Ibid.*

international developments have also been outlined. New federal legislation over the past 25 years with respect to mental health has been summarized.

The dimensions of community practices relative to the terms *therapeutic community* and *community care* have been elaborated with some emphasis on the patient's socialization within the community setting. New and emerging approaches to the solution of community care have been enumerated. The major thrusts in the control of mental illness have been discussed from the focal points of research (epidemiology), prevention and manpower.

Bibliography

Albee, George W.: *Mental Health Manpower Trends.* New York, Basic Books, Inc., 1959.

Albee, George W.: "Models, Myths, and Manpower." *Ment. Hyg.*, 52:168-80, 1968.

Baker, Frank, Schulberg, Herbert C., and O'Brien, Gregory: "The Changing Mental Hospital—Its Perceived Image and Contact with the Community." *Ment. Hyg.*, 53: 237–244, 1969.

Bellak, Leopold, and Barten, Harvey, eds.: *Progress in Community Mental Health.* Vol. I, New York, Grune and Stratton, 1969.

Bettis, Moody C., and Roberts, Robert: "The Mental Health Manpower Dilemma." *Ment. Hyg*, 53:163-175, April, 1969.

Buckley, Walter, ed.: *Modern Systems Research for the Behavioral Scientist.* Chicago, Aldine Publishing Company, 1968.

Caplan, Gerald: *Principles of Preventive Psychiatry.* New York, Basic Books Inc., 1964.

Collard, Joan: "The Public Health Nurse in After Care Programs." *Am. J. Pub. Health,* 56:210-217, February, 1966.

Cowen, Emory, Gardner, Elmer A., and Zax, Melvin, eds.: *Emergent Approaches to Mental Health Problems.* New York, Appleton-Century-Crofts, 1967.

Cowne, Leslie J.: "Approaches to the Mental Health Manpower Problem." *Ment. Hyg.,* 53:176-187, April, 1969.

Eisenberg, Leon: "Preventive Psychiatry." *Ann. Rev. Med.,* 13:343-357, 1962.

Flint, Robert T., and Spensley, Karen C.: "Recent Issues in Nursing Manpower: A Review." *Nursing Research, 18*:217-229, May-June, 1969.

Glasscotte, Raymond, *et al.: The Community Mental Health Center—An Interim Appraisal.* Washington, D.C., American Psychiatric Association, 1969.

Glasscotte, Raymond M., *et al.,* eds.: *The Psychiatric Emergency.* Washington, D.C., American Psychiatric Association, 1966.

Grace, Helen, and Davis, Lucille: "Primary Prevention: A Conceptual Model for Community Mental Health Nursing." *In* Bergersen, Betty S., *et al.* (eds.): *Current Concepts in Clinical Nursing.* St. Louis, C. V. Mosby Co., pp. 248-263.

Gruenbaum, Henry, ed.: *The Practice of Community Mental Health.* Boston, Little, Brown and Co., 1970.

Gruenberg, Ernest M.: *Evaluating the Effectiveness of Community Mental Health Services.* New York, Milbank Memorial Fund, 1966.

Hiestand, Dale L.: "Research Into Manpower for Health Service." *The Milbank Memorial Fund Quarterly,* Part II, Vol. XLIV, No. 4, October 1966.

Ishiyama, Toaru: "Staffing Patterns—A Solution to the Manpower Shortage?" *Ment. Hyg.,* 52:119-203, April, 1968.

Johannsen, Walter J.: "Attitudes toward Mental Patients." *Ment. Hyg.,* 53:218-227, April, 1969.

Kahn, J. H.: "Dimensions of Diagnosis and Treatment." *Ment. Hyg.,* 53:229-236, April, 1969.

Lapouse, Rema: "Problems in Studying the Prevalence of Psychiatric Disorder." *Am. J. Pub. Health, 57*:947-954, June, 1967.

Lapouse, Rema, and Monk, Mary A.: "An Epidemiologic Study of Behavior Characteristics in Children." *Am. J. Pub. Health., 48*:1134-1144, September, 1958.

Lapouse, Rema, and Monk, Mary A.: "A Method for Use in Epidemiologic Studies of Behavior Disorders in Children." *Am. J. Pub. Health., 54*:207-222, February, 1964.

Lawrence, P. J., ed.: *Mental Health and the Community.* Christchurch, New Zealand, 1963.

Loomis, Maxine E.: "The Clinical Specialist as a Change Agent." *Nursing Forum,* 7·136-145, No. 2, 1968.

Mackey, Richard A.: "Personal Concepts of the Mentally Ill Among Caregiving Groups." *Ment. Hyg., 53*:245-252, April, 1969.

Maris, Ronald: *Social Forces in Urban Suicide.* Homewood, Ill., The Dorsey Press, 1969.

McPartland, Thomas S., and Richart, Robert H.: "Social and Clinical Outcomes of Psychiatric Treatment." *Arch. Gen. Psychiat, 14·*179-184, February, 1966.

Monroe, Russell R., Klee, Gerald D., and Brody, Eugene B., eds.: *Psychiatric Epidemiology and Mental Health Planning: Psychiatric Research Report #22.* Washington, D.C., American Psychiatric Association, 1967.

National Commission on Mental Health Manpower: *Careers in Psychiatry,* New York, The Macmillan Co., 1968.

Norma, Edward C.: "Role of the Mental Health Consultee." *Ment. Hyg., 52*:304-308, April, 1968.

Ozarin, Lucy D.: "The Community Mental Health Center: Concept and Commitment." *Ment. Hyg., 52*:76–80, January, 1968.

Padilla, Elma, *et al.:* "The Public Image of Mental Health Professionals and Acceptance of Community Mental Health Services." *Am. J. Pub. Health, 56*:1524-1529, September, 1966.

Program Area Committee on Mental Health: *Mental Disorders: A Guide to Control Methods.* American Public Health Association, 1962.

Ray-Grant, Quentin: "Broad Horizons of Community Mental Health." *Journal of Psychiatric Nursing,* 5:109-120, March-April, 1967.

Redlich, F. C. and Pepper, Max: "Are Social and Community Psychiatry Subspecialties of Psychiatry?" *Am. J. Psychiat., 24*:37-44, April, 1968.

Reid, D. D.: *Epidemiological Methods in the Study of Mental Disorders.* Geneva, World Health Organization, 1960.

Roberts, Leigh M., Halleck, Seymour L., and Loeb, Martin B., eds.: *Community Psychiatry.* Madison, Wisconsin, University of Wisconsin Press, 1966.

Rubenstein, Robert, and Lasswell, Harold D.: *The Sharing of Power in a Psychiatric Hospital.* New Haven, Yale University Press, 1966.

Shneidman, Edwin S., and Farberow, Norman L.: *Clews to Suicide.* New York, McGraw-Hill Book Co., 1957.

Shumway, Sharon M., and Wisehart, Doris E.: "How to Know a Community." *Nursing Outlook, 17,* No. 9:63-64, September, 1969.

Singer, Richard G., and Blumenthal, Irving J.: "Suicide Clues in Psychotic Patients." *Ment. Hyg., 53*:346-350, July, 1969.

Stotland, Ezra: *The Psychology of Hope.* San Francisco, Jossey-Bass, Inc., 1969.

Susser, Mervyn: *Community Psychiatry: Epidemiologic and Social Themes.* New York, Random House, 1968.

Topf, Margaret, and Byers, Ruth Gordon: "Role Fusion on the Community Mental Health Multidisciplinary Team." *Nursing Research, 18*:270-275, May-June, 1969.

Ujhely, Gertud B.: "The Nurse in Community Psychiatry." *Am. J. Nursing, 69*:1001-1005, May, 1969.

Weiner, I. William: "The Effects of a Suicide Prevention Program." *Ment. Hyg., 53*:357-363, July, 1969.

Williams, Richard, and Ozarin, Lucy D., eds.: *Community Mental Health.* San Francisco, Jossey-Bass, Inc., 1967.

Suggestions for Further Reading

Anderson, Margaret, *et al.:* "Nursing and Social Work Roles in Cooperative Home Care and Treatment of the Mentally Ill." *Nursing Outlook, 11*:112-115, 1963.

Arnoff, Franklyn N.: "Realities and Mental Health Manpower." *Ment. Hyg.,* 52:181–189, 1968.

Arsenian, John: "Toward Prevention of Mental Illness in the United States." *Community Mental Health, 1*:320-325, 1965.

Barckley, Virginia: "The Nurse in Preventive Psychiatry." *Nursing Outlook, 8*:252-254, 1960.

Bulbalyan, Ann, Davidites, Rose Marie, and Williams, Florence: "Nurses in a Community Mental Health Center." *Am. J. Nursing, 69*:328-331, 1969.

Carter, Jerry W., Jr., ed.: *Research Contributions from Psychology to Community Mental Health.* New York, Behavioral Publications, Inc., 1968.

"Digest of Papers Forty-Seventh Annual Meeting, American Orthopsychiatric Association." *Am. J. Orthopsychiat., 40,* No. 2, 1970.

Evans, Frances Monet Carter: *The Role of the Nurse in Community Mental Health.* New York, The Macmillan Co., 1968.

Fagin, Claire M.: *Family Centered Nursing in Community Psychiatry.* Philadelphia, F. A. Davis Co., 1970.

Ishiyama, Toaru, *et al.:* "Does the Psychiatric Aide Have a Treatment Role?" *Ment. Hyg., 51*:115-118, 1967.

Jahoda, Marie: *Current Concepts of Positive Mental Health.* Joint Commission on Mental Illness and Health, Monograph Series No. I, New York, Basic Books, 1958.

Jarmusg, Robert T.: "Some Considerations in Establishing a Suicide Prevention Program." *Ment. Hyg., 53*:351-356, 1969.

Leininger, Madeleine: "Community Psychiatric Nursing: Trends, Issues and Problems." *Perspectives in Psychiatric Care, 7*:10-20, 1969.

McLean, Lenora J.: "Action and Reaction in Suicidal Crisis." *Nursing Forum, 8*:29-41, 1969.

Parad, Howard J., ed.: *Crisis Intervention: Selected Readings.* New York, Family Service Association of America, 1965.

Roose, Lawrence: "To Die Alone." *Ment. Hyg., 53*:321-327, 1969.

Rosenblum, Gershen and Hassol: "Training for New Mental Health Roles." *Ment. Hyg., 52*:81-86, 1968.

Tallent, Norman, Kennedy, George F., Jr., and Hurley, William T.: "A Program for Suicidal Patients." *Am. J. Nursing, 66*:2011-2016, 1966.

Wade, Mattie L., *et al.:* "How Public Health Nurses Promote Mental Health." *63*:81-83, 1963.

In Chapter 2, and again in Chapter 8, we emphasized that people, in our culture, satisfy most of their social needs in relationships with individuals or groups of individuals. Since most of our lives are spent in groups, it is imperative that we develop adequate skills and patterns of interaction within the framework of the group if we are to function with a minimum of grief and strife.

The skills involved in social accommodation and subordination become necessary for survival between the ages of six and nine years. This is usually the first time that the individual finds himself spending most of his time in a group of other individuals very much like himself. He begins to see himself in relation to the way these other individuals see him and respond to him. He begins also to learn what he can anticipate from these other individuals in the group and, in turn, what they anticipate from him. (See Chapter 4 for a more detailed discussion of this period of life.)

Group experiences are valuable learning experiences wherein an individual can not only develop skills in socialization but also develop greater self-understanding in relation to his needs, desires, conflicts and his usual pattern of coping with life situations. Through meaningful communication with other group members, including the nurse, an individual can clarify his thoughts and feelings, increase the continuity of his experiences and gain a different perspective of his problems.

Whenever a person's usual way of life is interrupted or circumstances require that other than minor changes in activities be made over an extended period of time, we have found that some form of group experience that promotes active participation is very helpful in facilitating readjustment. Since the person who is hospitalized is one of those who encounters this problem, group experiences are an important part of nursing care. In the material that follows, various aspects of this function of the nurse will be elaborated.

VALUES OF GROUP EXPERIENCES

Group experiences provide the patient with an opportunity to practice his social skills in playing new roles and in solving specific problems. Through these experiences the patient may also express his regressive tendencies in a socially acceptable manner. Regression to immature and infantile behavior is not sanctioned by our culture when one is engaged in serious work, but during recreation it is acceptable. These experiences also provide an opportunity for the release of tension and the expression of aggressive tendencies, as in striking a punching bag. There seems to be inherent in every individual a need for movement and a need for new experience, a change from the monotonous routines of daily living. The actual values of any group experience will, of course, depend upon the functioning level of each individual member and also the interaction level of the group. As the individual develops skills in group interaction, a sense of belonging, a sense of being one with the group, evolves, and the influence that each member has upon the behavior of other members increases.

Planning for Group Experiences

In planning group experiences, the nurse will use much the same approach as she does in meeting the patient's other needs for nursing care. Before any plan is implemented she must, first of all, have certain information. The amount of information required before the initiation of activities will depend somewhat upon how comfortable the nurse feels with the group. Perhaps the easiest way of acquiring this information is through a simple survey of facts about the patients. The following outline may prove helpful in assembling the data.

INFORMATION NECESSARY FOR PLANNING

Patient's name	Age
Interests and preferences	Dislikes
Occupation	Education
Religion	Economic status
Physical handicaps	Home
Characteristic overt pattern of behavior	Main problem he is attempting to solve
Special orders (for example, suicidal pre-	(for example, dependency)
cautions)	Current participation in activities

The next step to be taken by the nurse will be to look about the ward and determine what materials are available for activities. She will not only want to be aware of the equipment available for indoor and outdoor games but she will be alert to other materials that can be used creatively. She can also determine what materials can be requisitioned from the store or supply room. In some hospitals, the patients have access to a good many of their own things that they can use. Another source that is sometimes forgotten is discarded material about the hospital. For example, lard cans from the kitchen make attractive wastebaskets, and the repair shop may be discarding small amounts of leftover paint that could be used to paint the wastebaskets. If we but look about, we may find innumerable types of equipment and supplies that are either free or inexpensive. If the budget makes no provision for such activities, the administrator of the hospital will often solicit funds from available sources or donations from individuals in the community when the needs are called to his attention.

Determining what activities will be suitable and not in conflict with the structure provided by hospital environment is the next step the nurse will take. For example, it will not be feasible to secure old razor blades for patients to use in cutting out designs if several patients on the ward are extremely suicidal, just as it would not be practical to acquire an old metal ring to use as a basketball hoop for a dayroom that is quite small and already overcrowded. The nurse may remember that one of the patients mentioned that he wished the group had a place where they could post news events that would be of interest to the others, such as wishing someone "Happy Birthday" or congratulating someone when he is to go home. If other patients are equally stimulated, the nurse may capitalize on this interest by helping them to construct a clever and attractive bulletin board. Most of the needed materials can probably be found about the hospital. The nurse will not want to elicit the patients' interest in activities that cannot be carried out because of hospital regulations. For example, the nurse might stimulate interest in painting a mural on the walls, but if such an activity is not approved by hospital administration, it may eventually evoke hostility toward the patients involved.

When necessary information has been secured in relation to facts about the patients and their needs, the materials available, the needs of the ward that can plausibly be fulfilled by patient activity, and the framework in which the activities are to take place, the nurse will then be ready to analyze these data. She will interpret the information in terms of possible activities for individual projects and for group projects. It will then be necessary to determine which individuals will profit from the specific activity. In going over the information in regard to patients, the nurse will know almost automatically that Mr. J., who has very poor vision, would not enjoy reading the newspaper to his elderly roomate. She will also avoid asking Mrs. R., who is 84 years old, to play Ping-pong with a very active teen-ager. The nurse is most alert to the interests expressed by individual patients and will utilize them as the opportunity arises. These interests, however, may not always be verbalized but may be indicated in other ways. For example, a teen-age boy who has never developed much skill in reading may cast an occasional glance at the fatherly Mr. J. and move his chair closer as Mr. J. reads the sports news aloud. The nurse will also pay particular attention to the religious views of patients and will not encourage their participation in an activity that might evoke conflict. She will notice, too, whether Miss A. is apt to be overstimulated and hyperactive when she is in close contact with several others. She may also notice that Miss L., a very dependent person, is showing a few signs of being more assertive and may wish to provide the opportunity for her to make a few decisions in regard to activities for the day or the topic for discussion. In planning activities for groups the nurse will want to take into account the individual's need for practicing new skills in new roles; but she will be careful, too, not to place him in situations in which he will be overwhelmed or ridiculed. In helping to form group activities she will also avoid placing patients who are too antagonistic to one another in close contact. In some instances, it may be wise to let patients act out their conflicts with one another, but in others, the experience may be too traumatic for the patients. The nurse should consult the patient's physician whenever there is any doubt.

As we can see, there are many factors that must be taken into account before initiating activities if they are going to help the patient move forward toward the goal, recovery. However, as we become more skilled in this method of collecting and analyzing data, we think through these steps so rapidly that they seem almost automatic. We will also keep in mind that, in good planning, it often appears to the participant that no planning has taken place. When we enjoy an evening at a friend's home, it may not occur to us at the time that she has put much effort into the occasion because she seems so much at ease and so spontaneous. When we stop to consider that she prepared a very elaborate meal after working all day and had limited resources for entertaining her group, we realize that such a pleasant evening took considerable planning and effort but that we enjoyed it chiefly because of the spontaneity and our lack of awareness of what took place to make such an evening possible.

Implementing the Plan

After we have explored and assessed the possibilities, we have completed much of the groundwork and are ready to initiate action. We then consider who will initiate the activity and when, who will supervise it and how this shall be done. We will, at this point, wish to bring certain patients into the planning, and it may be that a patient can initiate the proposed activity. The patients may have many valuable suggestions that can be utilized. It is also important that we plan the time for the project to be undertaken. We will not want to suggest a party at a time when the patients ordinarily attend a movie, and we will not want to begin activities when we know that almost immediately they will be interrupted by the noon meal. It also will be useless to encourage Mrs. R. to engage in any activity when we know that it is about time for her son to make his weekly visit.

Whenever plans are initiated, someone from the staff must be available to supervise the activity. Equipment and materials must be made accessible to the group and must be accounted for when the activity is over. Interest, once it is aroused, should be maintained. Some patients will need encouragement, others may become too stimulated; but the alert nurse can usually modify plans to take these changes into account. The person supervising the activities will, at times, be a catalyst and, at other times, an active participant, depending upon what the circumstances of the moment dictate. The recording of observations for this period will be most helpful in planning future activities and will be valuable to the physician in his therapy with the patient.

THE "ACTIVATION" GROUP

In addition to these more structured, directive means of working with groups, in which the emphasis is on doing together and the goals are chiefly social and more group oriented, there is a less structured group wherein the goals are more individual and the nurse's role is less directive and primarily that of a participant observer. In this group, the activity is all intrapersonal and interpersonal without having any props, concrete or material objects to manipulate. We will call this group the "Activation" group, with the emphasis on the resolution of conflicts, the development of greater self-understanding, the reduction of anxiety and tension, and the development of more effective patterns of coping with stress and adapting to reality.

The size of the "Activation" group will vary from a minimum of four to a maximum of eight members. The meetings of the group will be scheduled for specific times and will usually last for one hour. It has proven effective for the nurse to tell the group members the purpose of the meetings. As in other units of interaction, there is no formula to tell the nurse exactly what to say, but the important thing is that she is comfortable in what she says. One nurse may say to her group, "We are going to meet twice a week to learn to better understand ourselves," whereas another may say, "We are going to get together to talk about how we feel in different situations."

In the first few meetings there will inevitably be an increase of tension and apprehension on the part of both the patients and the nurse, but this will gradually lessen as each member becomes more comfortable in the group situation. Although each member is expected to participate and to express his feelings in the group situation, there is a difference in the length of time it will take for all members to feel secure enough to express themselves. Assuming that there is a difference in the group members, some may be quiet and withdrawn, others friendly and responsive and still others may be hostile. The nurse will direct her remarks to a friendly member or one who is likely to respond, thus creating an atmosphere for further responses. Since we have learned from our experiences that people usually respond according to our expectations of them, the nurse's anticipations of the group members will, more or less, set the stage for their responses.

At first it may appear that the members are just "blowing off steam," but as the "Activation" group continues to meet and the channels of communication become more clear we will begin to see manifestations of group feeling and group identification evolving. The individual members begin to show more concern about other members and how they are feeling. They begin to find that, in spite of their differences, they have many things in common and begin to refer to "our" group, "we" feel, and such. Refer to Chapter 7 for more details about communication and interaction.

The nurse will function in the role of a stabilizer, a catalyst, a supporter, a reflector, an energizer, a validator and in other roles required by the group as they struggle to attain their goals. Just as the nurse encounters periods of silence in her interaction with one patient, she also will encounter silences in her interaction with the group. Here again, it is important for the nurse to learn to be comfortable in periods of silence and to develop a sense of timing in regard to when to interject a comment and when to remain silent.

The interaction within the group will be influenced by the individual members, their needs, their tolerance level for pain and stress, the degree to which they are motivated toward health and also the degree of understanding and the therapeutic skills possessed by the nurse. Throughout the group meetings an attitude of acceptance and permissiveness must prevail, and each individual member must feel that he is free to express himself, that he is accepted for what he is, that he will find support and other supplies as they are needed.

What will determine the characteristics of the group interaction, the goals of the group and the roles of a particular nurse within this group? The most important factor is the nurse herself and the degree to which she understands and accepts herself, for this understanding and acceptance set the limits for her understanding and acceptance of others. The motives that underlie the nurse's relationship to the group are extremely important—for example, whether she really wants to do something about these people and their stresses and conflicts or whether she merely wants to build up her own self-esteem. (See Chapter 8 for a more detailed discussion of motives in relationships.)

The degree to which the nurse is willing to look at her own interaction and to evaluate it in terms of what she is doing and why will greatly facilitate her development of greater self-understanding and therapeutic skills. While it is not always possible for the nurse to know and understand everything that is going on in her interaction with the group members at the time, a review of the situation in retrospect will enable her to validate and crystallize the processes and dynamics in the situation. (See Chapter 8 for a discussion of empathy and identification in relationships.)

CHARACTERISTICS OF AN EFFECTIVE
PLAN FOR GROUP EXPERIENCES

1. THE PLAN WILL BE FLEXIBLE AND ALLOW FOR CHANGE AND SPONTANEITY.   A plan that is not flexible enough to allow for minor changes will probably stifle creativeness. A group of patients, for example, making plans for invitations to the Christmas party may have a new and wonderful idea as one of the patients begins to design the invitations. If such an idea had been spontaneously accepted by the group, their creativity would be blocked if the nurse were to say, "I thought we agreed to design the invitations in the form of candles." In another instance, perhaps the committee planning the games for a

party had selected the ones they preferred when Miss B., a patient who is ordinarily quiet, suggested a game that could easily be played without any extra equipment. Everyone seemed interested, too, because Miss B. was actively participating. What would happen, then, if we were to say, "The next game that we are going to play is bingo"?

2. It Will Be Democratic in Principle. The plans that arouse the most interest are the ones that belong to everyone. If the patients are able to participate in activities, surely they are capable of assisting in formulating the plans. However, it may not be possible for everyone to contribute the same amount or to participate to the same degree.

3. It Will Be Practical. If satisfaction is to be attained, the plan must be one that is possible to achieve without threatening or overwhelming those concerned. It will not be feasible to plan activities for outdoor games in the wintertime if the patients do not have warm clothing.

4. It Must Be on the Level at Which the Patient Can Function. It may be necessary to initiate activities that are very simple. Perhaps Mrs. S. sits in a chair in the corner all day and refuses to engage in any games. It will first be necessary to arouse her interest, and the nurse may find that sitting beside her, slowly leafing through a magazine, and pointing out certain pictures will evoke a response from the patient. She may also try moving the patient's chair a little closer to activities each day, which may gradually arouse a spark of interest.

5. It Will Provide for a Gain That Is Greater Than Any Possible Loss. This characteristic may be illustrated in the plan for the patient who spends most of his time in fantasy. Since the patient apparently gains a great deal of satisfaction from his daydreams, any plan formulated to promote his participation with the group must offer greater satisfaction than that which he receives from fantasy.

6. It Will Provide for Variety. When plans for activities become monotonous they are no longer therapeutic unless monotony is desired, as, for example, for an individual who is hyperactive. Patients may enjoy a party occasionally, but if plans are made for one every night then such affairs may tend to become routine.

7. It Must Be Consistent in Principle. The characteristic of consistency is illustrated when the person assisting in the planning of the activities is permissive in all her relationships with the group. Patients usually like to anticipate the nurse's behavior and are apt to feel threatened if she is permissive at one time and not at others.

Summary

Group experiences have been discussed, and a methodology of approach for planning these experiences has been proposed. Providing for patients' needs in this respect is much the same as providing for any other need in that we must collect and analyze certain data, formulate a tentative plan of action and then implement and evaluate it.

The characteristics of an effective plan for group experiences will serve to evaluate the plan. An effective plan will (1) be flexible and allow for change and spontaneity, (2) be democratic, (3) begin on the level at which the patient can function, (4) be practical, (5) provide for a gain which is greater than any possible loss, (6) provide for variety, and (7) be consistent.

Group experiences have many values in that they provide the patient an opportunity to practice his social skills. They also offer an opportunity for expression of regressive and aggressive tendencies, as well as providing for the individual's need for movement and for change.

In addition to the value of group experiences orientated toward group goals and socialization, there was a discussion of "Activation" group experiences, which are orientated more toward the goals of the individual members. Through these experiences the individual develops greater self-understanding, more tolerance and concern for others, resolves inner conflicts and learns more effective ways of coping with the stresses of everyday life.

Some aspects of the nurse's role in the "Activation" group have been elaborated as well as some of the pressures that arise in group interaction. The importance of the nurse's self-understanding and acceptance has been emphasized, with suggestions for facilitating the development of greater self-understanding and the refinement of therapeutic skills.

Bibliography

Berne, Eric: *Principles of Group Treatment.* New York, Oxford University Press, 1966.
Berne, Eric: *The Structure and Dynamics of Organizations and Groups.* Philadelphia, J. B. Lippincott Co., 1963.
Bion, W. R.: "Experiences in Groups." *Human Relations, 1*:314-320, 487-496, 1948; 2:13-22, 1949.
Durkin, Helen E.: *The Group in Depth.* New York, International Universities Press, Inc., 1964.
Freud, Sigmund: *Group Psychology and Analysis of the Ego.* London, International Psychoanalytic Press, 1922.
Hinckley, Robert G., and Hermann, Lydia: *Group Treatment in Psychotherapy.* Minneapolis, University of Minnesota Press, 1951.
Powdermaker, Florence B., and Frank, Jerome D.: *Group Psychotherapy.* Cambridge, Mass., Harvard University Press, 1953.
Slavson, S. R.: *Recreation and the Total Personality.* New York, International Committee of Young Men's Christian Association, Association Press, 1948.
Whitaker, Dorothy S., and Lieberman, Morton: *Psychotherapy Through the Group Process.* New York, Atherton Press, 1964.

326 PSYCHIATRIC-MENTAL HEALTH NURSING IN COMMUNITY SETTINGS

Suggestions for Further Reading

Ackerman, Nathan W.: "The Family Approach and Levels of Intervention." *Am. J. Psychotherapy, XXII*:5-14, 1968.
Berthiaume, Aileen B.: "Observing Is More than Watching." *Nursing Outlook, 5*:290-292, 1957.
Brown, Frances G.: Therapeutic Group Discussions. *Am. J. Nursing, 58*:836-839, 1958.
Copp, Laurel, and Copp, John Dixon: "Look to the Pattern of Relationships." *Am. J. Nursing, 60*:1285-1286, 1960.
Dade, Lucy S.: "Diversional Activities for Patients." *Am. J. Nursing, 47*:384-386, 1947.
Edman, Irwin: "Bibliotherapy." *Am. J. Nursing, 47*:668, 1947.
Fernandez, Theresa M.: "How to Deal with Overt Aggression." *Am. J. Nursing, 59*:658-660, 1959.
Fries, Olive H., and McLellan, Mary Lou: "Helping Patients Get Well." *Nursing Outlook, 7*:654-655, 1959.
George, Gloria R., and Gibson, Robert W.: "Patient Staff Relationships Change with Environment" *Ment. Hosp. 10*:18-19, 1959.
Gregory, Elizabeth M · "How to Help a Patient During an Emotional Crisis" *Nursing World, 132*:8-11, 1958.
Hart, Betty L., and Rohweder, Anne W.: "Support in Nursing" *Am. J. Nursing, 59*:1398-1401, 1959.
Hartlage, Lawrence C.: "Mobilizing Group Forces to Modify Behavior of Long-term Patients." *Perspectives in Psychiatric Care, 2*:35-38, 1964.
Hayter, Jean: "Reassure the Patient." *Nursing World, 134*:21-32, 1950.
Hibarger, Victoria E., Blanchard, William H., and Glogow, Eli: "Nurses Use the Group Process." *Am. J. Nursing, 55*:334-336, 1955.
Knowles, Lois N.: "How Can We Reassure Patients?" *Am. J. Nursing, 59*:834-835, 1959.
Lamb, Josephine T.: "Freedom for Patients in Mental Hospitals." *Am. J. Nursing, 58*:358-360, 1958.
Marshall, Margaret A.: "Hopelessness." *Nursing World, 133*:30-31, 1959.
Martinez, Ruth E.: "The Nurse as Group Psychotherapist." *Am. J. Nursing, 58*:1681-1682, 1958.
Mintz, Elizabeth E.: "Terapy Techniques and Encounter Techniques." *Am. J. Psychotherapy, XXV*:104-109, 1971.
Morgan, Margaret: "Pulling Strings." *Am. J. Nursing, 47*:623, 1947.
Morimoto, Francoise R.: "Socializing Role of Psychiatric Ward Personnel." *Am. J. Nursing, 54*:53-55, 1954.
Norris, Catherine M.: "The Nurse and the Crying Patient." *Am. J. Nursing, 57*:323-327, 1957.
Papanek, Helene: "Therapeutic and Antitherapeutic Factors in Group Relations." *Am. J. Psychotherapy, XXIII*:396-404, 1969.
Pullinger, Walter F., Jr.: "Remotivation." *Am. J. Nursing, 60*:683-685, 1960.
Rohweder, Anne W., and Hart, Betty L.: "How Attitudes Are Taught and Caught." *Am. J. Nursing, 60*:806-809, 1960.
Schwartz, Doris: "Uncoöperative Patients." *Am. J. Nursing, 58*:75-77, 1958.
Slavson, S. R.: *Recreation and the Total Personality.* New York, International Committee of Young Men's Christian Association, Association Press, 1948, pp. 1-70, 86-102, 141-165.
Sommer, Robert: "Working Effectively with Groups." *Am. J. Nursing, 60*:223-226, 1960.
Speroff, B. J.: "Empathy Is Important in Nursing." *Nursing Outlook, 4*:326-327, 1956.
Wauda, Lottie. "Waste Materials in Occupational Therapy." *Am. J. Nursing, 46*:257-258, 1946

Part Five   The Teaching-Learning Milieu for Psychosocial Nursing

Chapter 26   The Student-Patient-Teacher Constellation

As has been implied throughout the previous material, the psychiatric patient, regardless of his diagnosis or his overt behavioral manifestations, is more like other people than he is unlike them. He may differ, just as all people do, in his inherent potential, in the quality and kind of experiences he has had, in the degree of warp and areas of vulnerability that he has developed, in the overt expression of his needs and his desires, in his attempts to cope with reality as he sees it and to maintain his existence at whatever level he has found it possible.

To all outward appearances, the psychiatric patient is chronologically an adult, just as many of his colleagues are who are functioning in society and hanging on by the skin of their teeth. What he really wants is what everyone wants: a chance to "become," to feel adequate and capable, to find some rhyme or reason for his existence, to experience a minimum of anxiety and to achieve a level at which he can to some degree be productive in some area.

The blossoming of an individual is not an accumulation of knowledge and experience like bricks placed one upon the other to build a wall. It is the "person" within this individual who must be nurtured and helped to mobilize and achieve his potential. Just as the family provides the basic context of growth and experience, success or failure, so does it provide the context for health or illness. More and more emphasis is being given to a study of the family members in their reciprocal role relationships and how curative experiences can be provided for the whole group. Since the family unit is made up of individuals, who to various degrees have become "persons," who have structured multiple roles during each cycle of development (see Chapter 4) the members of the family will continue to have reciprocal interaction and influence.

It has become more and more evident that the adult who is dissatisfied, who is constantly harried by apprehension and who feels inadequate and incompetent is still trying to solve or complete some of the tasks that should have been completed when he was a child. This statement is not new and has been said in a thousand different ways down through the centuries. Its meaning is slowly getting through to more people as reflected in the demands for more adequate facilities for the detection and treatment of the problems of children and for the education of parents.

How does the psychiatric nurse — or any nurse, for that matter — fit into this scheme of ever-expanding problems that reach far beyond the walls of the traditional hospital? The nurse, to the degree that she is a maturing autonomous person, will be able to provide the kinds of experiences that are required for the growth of her patients. If she really understands the material presented in the first chapters and has some understanding of her own needs, her patterns of interaction, communication and other means of seeking satisfaction and security, and if she is motivated to develop further awareness and understanding, the nurse will inevitably experience surges of growth as she has positive experiences in the supervisory process. Positive experiences do not necessarily imply pleasant experiences, because it is often painful to look at oneself and what goes on in one's everyday situations. These experiences are positive because they lead to forward movement and are necessary for growth and ultimate self-realization.

We seldom stay on a plateau for long if we are really living: we either move backward (regress) or we move forward (progress), because life in all of its manifestations is dynamic. The psychiatric hospital has been called a "school for living," although it has more often become a "school for existing." We are all familiar with the tradition and heritage of the psychiatric hospital, and it is easy to see how it has fallen into decay. If a psychiatric hospital can be considered a "school for living," what implications does this have for a school of nursing?

We have seen many students who have been, or at least are on their way to becoming, "real" persons who are "living," but by the time they complete their programs they are ready for the ranks of the "armored cars who push each other around." Just as children use their parents as models, students use their teachers as models. This is something we cannot control; it just happens.

Since students, just as patients, are a subclassification of people, they too have the same basic needs, although their overt expression, their patterns of activity and their degree and extension of warp may differ. The environment or atmosphere essential for growth at any level is basically the same, although additional ingredients may be necessary as growth ensues (see the chapters on *Early Development, Interaction and Communication*). As has been said over and over again, assuming that the basic biologic needs are met, it is the quality of the environment—which is created by people—that is so vital to the flowering of the "person."

Freedom and responsibility seem to pose increasing problems in contemporary living. How often do we hear the questions or comments: "Why aren't people more responsible? Nobody seems to care any more." "The important thing is not how you play the game but whether or not you get caught." "Why should we be concerned about that? Let somebody else take care of it." All these statements seem to reflect the estrangement and depersonalization in our modern society.

With all our scientific knowledge and the surging ahead of mechanization, there seems to be a tendency for man to become more and more mechanical and to function automatically, as if he too were a machine. If our aim is to promote the development of robots who can carry on the tasks of living without "giving us any troubles," we have been going in the right direction. On the other hand, if our aim is the development of free autonomous persons who are capable of independent thinking, interacting on a level of interdependence, and assuming responsibility, we have to make the decision and proceed accordingly rather than to continue on the assumption that our "good" intentions will solve the problem.

The basic pattern of growth is the same, whether it occurs in infancy, adolescence or adulthood. One either continues to grow or one stagnates. One can, however, become a responsible adult only to the degree that one has had the freedom "to be" as an infant and child. We have recently seen more and more interest expressed in guaranteeing the rights provided us by the Constitution. We have a Bill of Rights for patients, a Bill of Rights for the senior citizen, and so on, but we tend to forget some of the rights inherently ours, such as the right of self-determination, the right to be oneself. To the degree that these rights have not been provided for in the life of a person, he has to really experience situations wherein they are provided, if inner change is to occur and he is to mobilize his potential and move forward.

It is fairly widely accepted now in educational circles that learning results in a change of behavior and that the anticipated changes in behavior become our educational objectives. Whether we really believe this or merely give lip service to it determines the quality of the climate or atmosphere we foster in learning situations for students during both undergraduate and graduate study.

What the patient wants in his nurse is similar to what the student wants in his teacher: someone who will accept the patient as a person and who is comfortable enough with himself to allow the patient the freedom to be himself in their interaction. Acceptance of a person does not imply either approval or disapproval of his activities. Everyone, except those with a severe degree of pathology, has his own built-in function of disapproval, which is usually much stronger than his function of approval. To become an autonomous person, one must eventually learn to evaluate one's own behavior critically. In precise use, according to Webster, *critical* implies an effort to see a thing clearly in order to evaluate it fairly. If this were always the true intention when we "help" someone look critically at a situation he has experienced in order for him to learn from his activities, we would not evoke so many responses of resentment, defensiveness and often overt hostility. We have to learn to be critical without condemning, blaming, denouncing, censuring or disapproving; these elements are responsible for most negative reactions. We have often clouded the issue by labeling our action as "constructive" criticism and saying, when students or patients do not react as we desire, that there is something "wrong" with them. As stated previously, "good" intentions are not enough to heal our depersonalized world. We have to become aware of the true motives that underlie our actions and determine just how constructive we really are.

We often tell students to give patients support in order to offer them reassurance, but how many times do we clarify what support or reassurance means and how we can go about providing it? Neither support nor reassurance is something we can put by the spoonful on a tray and serve; it is something found within the person and communicated primarily on a nonverbal level. To *assure* means to make safe, to secure against change or risk, while *assurance* is a state of being sure, confident, self-reliant or certain. On the other hand, *reassurance* means to assure anew, to restore confidence, while *support* means to sustain, to comfort or to strengthen. Thus, it goes without saying that one can offer reassurance only to the degree that one is sure, confident and self-reliant. It is the reflection of this state that may offer others an opportunity to feel less threatened and less helpless. If we have a minimum of tension and are free from anxiety, the comfort of the other person may also be facilitated. We must continually examine our own situations of interaction and discover when and under what circumstances we experience stress and become uncomfortable or anxious, before our awareness shrinks to the degree that we miss all the significant clues in the situation. When we are in a situation with someone who is anxious, do we also become anxious and further exaggerate and distort the situation, or are we an autonomous person who can be genuine and at the same time help neutralize and clarify the feelings of the anxious person.

Anyone, whether he is a patient, student or teacher, needs someone with whom he can validate—that is, someone with whom he can share his ideas, feelings and other experiences and determine whether they are founded on reality or fantasy. Experiences in true validation lead to experiences in true collaboration, which is the ultimate in interpersonal interaction. As the student and the patient grow, so grows the teacher.

Summary

The student-patient-teacher constellation has been explored and the similarities of the person in each role have been emphasized. The degree of growth and expansion of a person in any one of these roles is directly related to that of the persons in the other two roles. In any "helping" relationship, it is vital that the essential ingredients for growth be present if any mobilization of potential and any forward movement is to evolve. Only as the needs of the student are provided for, and she moves forward, will she be able to provide for the needs of the patient so that he may move forward also.

Suggestions for Further Reading

Erikson, Erik H.: *Insight and Responsibility.* New York, W. W. Norton & Co., Inc., 1964, Chapters III and VI.
Jersild, Arthur T.: *The Psychology of Adolescence.* New York, Macmillan Co., 1963, pp. 342-350.
Lidz, Theodore: *The Person.* New York, Basic Books, Inc., 1968.
Rogers, Carl R.: *Client-Centered Therapy.* Cambridge, Mass., Riverside Press, 1951, Chapter 9.
Rosenblith, Judy, and Allinsmith, Wesley: *The Causes of Behavior.* Boston, Allyn and Bacon, Inc., 1962.
Weigert, Edith: *The Courage to Love.* New Haven, Yale University Press, 1970.

Chapter 27   Stress Situations in the Student's Social System

As the student nurse learns the values and norms of the nursing profession, her behavior changes, and sometimes, in the enculturation process, the student will encounter a number of stress factors. It may help the student to know that she is not unique in experiencing stress: stress situations are experienced by other nursing students and are also encountered in other disciplines in the health professions. As students "grow up," it may not be desirable to alleviate all stress because, to a certain degree, stress may be necessary for motivation. Too much stress, on the other hand, is undesirable. This chapter is directed especially to college students, since it is this type of student with which the authors work. Noncollege students, however, may also recognize factors that are applicable to themselves.

The nurse makes up a part of the patient's dynamic environment. When the nurse encounters stress, she is affected in some way, and often these behavioral changes are reflected in her work with patients.

The nurse is a part of the hospital social system, and this chapter may help the nurse to have a better understanding as to how she became a part of nursing and thus a part of the social system in a hospital. Graduate students may wish to compare the enculturation process of other disciplines in the health professions with that of nursing. Often such a comparative study will provide insights essential to understanding the roles of colleagues from other fields and their special interest in the psychiatric patient.

IDENTIFICATION OF STRESS FACTORS

Since stress factors in the education of various types of profession-al students within the health field seem to have some commonalities with stress-producing elements in collegiate nursing education, a sur-vey of the pertinent literature was made in order to provide a few clues to the identification of stress factors in collegiate nursing education.

Stress factors in any emerging profession are great, and particu-larly so in a field that makes application of the sciences basic to the understanding of man. Nursing is such a profession. While there are many changes outside the profession that produce drastic changes in it, there are simultaneously many changes from within.

DEFINITION OF TERMS

A *stress factor* is any element or situation encountered by the colle-giate nursing student in the enculturation process of becoming a nurse and is also one that is described by the student as being stressful.

An *innovation* is the actual implementation of a new idea.

The degree of *alleviation of stress* is the extent to which stress has been reduced, as evaluated by the student. A student may choose between several situations and rank each according to the amount of stress generated in herself.

STRESS FACTORS IN MEDICAL SCHOOLS

Bloom[1] states that to acquire greater detachment in the face of emotion-laden experiences is one of the primary problems of medical students during the first two years. As medical students pass from working with dead animals to cadavers, live animals, and finally to patients, they learn the process of detachment and regard each of the phases as one step closer to being doctors. Medical students, like colle-giate nursing students, begin with a motivation to help people, and each develops a kind of cynicism as the educational program progress-es. In both instances, there appears to be a disenchantment phase. Bloom[2] points out that, for the physician, the internship and residency contribute more to socialization of the profession than any other expe-rience. Bloom also credits the school environment as being a vitally important influence on the professional.

According to Becker,[3] medical students spend a great deal of time

---

[1]Samuel W. Bloom: "The Process of Becoming a Physician." *Ann. Am. Acad. Polit. & Social Sci., 346*:77-87, March, 1963.

[2]*Ibid.*, p. 87.

[3]Howard S. Becker and Blanche Geer: "The Fate of Idealism in Medical Schools." *Am. Soc. Rev. 23*:50-56, February, 1958.

learning to live with uncertainty. They must learn that there are no immediate answers for many things. Becker also finds support for the fact that medical students never lose their idealism but simply find it irrelevant to their daily concerns in the school. The idealism simply lies dormant and is put to use when an appropriate situation presents itself.

INTERDISCIPLINARY APPROACHES

Abandoned by medicine in its infancy, nursing clutched at most anything until it started to grow up. In some cases, nursing looked to dentistry for leadership in the natural sciences, and like dentistry, was preoccupied with techniques rather than theory. Nursing has had to learn from other disciplines and has perhaps leaned too heavily on the social sciences. For while the social sciences are exceedingly important, they are of little immediate value applied to a patient who has an obstructed airway. Nursing is now trying to swing the pendulum back into balance.

Dentistry has had a similar history in its relationship with medicine. A visiting dentist once commented to the dean of a school of dentistry that the medical and dental schools of the university were separated by only a narrow street. The dean answered that, although the street appeared narrow, the distance across it was wider than any in the whole world.[4]

In a few universities in the country, some headway has been made in solving these problems of relationships. The medical and dental schools use the same selection process in admitting students, and dental students are required to have the same pre-professional program as medical students. The students of both schools then share the same basic science courses given during the first two years in professional school.

In other universities, similar relationships between nursing and medicine have been improved by assigning the student nurse, student physician, and other appropriate professional students to a family that they all follow through their professional schooling.

THE PUBLIC IMAGE OF THE NURSE

Ross[5] states that, on the whole, nurses seem more aware than members of other professions of the changes that their profession is undergoing and will undergo in the future. The author further states that this awareness is manifested in restlessness and dissatisfaction. Ross[6] believes that the greatest dilemma in nursing is to reconcile the

---

[4]A. Leroy Johnson: *Dentistry, As I See It Today.* Boston, Little, Brown and Co., 1955, p. 24.

[5]Aileen D. Ross: *Becoming a Nurse.* Toronto, Macmillan Co., 1961, p. 397.

[6]*Ibid.,* p. 398.

new conception with traditional functions that doctors and the public still associate with the nurse but which, in actual practice, are being turned over to nurse technicians and other such hospital workers.

Although Ross offers no specific reasons for manifestations of restlessness and dissatisfaction, the writer suggests that, because of the newness of every aspect of the nurse role, it is only natural that nursing is as self-conscious as any teen-age young lady trying to become a woman.

DEATH AND DISGUSTING TASKS

Jahoda[7] asserts that caring for patients who have incurable diseases is one of the nurse's most distressing tasks. Nurses, she continues, are confronted with the threat and reality of suffering and death, and their work by ordinary standards is distasteful, disgusting and frightening.

EXPRESSIVE AND INSTRUMENTAL FUNCTIONS

Skipper and Sakumoto[8] found that nurses tended to maximize expressive functions more than physicians but that they did not stray too far from instrumental activities. Nurses believe that terminal patients should receive considerable attention, while physicians tend to feel that such patients should receive less attention. The authors conclude that placing primary function on one type of activities to the relative or total exclusion of the other is not justified.

SKILL HIERARCHY IN NURSING

Benne and Bennis[9] speak of the blurred self-image in nursing. They mention that the nurse's self-image of real nursing is bedside nursing. They suggest that nursing might also have a skill hierarchy and promote unusually good bedside nurses to some such classification as distinguished nurse.

DECISION MAKING IN NURSING

Coser,[10] by relating the attitudes of surgical nurses to the ward social structure, confirms Merton's formulation that some social struc-

[7]Marie Jahoda: "Nursing as a Profession." *Int. Nursing Rev., 8*:10-21, May-June, 1961.

[8]James K. Skipper and Raymond E. Sakumoto: "The Nurse-Role: An Instrumental and/or Expressive Function." *Canadian Nurse, 59*:140, February, 1963.

[9]Kenneth D. Benne and Warren Bennis: "What Is Real Nursing? Role Conflict in Nursing." *Canadian Nurse, 57*:122, February, 1961.

[10]Rose Laub Coser: "Authority and Decision in a Hospital." *Am. Soc. Rev., 23*:63, February, 1958.

tures exert a definite pressure upon certain persons in the society to engage in nonconformist rather than conformist conduct.[11] Coser believes that ritualism or innovation is largely a function of the specific social structure rather than merely a "professional" or "character trait." In Coser's study, the physician's expectations on the surgical unit indicated that they wished a nurse with considerable foresight, whereas the physicians on the medical units emphasized the nurses' ritualistic abilities. The surgical nurses in Coser's study had considerably more autonomy and initiative than the medical nurses. Surgical nurses had far more power and made a considerable number of decisions. That the surgeons are in the operating rooms for a good part of the day forces the surgeon to rely on the surgical nurse. The nurses in this study were also willing and ready to use the informal social system to innovate.

CHARACTERISTIC PATTERN OF NURSING STUDENTS' NEEDS

Levitt, Lubin and Zuckerman,[12] in a study comparing student nurses, college women and graduate nurses, indicate that the student nurse has a characteristic personality of needs. The less assertive or more feminine needs, such as nurturance and abasement, are predominant. It is also affirmed that the perception of the nurse's role in society is one in which she is seen as deriving inner satisfaction rather than succeeding along more conventional lines.

CAREER CHOICE

Davis and Olesen[13] state that the fostering of high degrees of vocational commitment in our society is associated typically with such attributes as maleness, a middle-class achievement orientation and potential professional status. These authors found that nursing students experience considerable stress because of the difficulty they have in psychologically integrating the student nurse role with the concurrently emerging identity of adult womanhood. Davis and Olesen point out further that unless one is willing to pay for deviant adaptation to traditional norms, the collegiate nurse must effect viable combinations among roles that are often conflicting—companion, sexual partner, mother, orchestrator of family and outside worker. For this reason, as

[11]Robert K. Merton: *Social Theory and Social Structure.* Chicago, The Free Press of Glencoe, 1957, 131–160.

[12]Eugene Levitt, *et al.:* "The Student Nurse, the College Woman, and the Graduate Nurse: A Comparative Study." *Nursing Res., 11*:80–82, Spring, 1962.

[13]Fred Davis and Virginia Olesen: "Initiation Into a Woman's Profession: Identity Problems in the Status Transition of Coed to Student Nurse." *Sociometry, 26*:89-101, March, 1963.

the authors state, the nursing student's choice of career is more tentative and more ambivalent than that of the male. While all middle-class girls, to some degree, face the same problem, the student in transition from coed status to student nurse status encounters perhaps more stress than any other occupational group. The problem for these girls seems concerned with reconciling nursing values and demands with already integrated middle-class norms and values in relation to the adult female role.

Davis and Olesen found that the collegiate nursing student "in transition" has highly ambivalent feelings regarding her adequacy and a certain early disenchantment with her career choice. The students anticipate meeting medical and other students in the health professions, and they expect the atmosphere to differ little from that of the liberal arts campus. However, medical students, if they notice the student at all, think of her as a nurse and not as a college-educated person eligible for marriage. The authors further point out that the student is not prepared to be subsumed under an occupational classification by a young man, especially when his social background is so similar to her own.

Another stress factor enumerated by Davis and Olesen[14] is the immersion in an all-female milieu. Therefore, the interaction roles are those which put a premium on getting on with women. Such an immersion, according to Davis and Olesen, signifies a kind of regression to an earlier maturation stage of latency.

The impact of nursing itself upon the student is, of course, still another stress factor.

ATTRITION RATE IN SCHOOLS OF NURSING

In a study on causes of student withdrawal from nurse training, Teal and Fabrizio[15] found that those who remained in training stood higher in their high school graduating class than those who dropped out. Students who dropped out also seemed to experience more difficulty with liberal arts courses, while nursing courses tended to present the second major difficulty. Then, too, students tended to drop out near the end of the first year of school. A greater number of dropouts had other post-secondary education, indicating some possible indecision about a career goal. Those who stayed in training felt that they

---

[14]Fred Davis and Virginia Olesen: "Initiation Into a Woman's Profession: Identity Problems in the Status Transition of Coed to Student Nurse." Sociometry, 26:94-95, March, 1963.

[15]Gilbert Teal and Ralph A. Fabrizio: "Causes of Student Withdrawal from Nurse Training." Stamford, Conn., Public Service Research, Inc., 1964 (mimeographed), pp. 9-27.

were well prepared in high school and also believed that they studied very hard in secondary school.

In general, in the aforementioned study, students thought that none of their courses should be eliminated or condensed but that clinical courses and fine arts should be expanded. Only a few thought that courses in natural sciences should be expanded. When students needed help, a greater percentage of retainees sought help from instructors or friends and relatively few sought the help of "deans" or "school counselors." In regard to the dropouts, only a few sought help and were satisfied with the help they received. In general, all students found nursing much harder than they expected, and the authors suggest that they do not have a clear picture of what nursing education entails.

Most retainees in the study, when asked if they would choose nursing if they had it to do all over again, replied in the affirmative. Most students thought that their picture of nursing education was now much different than prior to entrance. Their picture of what a graduate nurse does also changed greatly between entrance and graduation.

In the same study, students were also asked why they selected a particular school. The most important reasons were given by students in the following order: (1) good reputation or accreditation, (2) preferable type of program and/or courses, (3) "close to home," (4) appealing school atmosphere (i.e., friendly, large, small), and (5) recommendation of others.

OUTMODED TRADITIONS

Budzyna[16] believes that because of the rapidly changing social order, which makes its mark on nursing, the outmoded traditions must be handled reverently and set aside with honor by the individual members of the profession. The author further states that her study indicated that there was considerable latitude in the practice of nursing and that some degree of standardization must occur if nursing folkways are to function in a uniformly organized fashion.

THE FUTURE NURSE INNOVATOR

If the student cannot handle the stress situations encountered in becoming a nurse, then the anxiety generated may affect others with

[16]Anna Helen Budzyna: "Culture Lag in the Concepts of Nursing." *Nursing Res.*, *10*:132-140, Summer, 1961.

whom she has interpersonal contacts. As seen in the previous chapter, such factors may bring about some undesirable patient responses. Many undergraduate students make remarkably good adjustments, and with more help from instructors in developing innovations to make nursing more rewarding, the degree of stress might be reduced significantly. Graduate students interested in research may wish to generate hypotheses with respect to the effects of certain innovations upon a specific stress factor listed in the aforementioned section.

It is also hoped that students will begin to look at nursing as a science. It is hoped that students, rather than only performing techniques in accord with the hospital procedure book, will also look at the underlying principles and theories relevant to nursing practice. It is of considerable concern to a good many nurse educators that student nurses do not seem interested in the relationship of the natural and social sciences in nursing. While it is commendable that students are eager to work with patients, it would appear that more eagerness to acquire the knowledge needed to attain the degree of perfection students seem to desire in administering patient care would also be appropriate. Perhaps students could help nurse educators examine the situation more closely to discover why they do not seem to be so interested in the underlying knowledge basic to patient care.

As the student becomes a nurse engaged in her chosen career, she will then be in a position to bring about significant changes in the social system. For such innovations to be successful, the innovator must have a broad background in liberal education.

Summary

The student is an important part of both the hospital and patient social system. In the enculturation process of becoming a nurse, the student will encounter many stress-producing situations, as well as innumerable satisfying experiences. Students often think something is wrong with themselves because they feel a certain way and are surprised to find that other students feel the same way. Student nurses are even more surprised to find that students in other health disciplines have similar experiences.

A few stress factors encountered by students in medicine have been enumerated and some of the research findings have been summarized with reference to stress factors in the enculturation process of becoming a nurse in a collegiate setting.

The enculturation process in the professionalization of various health disciplines often generates anxiety within the individual student and thus is reflected in patient behavior. It behooves the leaders in nursing to implement innovations for the alleviation of too much stress; however, social change is often slow to occur, and much will be left to be done by today's students, who will be the leaders of the future.

Bibliography

Becker, Howard S. and Geer, Blanche: "The Fate of Idealism in Medical School." *Am. Soc. Rev., 23*:50-56, February, 1958.

Benne, Kenneth D., and Bennis, Warren: "What is Real Nursing?: Role Conflict in Nursing." *Canadian Nurse, LVII:57*:122, February, 1961.

Bloom, Samuel W.: "The Process of Becoming a Physician." *Ann. Am. Acad. Polit. & Social Sci. 346*:77-87, March, 1963.

Bucher, Rue, and Strauss, Anselm L.: "Professions in Process." *Am. J. Sociology, 66*:325-334, January, 1961.

Budzyna, Anna Helen: "Cultural Lag in the Concepts of Nursing." *Nursing Res., 10*:132-140, Summer, 1961.

Coser, Rose Lamb: "Authority and Decision in a Hospital." *Am. Soc. Rev., 23*:56-63, February, 1958.

Darly, Ward: "The Professions and Professional People." *Nursing Forum, 1*:83-89. Winter, 1961-62.

Davis, Fred, and Olesen, Virginia: "Initiation into a Woman's Profession: Identity Problems in the Status Transition of Coed to Student Nurse." *Sociometry, 26*:89-101, March, 1963.

De Looff, Dorothy and Mowla, K.: "The Role of the Nurse in a Changing Society." *Internat. Nursing Rev., 8*:57-61, November-December, 1961.

Eron, Leonard D.: "The Effect of Nursing Education on Attitudes." *Nursing Res., 4*:24-27, 1955.

Etzioni, Amita, ed.: *The Semi-Professions and Their Organization.* New York, The Free Press, 1969.

Falardeau, Jean-C.: "The Role of the Nurse in a Changing Society." *Canadian Nurse, 58*:244-247, March, 1962.

Gunter, Laurie M.: "Notes on a Theoretical Framework for Nursing Research." *Nursing Res., 11*:219, Fall, 1962.

Hassenplug, Lulu: "The World of Nursing. . . . 2000 A.D." *Am. J. Nursing, 62*:100, August, 1962.

Jahoda, Marie: "Nursing as a Profession." *Internat. Nursing Rev., 8*:10-21, May-June, 1961.

Johnson, A. Leroy: *Dentistry, As I See It Today.* Boston, Little, Brown and Co., 1955.

Katz, Elihu and Menzel, Herbert: "Social Relations and Innovation in the Medical Profession: The Epidemiology of a New Drug." In E. Gartley Jaco, ed., *Patients, Physicians and Illness.* Chicago, Free Press of Glencoe, 1958.

Kuntz, Richard A., and Flaming, Karl H.: "Professionalism." *Am. J. Nursing, 63*:75, January, 1963.

Levitt, Eugene *et al.*: "The Student Nurse, the College Woman, and the Graduate Nurse: A Comparative Study." *Nursing Res., 11*:80-82, Spring, 1962.

Major, Dorothy M.: "A Profession. . . . Its Growth and Development." *Nursing Outlook, 11*:33, January, 1963.

Mauksch, Hans O.: "Becoming a Nurse: A Selective View." *Ann. Am. Acad. Polit. & Social Sci., 346*:88-98, March, 1963.

Merton, Robert K.: *Social Theory and Social Structure.* Chicago, Free Press of Glencoe, 1957, pp. 131-160.

Merton, Robert K., Reader, George G., and Kendall, Patricia L.: *The Student Physician.* Cambridge, Mass., Harvard University Press, 1957.

Mullane, Mary: "Proposals for the Future of Nursing." *Nursing Forum, 1*:73, Fall, 1962.

Olesen, Virginia, and Whittaker, Elvi: *The Silent Dialogue.* San Francisco, Jossey-Bass, Inc., 1968.

O'Malley, Claire D.: "Nursing in a Space Age Hospital." *Am. J. Nursing, 62*:54, December, 1962.
Pellegrino, Edmund D.: "The Changing Role of the Professional Nurse in the Hospital." *Hospitals, 35*:56–62, December 16, 1961.
Rogers, Martha: "Comments on the Theoretical Basis of Nursing Practice." *Nursing Science, 1*:11, April-May, 1963.
Ross, Aileen D.: *Becoming A Nurse.* Toronto, Macmillan Co. of Canada Ltd., 1961.
Schulman, Sam: "Basic Functional Roles in Nursing: Mother Surrogate and Healer." In E. Gartley Jaco, ed., *Patients, Physicians, and Illness.* Chicago, Free Press of Glencoe, 1958.
Skipper, James K., and Sakumoto, Raymond E.: "The Nurse-Role: An Instrumental and/or Expressive Function." *Canadian Nurse, 59*:139, February, 1963.
Teal, Gilbert, and Fabrizio, Ralph A.: "Causes of Student Withdrawal from Nurse Training." Stamford, Conn., Public Service Research, Inc. (mimeographed), 1964.
Tyron, Phyllis A., and Leonard, Robert C.: "Nursing Procedure." *Nursing Forum, 3*:79-89, No. 2, 1964.

Suggestions for Further Reading

Bloom, Samuel W.: "The Process of Becoming a Physician." *Ann. Am. Acad. Polit. & Social Sci., 344*:77-87, March, 1963.
Coser, Rose Laub: "Authority and Decision in a Hospital." *Am. Soc. Rev., 23*:56-63, February, 1958.
Davis, Fred, and Olesen, Virginia: "Initiation into a Woman's Profession: Identity Problems in the Status Transition of Coed to Student Nurse." *Sociometry, 24*:89-101, March, 1963.
Dickoff, James, and James, Patricia: "Power." *Am. J. Nursing, 68*:2128-2132, October, 1968.
Psathas, George: *The Student Nurse in the Diploma School of Nursing.* New York, Springer Publishing Co., 1968.
Ross, Aileen D.: *Becoming A Nurse.* Toronto, Macmillan Co. of Canada, Ltd., 1961.
Yamamoto, Kaoru: *The College Student and His Culture.* Boston, Houghton Mifflin Co., 1968.

Appendix

CODE FOR NURSE-PATIENT INTERACTION

Code Categories	*Code Translation*
1. NTrP	Nurse tranquilizes patient.
2. PHEN	Patient expresses hostility about environment to nurse.
3. PHFaN	Patient expresses hostility about family to nurse.
4. PHN	Patient hostile to nurse.
5. NOfSuP	Nurse offers suggestions to patient.
6. NOfSP	Nurse offers service to patient.
7. POfSuN	Patient offers suggestions to nurse.
8. NOfTP	Nurse offers thing to patient.
9. NOfThP	Nurse offers therapeutic service or statement to patient.
10. PCmN	Patient commands nurse.
11. PApN	Patient approves nurse.
12. NApP	Nurse approves patient.
13. PReApN	Patient requests approval of nurse.
14. NAmP	Nurse arranges next meeting with patient.
15. PIntN	Patient expresses interest in nurse.

Code Categories	Code Translation
16. NGIP	Nurse gives information to patient.
17. PGIN	Patient gives information to nurse.
18. NGSP	Nurse gives service to patient.
19. PGIPcN	Patient gives information about physical complaint to nurse.
20. NGPhSP	Nurse gives physical service to patient.
21. NReIP	Nurse requests information of patient.
22. PReIN	Patient requests information of nurse.
23. PReSN	Patient requests service of nurse.
24. NReIPcP	Nurse requests information about patient's physical condition.
25. PReCnPcN	Patient requests concern of nurse in regard to his physical complaint.
26. PReTrN	Patient requests tranquilizing statements of nurse.
27. PReTN	Patient requests thing of nurse.
28. PVAxN	Patient verbalizes anxiety to nurse.
29. PRpN	Patient responds positively to nurse.
30. NRpP	Nurse responds positively to patient.
31. PRnN	Patient responds negatively to nurse.
32. PRwaN	Patient responds warmly to nurse.
33. NRwaP	Nurse responds warmly to patient.
34. NRsilP	Nurse responds silently to patient.
35. PRsilN	Patient responds silently to nurse.
36. NRoP	Nurse's response to patient was indeterminate.
37. NSiP	Nurse signals patient.
38. PSiN	Patient signals nurse.
39. PSiAxN	Patient signals anxiety to nurse.
40. NCnP	Nurse shows concern about patient.
41. PCnPtN	Patient expresses concern about another patient to nurse.
42. NGThP	Nurse gives therapeutic service to patient.
43. PAaN	Patient affirms adequacy to nurse.
44. PPaN	Patient participates in action with nurse.
45. PHuN	Patient initiates humor with nurse.
46. NHuP	Nurse initiates humor with patient.
47. PChitN	Patient chit chats with nurse.
48. PConf1N	Patient confides somewhat in nurse.
49. PConf2N	Patient confides to a great extent in nurse.
50. PMe	Patient misuses equipment.
51. NExEn	Nurse exits and enters.
52. NStP	Nurse sits with patient.
53. PWeN	Patient expresses "weness" — togetherness — to nurse.

Code Categories	Code Translation
54. PtFcRl	Other patients facilitate the nurse-patient relationship.
55. PtBRl	Other patients block the nurse-patient relationship.
56. PtORl	The effect of other patients on the nurse-patient relationship was indeterminate.
57. PHPtN	Patient expresses hostility about another patient to the nurse.
58. PFPtN	Patient expresses friendliness about another patient to nurse.
59. PgFcRl	Personnel general facilitates nurse-patient relationship.
60. PgBRl	Personnel general blocks nurse-patient relationship.
61. PgORl	The effect of personnel general on the nurse-patient relationship was indeterminate.
62. PHPgN	Patient expresses hostility about personnel general to nurse.
63. PFPgN	Patient expresses friendliness about personnel general to nurse.

Index

Observation(s) (*Continued*)
definition of, 79–80
interpretation of, 128
participant, method of, 134
process of, 80–81
skills in, 79–87
factors hindering, 83–84
Oedipal phase, of childhood, biosocial development during, 53–55
Old age. See *Aged.*
Oral activities, in infancy, 45
Organization, of hospital hierarchy, 272
Orientation, of individual. See *Biosocial development and orientation.*
Overt response, definition of, 14
Oxanamide, 173, 174
Oxazepam, 173, 254

Pacatal, 161, 164
Paranoia, suspicion in, 209
Pargyline, 168, 171
Parnate, 168, 171
Patient(s)
aged. See *Aged.*
approach toward, 96
behavior of. See also *Behavior.*
coding of, 135, 345–347
communications with, 96–103
conversation with, 100, 101–103
data on, classification of, 125
collection of, 125
advanced method of, 133–140
for group experiences, 319
mobility of, and nursing care, 285
psychiatric. See *Psychiatric patient(s).*
suggestions to, 99
Pavlov, Ivan, 182
Peers, of child, in juvenile period, 56
Perception, behavior and, 22
Perrow, Charles E., 275
Personal hygiene, of psychiatric patient, 146–148
Personality, adjustment and, 27–42
Persuasion, as tool in communication, 96
Pertofrane, 168, 170
Pharmacologic agents, in psychiatric therapy, 160–175. See also *Drug(s).*
Pharmacologic convulsive therapy, 158–160
Phenaglycodol, 173, 174
Phenelzine, 168, 170
Phenothiazine derivatives, 161
aliphatics, 160, 161
piperazines, 161, 164
piperidines, 161, 164
Phobic period, normal, 55

Physical aspects, of patient environment, nursing role and, 268
Physiochemical therapy, nursing functions in, 155–179
Pinel, Philippe, 297
Piperazines, 161, 164
Piperidines, 161, 164
Pipradol, 168, 172
Plato, 295
Population, aging, implications of, 68
changes in, 67
Prevention, of mental illness, types of, 309
Privacy, for aged patient, 240
Prochlorperazine, 161, 164
Projection, definition of, 37
Promazine, 160, 164
Protection, of patient, aged, 238
and therapeutic environment, 269
lack of, in deprived milieu, 281
Psychiatric hospital(s)
admission of patient to, 151
care of keys in, 149
day, 181
development of, 296
for outpatients, 181, 184
night, 181
organization of, roles and, 272
psychosocial milieu of, 267–278
relation of, to community, 274–276
social structure in, 272–274
formal, 272
informal, 273
Psychiatric patient(s)
addicted, 251–258
aged, 244–246
and socio-environmental milieu, 189–292
antisocial, 259–266
autistic, 197–207
clothing of, 153
complaints of, 286
diagnostic tests for, 151–153
distrustful, 209–215
eating habits of, 150. See also *Food intake.*
elated, 229–235
energy restoration in, 150–151
environment of, for insulin therapy, 156
high-visibility nursing functions and, 143–188
history of beliefs regarding, 295–304
homicidal, 149
hospital admission of, 151
hygiene of, 146–148
in deprived milieu, 280
responses to nurse requests in, 288
in group experiences with nurse, 317–326
legislation regarding, 152, 301–302